This book is to be returned on or before
the last date stamped below.

A.A.O.S.
Symposium on
Reconstructive surgery
of the knee

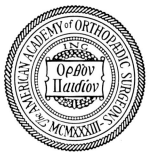

American Academy
of
Orthopaedic Surgeons

Symposium on

Reconstructive surgery of the knee

Rochester, New York
May 1976

with 346 illustrations

The C. V. Mosby Company

Saint Louis   1978

The C. V. Mosby Company
11830 Westline Industrial Drive, St. Louis, Missouri 63141

Library of Congress Cataloging in Publication Data

Main entry under title:

Symposium on reconstructive surgery of the knee,
   Rochester, New York, May 1976.

   Papers presented at a course sponsored by the
Committee on Rehabilitation of the American Academy of
Orthopaedic Surgeons.
   Bibliography: p.
   Includes index.
   1. Knee—Surgery—Congresses. 2. Arthroplasty—
Congresses. I. American Academy of Orthopaedic
Surgeons. Committee on Rehabilitation.
RD561.S95   617'.582   78-6486
ISBN   0-8016-0132-0

CB/CB/B   9   8   7   6   5   4   3   2   1

Contributors

Robert H. Arbuckle, M.D.

Clinical Fellow in Orthopaedic Surgery, Harvard Medical School; Chief Resident in Orthopaedic Surgery, Peter Bent Brigham Hospital, Boston, Massachusetts

Edmund Y. S. Chao, Ph.D.

Director, Biomechanics Laboratory, Department of Orthopedics, Mayo Clinic, Rochester, Minnesota

H. Royer Collins, M.D.

Director of Clinical Research, National Athletic Health Institute; Orthopedic Surgeon, Sports Medicine, Inglewood, California

Kenneth E. DeHaven, M.D.

Assistant Professor of Orthopaedics and Head, Section of Athletic Medicine, University of Rochester School of Medicine and Dentistry, Rochester, New York

Nas S. Eftekhar, M.D.

Associate Clinical Professor of Orthopaedic Surgery, College of Physicians and Surgeons, Columbia University; Associate Attending at Columbia-Presbyterian Medical Center, New York, New York

C. McCollister Evarts, M.D.

Chairman and Dorris Hudgins Carlson Professor of Orthopaedics, Department of Orthopaedics, University of Rochester School of Medicine and Dentistry, Rochester, New York

A. Hadjipavlou, M.D., F.R.C.S.(C)

Consultant, Queen Mary Veterans' Hospital; Orthopaedic Surgeon, Santa Cabrini Hospital, Montreal, Quebec, Canada

Mason Hohl, M.D.

Clinical Professor, Department of Surgery/Orthopaedics, University of California, Los Angeles, California

Lanny L. Johnson, M.D.

Clinical Associate Professor of Surgery, College of Human Medicine, Michigan State University, East Lansing, Michigan

Robert J. Johnson, M.D.

Associate Professor, Department of Orthopaedic Surgery, University of Vermont College of Medicine, Burlington, Vermont

Herbert Kaufer, M.D.

Professor, Section of Orthopaedic Surgery, Department of Surgery, University of Michigan, University Hospital, Ann Arbor, Michigan

Donald B. Kettelkamp, M.D.

Professor and Chairman of Orthopaedic Surgery, Indiana University School of Medicine, Indianapolis, Indiana

Martin W. Korn, M.D.

Clinical Assistant Professor of Orthopaedics, Department of Orthopaedics, University of Rochester School of Medicine and Dentistry, Rochester, New York

Robert L. Larson, M.D.

Senior Clinical Instructor of Orthopaedics, University of Oregon Medical School, Portland, Oregon; Chief, Orthopaedic Section, Sacred Heart General Hospital; Director of Athletic Medicine, Athletic Department, University of Oregon, Eugene, Oregon

Robert E. Leach, M.D.

Professor and Chairman of Orthopedics, Department of Orthopedics, Boston University School of Medicine, Boston, Massachusetts

Larry S. Matthews, M.D.

Associate Professor, Section of Orthopaedic Surgery, University of Michigan, University Hospital, Ann Arbor, Michigan

David G. Murray, M.D.

Chairman, Department of Orthopedic Surgery, State University of New York, Upstate Medical Center, Syracuse, New York

Carl L. Nelson, M.D.

Professor and Chairman, Department of Orthopaedics, University of Arkansas for Medical Sciences, Little Rock, Arkansas

James A. Nicholas, M.D.

Director of Orthopedic Surgery and Founding Director, Institute of Sports Medicine and Athletic Trauma, Lenox Hill Hospital; Clinical Professor of Orthopaedic Surgery, Cornell University Medical College, New York, New York

Richard L. O'Connor, M.D.

West Covina Hospital, West Covina, California

Harold E. Olsson, M.D.

Department of Radiology, Providence Hospital, Seattle, Washington

Malcolm H. Pope, Ph.D.

Research Professor, Department of Orthopaedic Surgery, University of Vermont College of Medicine, Burlington, Vermont

Eric L. Radin, M.D.

Associate Professor in Orthopedic Surgery, Harvard Medical School, Boston, Massachusetts; Lecturer in Mechanical Engineering, Massachusetts Institute of Technology, Cambridge, Massachusetts

Stephen C. Robinson, M.D.

Naval Regional Medical Center, Long Beach, California

A. A. Savastano, M.D.

Surgeon-in-Chief, Department of Orthopedic Surgery, Rhode Island Hospital; Clinical Professor of Orthopedic Surgery, Brown University Medical School, Providence, Rhode Island

David Segal, M.D.

Director of Orthopedics, Boston City Hospital; Associate Professor of Orthopedics, Boston University School of Medicine, Boston, Massachusetts

James A. Shaw, M.Eng.

Department of Orthopedic Surgery, State University of New York, Upstate Medical Center, Syracuse, New York

Theodore N. Siller, F.R.C.S.(C), F.A.C.S.

Demonstrator in Surgery, Department of Surgery, McGill University; Consultant in Orthopaedics, Queen Mary Veterans' Hospital; Associate, Department of Orthopaedics, Reddy Memorial Hospital, Montreal, Quebec, Canada

Clement B. Sledge, M.D.

Professor of Orthopedic Surgery, Harvard Medical School; Surgeon-in-Chief, Robert B. Brigham Hospital; Orthopedist-in-Chief, Peter Bent Brigham Hospital, Boston, Massachusetts

David A. Sonstegard, Ph.D.

Associate Professor, Department of Applied Mechanics and Engineering Sciences and Department of Surgery, University of Michigan, Ann Arbor, Michigan

Robert M. Spitzer, M.D.

Department of Radiology, Rochester General Hospital, Rochester, New York

John D. States, M.D.

Chairman, Department of Orthopaedics, Rochester General Hospital; Professor, Department of Orthopaedics, University of Rochester School of Medicine and Dentistry, Rochester, New York

William H. Thomas, M.D.

Clinical Instructor in Orthopedic Surgery, Harvard Medical School; Surgeon, Robert B. Brigham Hospital, Boston, Massachusetts

Peter S. Walker, Ph.D.

Director, Product Development, Howmedica, Inc., Orthopaedics Division, Rutherford, New Jersey

Stephen Wasilewski, M.D.

Resident, Department of Orthopedics, Boston University School of Medicine, Boston, Massachusetts

Theodore R. Waugh, M.D.

Professor and Chief, Department of Orthopaedic Surgery, New York University–Bellevue Medical Center, New York, New York

Alan H. Wilde, M.D.

Chairman, Department of Orthopaedic Surgery, Cleveland Clinic Foundation, Cleveland, Ohio

V. A. Zecchino, M.D.

Clinical Instructor of Orthopedic Surgery, Brown University Medical School, Providence, Rhode Island

Preface

The papers contained in this text represent the efforts of faculty members who participated in the course "Reconstructive Surgery of the Knee" sponsored by the Committee on Rehabilitation of the American Academy of Orthopaedic Surgeons in Rochester, New York, May 17-20, 1976.

Individual authors provide a thorough analysis and their views concerning a wide variety of knee joint disorders. Discussions on the anatomy and function of the knee joint and diagnostic procedures utilized in the management of the knee joint disorders are presented. Common problems of the knee joint are discussed, and surgical procedures for various disorders are reviewed. Ligamentous reconstruction of the knee and total knee joint reconstruction are included. The volume concludes with discussions of complications and results.

C. McCollister Evarts, M.D., Editor

for the Committee on Continuing Education

Contents

PART ONE

Form and function of the knee

1. Functional anatomy of the meniscus

Robert J. Johnson
Malcolm H. Pope

It is not the purpose of this chapter to evaluate in detail the anatomic features of the menisci, but a few salient points will be made. Fig. 1-1 demonstrates diagrammatically the superior surface of the tibia with the menisci in place. The medial meniscus is C shaped because its anterior horn is attached far anteriorly and slightly below the front edge of the articular surface of the tibia. It is quite wide posteriorly and narrow anteriorly. When viewed from above, the lateral meniscus is more circular and of a consistent width. The anterior horn of the lateral meniscus and the posterior horns of both menisci are inserted into the intracondylar eminence. Although the lateral collateral ligament is not attached to the lateral meniscus, the midportion of the lateral capsular ligament is attached to the meniscus as far posteriorly as the recess for the popliteus tendon. This, in effect, is equivalent to the well-documented attachment of the deep medial collateral ligament (medial capsular ligament) to the medial meniscus. It is recognized that the popliteus sends a strong slip of muscle into the posterior horn of the lateral meniscus, but the semimembranosus also has a direct insertion into the posterior portion of the medial meniscus. The anterior horns of the menisci are attached by fibrous bands to the patella in such a fashion as to draw the menisci forward as the knee is extended by the quadriceps mechanism.[10] The ligaments of Humphrey (anterior meniscofemoral) and Wrisberg (posterior meniscofemoral) extend from the posterior horn of the lateral meniscus into the medial femoral condyle, respectively, just anterior and posterior to the posterior cruciate ligament.

The anatomic configuration of the menisci certainly suggests that these structures serve a vital mechanical function within the knee. However, Sutton in 1897 stated that the menisci were merely functionless remnants of muscle origin.[11] Many investigators since that time have oberved that following meniscectomy the menisci are replaced by fibrous scar tissue that mimics their original configuration. Observations such as these probably led to the attitude among most orthopaedists that the menisci were essentially expendable structures. Yet many inves-

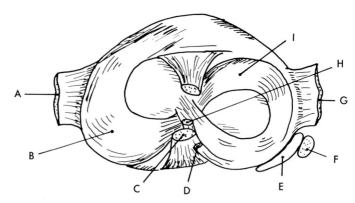

Fig. 1-1. Superior view of tibial plateau with menisci intact and ligaments transected. *A,* Medial capsular ligament (deep medial collateral ligament). *B,* Medial meniscus. *C,* Posterior cruciate ligament. *D,* Ligament of Wrisberg. *E,* Recess for passage of popliteus tendon. *F,* Lateral collateral ligament. *G,* Middle one third of lateral capsular ligament. *H,* Ligament of Humphrey. *I,* Lateral meniscus. (Modified from Helfet, A. J.: The management of internal derangements of the knee, ed. 1, Philadelphia, 1963, J. B. Lippincott Co., p. 11.)

tigators through the years have revealed significant anatomic and mechanical changes within the knee following meniscectomy.* These changes demonstrate that the knee is functionally altered by the absence of a meniscus. Some would argue that the injury producing damage to the mensicus is responsible for the changes observed postoperatively and that the excision of the meniscus itself has no ill effect. Although there is no possible way to know exactly what is responsible for the postoperative changes in humans, the work of King[11] and most recently that of Cox et al.[3] clearly demonstrate that removal of previously undamaged menisci in dogs rapidly leads to the development of severe degenerative changes.

Several meniscal functions have been previously proposed. These include the following:

1. Provision of stability
2. Provision of shock absorption
3. Provision of increased congruity
4. Aiding in lubrication
5. Prevention of synovial impingement
6. Limitation of extremes of flexion and extension
7. Transmission of loads across the joint
8. Reduction of contact stress

We will discuss several of these at length.

---

*References 1, 4, 5, 7-9, 11-13, 21.

KNEE JOINT STABILITY

In 1974 Johnson et al.[9] evaluated 99 patients who had undergone meniscectomy; the mean follow-up was 17 years. Preoperatively only 3 of these patients were known to have mild medial collateral ligament instability. At the time of follow-up 37 of these individuals had readily demonstrable anteromedial rotational instability. How many of these patients had rotational instability at the time of their surgery was impossible to establish because this phenomenon was not described by Slocum and Larson[19] until many years after the patients' operations. Although 24 of the patients had some medial collateral or anterior cruciate instability at the time of follow-up, 13 had no other clinically demonstrable instability. This suggested that the menisci may serve an important role in controlling rotational stability of the knee or that removal of the meniscus may in some way jeopardize the medial capsular ligament's role in preventing anteromedial rotational instability.

Wang and Walker[23] recently reported their findings concerning the role of the meniscus in relationship to rotatory laxity of the knee. They studied unloaded human cadaver knees at 25° of flexion before and after removal of both menisci. They defined two types of rotatory laxity, primary and secondary. The former occurred at torques up to 0.5 Nm and represented the looseness of the joint before significant resistance was encountered. The latter occurred at torques between 0.5 Nm and 5 Nm and represented significant resistance prior to plastic failure of soft tissue structures. In their study this failure was found to occur at approximately 12.5 Nm. Under such loads the ligaments were stretched but not totally disrupted and, as might be expected, they found greater rotational instability after such ligamentous failure. They determined primary and secondary rotatory laxity of eight human knees before and after removal of both menisci. A 14% increase in primary rotatory laxity and a 2% increase in secondary laxity were observed. Although they thought that the increase in secondary laxity was not significant, they concluded that the menisci serve to restrict primary rotatory laxity, perhaps by acting as space-filling buffers.

More recently Hsieh and Walker[6] evaluated the anteroposterior laxity of human knee specimens fixed in positions of 0° and 30° of flexion with and without loads applied to the joints. They found that meniscectomy had little effect on laxity in the anteroposterior plane in the otherwise intact knee. However, after sectioning the cruciate ligaments and repeating these same anteroposterior loads before and after removal of the menisci, they determined large differences in anteroposterior stability. They concluded that the menisci apparently play an important role in preventing this instability when cruciate function has been lost. This may well account for the frequent development of a torn meniscus after apparently isolated disruption of the anterior cruciate ligament. In our experience, untreated tears of the anterior cruciate almost invariably lead to episodes of instability (pivot shift syndrome) and, later still, torn menisci.

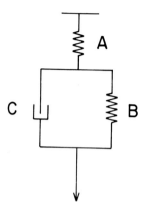

Fig. 1-2. Model of meniscus. *A,* Series of elastic element. *B,* Parallel elastic element. *C,* Parallel dashpot or damper. If a load is applied to model, dashpot provides enhanced resistance at higher rates of loading (as does the barrel of a syringe).

SHOCK ABSORPTION

Radin et al.[15] have demonstrated the role of energy absorption in the onset of osteoarthritic changes. In a subsequent paper, Radin and Paul[16] observed that the articular cartilage itself has little force-attenuating ability, primarily because of its relative thinness. Thus other structures such as the subchondral bone and the menisci are required to absorb shock within the joint.

The menisci can be represented rheologically by a model consisting of two springs and a dashpot (Fig. 1-2). Such a model has the capability of absorbing energy. A prime consideration in impact absorption is the ability to undergo deflection, and in this respect the menisci have an excellent geometry. The deflection of the ligaments and the capsular attachments of the meniscus are also of importance in this regard. Krause et al.[12] found the menisci to absorb energy most efficiently at relatively low loading rates, but even at higher rates of loading the amount of energy absorption was probably still significant.

CONGRUITY

The lack of congruence of the articular surface is corrected by the presence of the menisci. The space filled by the menisci is analogous to the space left by a sphere resting on a plane. Virchow has called this the socket-forming function.[20]

LUBRICATION

MacConaill[14] observed many years ago that menisci, or articular discs, are present in joints in which motion occurs about an axis perpendicular to the articular surfaces. They are likely to be present in those joints in which the articular surfaces are relatively flat and screwlike motion occurs. MacConaill[14] described the menisci as simple mechanical devices that act as Mitchell thrust blocks and thus aid in providing lubrication to the joint. However, it is not likely that the structure of the meniscus can act in this fashion because of the low relative speeds between surfaces in the joint. It is probably more realistic to state that the menisci do provide efficiency for joint lubrication by simply acting as space-filling buffers, so that joint fluid between the femoral and tibial surfaces can be kept in place more readily. MacConaill[14] found the coefficient of friction within the joint to rise 20% after meniscectomy.

SYNOVIAL IMPINGEMENT

The space-filling effect of the menisci has been suggested as a means of preventing impingement of the synovium betweeen the articular surfaces. However, we know of no published reports of such sequelae following meniscectomy.

LIMITS OF EXTREMES OF FLEXION AND EXTENSION

It is common knowledge that in full extension the menisci are forced far forward within the joint. In this compact, screwed-home position the anterior horns of the menisci act as a buffer to further hyperextension of the joint. Likewise, in flexion when the menisci are forced far posteriorly in the joint, they probably serve to prevent further flexion of the knee.

LOAD TRANSMISSION

In 1948 Fairbank[5] described three radiographic changes that he frequently noted following meniscectomy. These included an osteophytic ridge on the femoral condyle, joint space narrowing, and flattening of the femoral condyle at the site of the meniscectomy (Fig. 1-3). In a study of the late results after meniscectomy Johnson et al.[9] observed that 74% of 99 postmeniscectomy knees had at least one of "Fairbank's changes" at the time of follow-up, but these changes were present in only 6% of the opposite, unoperated knees of the same individuals. Fairbank[5] attributed these changes to loss of the weight-bearing function of the meniscus. He believed that these changes were not consistent with those of osteoarthritis and, for that matter, were not even precursors of such arthritis. The functional results of meniscectomy were not observed by Fairbank to be altered by the presence of these changes. However, both Huckle[7] and Johnson et al.[9] noted that increased numbers of Fairbank's changes at the time of follow-up were associated with poorer recovery.

These observations, coupled with a close evaluation of the microscopic structure of the meniscus, can only lead one to conclude that the menisci do in fact assist in the transmission of load from the femur to the tibia. Fig. 1-4 is taken from the work of Bullough et al.[2] and demonstrates the relative orientation of the collagen fibers within the meniscus. The majority of these fibers are aligned in a circumferential fashion. This would indicate that the meniscus is designed to resist those forces that tend to elongate it or to extrude it from the joint when

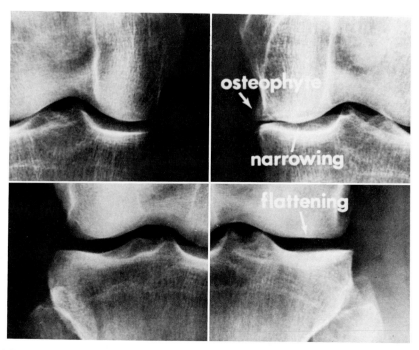

Fig. 1-3. Roentgenographic changes following meniscectomy described by Fairbank.[5] Upper two photographs compare medial compartments of knees of one patient who had medial meniscectomy. Lower two photographs show lateral compartments of knees of patient who had lateral meniscectomy. (From Johnson, R. J., Kettlekamp, D. B., Clark, W., and Leaverton, P.: J. Bone Joint Surg. **56-A:**721, 1974.)

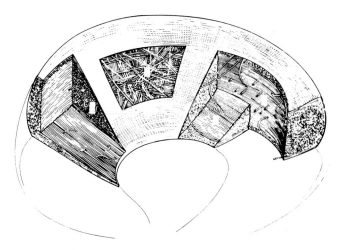

Fig. 1-4. Reconstruction of collagen pattern within meniscus. (From Bullough, P. G., Munuera, L., Murphy, J., and Weinstein, A. M.: J. Bone Joint Surg. **52-B:**565, 1970.)

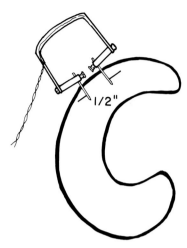

Fig. 1-5. Humpback strain transducer as it was inserted into anterior horn of medial meniscus.

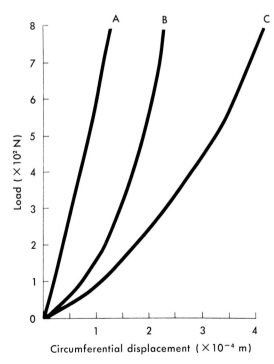

Fig. 1-6. Circumferential displacement of human medial meniscus. Average peripheral displacement for menisci of three human knees tested at A, no flexion and 5° of external rotation; B, 45° of flexion and no external rotation; and C, no flexion and no external rotation. Peripheral displacement was measured by transducer shown in Fig. 1-5. (From Krause, W. R., Pope, M. H., Johnson, R. J., and Wilder, D. G.: J. Bone Joint Surg. **58-A**:603, 1976.)

the femur is bearing weight on the tibia. Because the menisci are most firmly attached at their anterior and posterior horns, they would be expected to elongate as weight is borne by the joint. If they are simply passive space fillers at the margins of the joint, no such elongation would occur when weight was applied.

Therefore an experiment was designed to determine if the menisci do in fact elongate during weight bearing.[12] Human cadaver knees were utilized and tested using a humpback strain transducer (Fig. 1-5), which was placed in the anterior aspect of the medial meniscus as the load was applied by an Instron Universal Testing Machine. This device was capable of applying loads at various strain rates to whole human knee specimens mounted by clamps firmly attached to the femur and tibia. If any elongation occurred within the meniscus during loading, the two limbs of the transducer were forced to separate. Typical results are depicted in Fig. 1-6 and represent the results of three tests on the same human knee. The circumferential displacement (elongation) of the meniscus is depicted on the horizontal axis and the load (in newtons) on the vertical axis. In each case the meniscus was elongated as the load was applied. This directly revealed that the meniscus was resisting the load applied from the femur to the tibia. In this regard, one can draw an analogy between the collagen fiber orientation in the

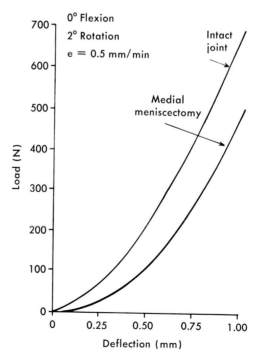

Fig. 1-7. Load-deflection graph of human knee (right knee) at no flexion and 2° rotation at loading rate of 0.5 mm/min, showing result before and after medial meniscectomy.

meniscus and the cable wrapped around the barrel of an ancient cannon to withstand the hoop or circumferential stresses generated as the gunpowder exploded.

Krause et al.[12] also evaluated the effect of meniscectomy on the transmission of load across the knee in both canine and human specimens. The results of this study were again obtained from testing complete specimens in the Instron compression testing machine both before and after meniscectomies. The load was measured in newtons and the deflection in this case was the compressive deflection of the entire knee specimen as weight was applied (Fig. 1-7). In the intact knee with both menisci present, when a load of approximately 700 N was applied, the compressive deflection of the whole knee was 1 mm. After this was established, a medial meniscectomy was performed on the specimen and the same test was repeated exactly. This time, when the compressive deflection had reached 1 mm, only approximately 500 N was being applied. From experiments such as this it was concluded that the menisci transmit weight, thereby protecting the articular cartilage and the subchondral bone. It was observed in dogs that the menisci transmit approximately 65% of the load, whereas in humans the menisci transmit between 30% and 55% of the load.

Several other investigators have recently presented reports confirming the weight-bearing function of the menisci.[17,18,22]

CONTACT STRESS

We also evaluated the effect of meniscectomy on contact stress.[12] Stress, of course, is measurement of the load per unit area. This implies a knowledge of the area of contact within the knee, and to determine this we used dye techniques before and after meniscectomy to measure exactly the areas of contact. When this was done the results given in Table 1-1 were obtained. The amount of stress increased nearly threefold after meniscectomy. It should be noted that this computation is for the average stress and that the peak stress in the localized area at the center of the contact zone could be considerably higher. Fig. 1-8 shows one hypothesis for the interaction of the increased contact stress in the development of Fairbank's changes previously described.

Table 1-1. Mean stress across joint

Species	Number of subjects	Angle of flexion	Load (newtons)	Contact area ($\times 10^{-4}$ m^2)	Stress (10^5 N/m^2)
Dog	1	60°			
Menisci intact			89.0	2.77	3.21
After meniscectomy			64.8	0.64	10.04
Human	3	0°			
Menisci intact			1000.0	20.84	4.80 ±0.82
After meniscectomy			680.0	5.88	11.56 ±2.06

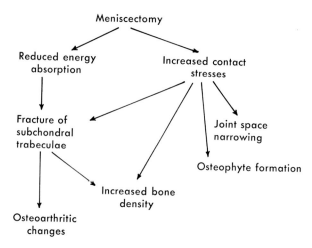

Fig. 1-8. Summary of effects of meniscectomy and their possible influence on Fairbank's changes.

CONCLUSION

The findings presented in this chapter can leave no doubt that the menisci serve several important mechanical functions within the knee. Present knowledge of these functions is at best superficial, and much work is still to be accomplished before they can be totally understood. We believe that a torn meniscus that is producing such clinical manifestations as localized pain, locking, and recurrent effusions should be removed. However, every effort should be made to avoid removing normal menisci.

References

1. Appel, H.: Late results after meniscectomy in the knee joint. A clinical and roentgenologic follow up investigation, Acta Orthop. Scand. Suppl. **133**:1, 1970.
2. Bullough, P. G., Munuera, L., Murphy, J., and Weinstein, A. M.: The strength of the menisci of the knee as it relates to their fine structure, J. Bone Joint Surg. **52-B**:564, 1970.
3. Cox, J. S., Nye, C. E., Schaefer, W. W., and Woodstein, I. J.: The degenerative effects of partial and total resection of the medial meniscus in dogs' knees, Clin. Orthop. **109**:178, 1975.
4. Dandy, D. J., and Jackson, R. W.: The diagnosis of problems after meniscectomy, J. Bone Joint Surg. **57-B**:349, 1975.
5. Fairbank, T. J.: Knee joint changes after meniscectomy, J. Bone Joint Surg. **30-B**:664, 1948.
6. Hsieh, H., and Walker, P. S.: Stabilizing mechanisms of the loaded and unloaded knee joint, J. Bone Joint Surg. **58-A**:87, 1976.
7. Huckle, J. R.: Is meniscectomy a benign procedure? A long-term follow up study, Can. J. Surg. **8**:254, 1965.
8. Jackson, J. P.: Degenerative changes in the knee after meniscectomy, Br. Med. J. **2**:525, 1968.
9. Johnson, R. J., Kettelkamp, D. B., Clark, W., and Leaverton, P.: Factors affecting late meniscectomy results, J. Bone Joint Surg. **56-A**:719, 1974.

10. Kaplan, E. B.: Factors responsible for the stability of the knee joint, Bull. Hosp. Joint Dis. **18:**51, 1957.
11. King, D.: The function of semilunar cartilages, J. Bone Joint Surg. **18:**1069, 1936.
12. Krause, W. R., Pope, M. H., Johnson, R. J., and Wilder, D. G.: Mechanical changes in the knee after meniscectomy, J. Bone Joint Surg. **58-A:**599, 1976.
13. Lagergren, K. A.: Meniscus operations and secondary arthrosis deformans, Acta Orthop. Scand. **14:**280, 1953.
14. MacConaill, M. A.: The movements of bones and joints. 3. The synovial fluid and its assistants, J. Bone Joint Surg. **32-B:**244, 1950.
15. Radin, E. L., Parker, H. G., Pugh, J. W., Steinberg, R. S., Paul, I. L., and Rose, R. M.: Response of joints to impact loading. III, J. Biomech. **6:**51, 1973.
16. Radin, E. L., and Paul, I. L.: Does cartilage compliance reduce skeletal impact loads? Arthritis Rheum. **13:**139, 1970.
17. Seedholm, B. B., Dowson, D., and Wright, V.: Functions of the meniscus—A preliminary study. In Proceedings of the British Orthopaedic Research Society, J. Bone Joint Surg. **56-B:**381, 1974.
18. Shrive, N.: The weight-bearing role of the menisci of the knee. In Proceedings of the British Orthopaedic Research Society, J. Bone Joint Surg. **50-B:**381, 1974.
19. Slocum, D. B., and Larson, R. L.: Rotatory instability of the knee. Its pathogenesis and a clinical test to demonstrate its presence, J. Bone Joint Surg. **50-A:**211, 1968.
20. Steindler, A.: Kinesiology of the human body, ed. 1, Springfield, Ill., Charles C Thomas, Publisher, 1955, p. 340.
21. Tapper, E. M., and Hoover, N. W.: Late results after meniscectomy, J. Bone Joint Surg. **51-A:**517, 1969.
22. Walker, P. S., and Erkman, M. J.: The role of the menisci in force transmission across the knee, Clin. Orthop. **109:**184, 1975.
23. Wang, C. J., and Walker, P. S.: Rotatory laxity of the human knee, J. Bone Joint Surg. **56-A:**161, 1974.

2. Knee joint stability without reference to ligamentous function

Robert J. Johnson
Malcolm H. Pope

When one thinks of the subject of knee joint stability, ligamentous function usually comes to mind. Almost all discussions of the knee afflictions of athletes, and many of those involving individuals with arthritis, deal with the problems of ligamentous dysfunction. Yet careful consideration dictates evaluation of several other factors that contribute to knee joint stability or the lack of it.

JOINT SURFACE TOPOGRAPHY

The inherent stability provided solely by the contours of the proximal tibia and distal femur are at best very poor. The rounded distal femur is required to rest on the relatively flat surface of the tibia. Although a superficial evaluation might suggest that there is no possibility of any stability being provided by the bones themselves, the intercondylar eminence of the tibia does provide some potential for stability. Fig. 2-1 shows an idealized intercondylar eminence that provides a solid ridge from the front of the tibia to the back. This configuration would allow only anterior and posterior motion of the tibia and femur relative to one another. However, the intercondylar eminence more closely resembles the peg depicted in Fig. 2-2. Thus there can be rotation about the tibial spines as well as motion in the anteroposterior plane. Shear in the medial and lateral directions is quite effectively checked by this model.

Fig. 2-3 shows that the intercondylar eminence is in reality roughly conical in shape when viewed from the front and thus still can play a role in controlling the amount of rotation that is possible within the joint. On the left the knee is in neutral rotation and the femur sits well down on the top of the tibia. On the right the knee has been externally rotated several degrees. As long as the capsule and ligaments are intact, the femur must necessarily ride up on the intercondylar eminence. This elevation of the femur and all the body mass above the level of the knee absorbs energy and thus minimizes the amount of load that the capsule and ligaments must control as rotation occurs.

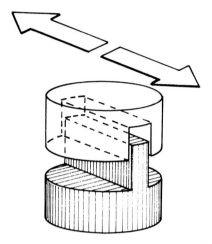

Fig. 2-1. Idealized intracondylar eminence of knee resembling a ridge. (From Kapandji, I. A.: The physiology of the joints. Vol. 2, lower limb, ed. 2, Edinburgh, 1970, Churchill Livingstone.)

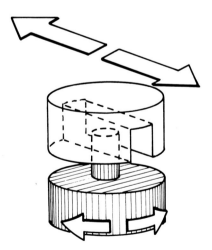

Fig. 2-2. Idealized intracondylar eminence of knee resembling a peg. (From Kapandji, I. A.: The physiology of the joints. Vol. 2, lower limb, ed. 2, Edinburgh, 1970, Churchill Livingstone.)

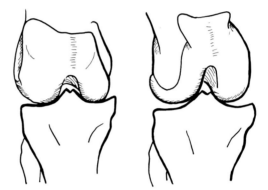

Fig. 2-3. On left is anatomic drawing of knee flexed approximately 45° with no rotation of femur relative to tibia. Drawing on right depicts knee flexed 45° but tibia externally rotated several degrees relative to femur.

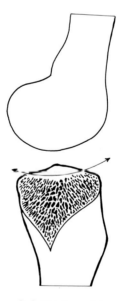

Fig. 2-4. Sagittal section through medial tibial condyle. (From Kapandji, I. A.: The physiology of the joints. Vol. 2, lower limb, ed. 2, Edinburgh, 1970, Churchill Livingstone.)

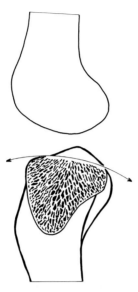

Fig. 2-5. Sagittal section through lateral tibial condyle. (Modified from Kapandji, I. A.: The physiology of the joints. Vol. 2, lower limb, ed. 2, Edinburgh, 1970, Churchill Livingstone.)

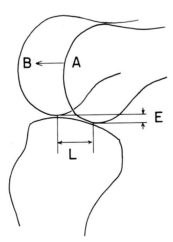

Fig. 2-6. Lateral view of knee demonstrating relative motion of femur on tibia. (From Kapandji, I. A.: The physiology of the joints. Vol. 2, lower limb, ed. 2, Edinburgh, 1970, Churchill Livingstone.)

The contours of the tibial plateau are not planar. When the medial femoral condyle is observed in sagittal section as depicted in Fig. 2-4, concavity is observed. In effect, this provides what appears to be a slight socket to receive the distal end of the femur. However, McLeod[8] has demonstrated in his studies of tibial plateau topography that the medial tibial plateau is always convex when viewed in the coronal plane. Fig. 2-5 shows the lateral tibial plateau in sagittal section. Here, again, no inherent stability is to be expected from the convexity that is observed. McLeod's work,[8] however, shows that in the coronal plane there is always slight concavity. Thus neither side of the tibial plateau provides topography that can offer much assistance in stabilizing the knee. Yet careful analysis of the lateral aspect of the knee (Fig. 2-6) suggests that in certain circumstances even the convex tibial plateau may actually help protect the ligaments and capsule. In this diagram, if the femur of the flexed knee is initially in the more posterior position (A) and then displaced anteriorly as in rotation through the distance L to come to rest in the more anterior position (B), it will necessarily ride upward on the tibial condyle over the distance E. Such movement absorbs energy and reduces the requirements of the ligament and capsule to stabilize the knee. Needless to say, if the rotation depicted in Fig. 2-6 were reversed from position B to position A, stability would be jeopardized because the femur would be passing down the slope that has the vertical height E.

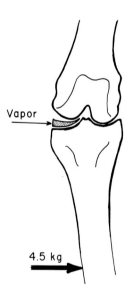

Fig. 2-7. Anterior view of knee and leg depicting a moment of 4.5 kg being applied to medial aspect of distal tibia. Moment has overcome effect of atmospheric pressure and thus vaporization has occurred in medial compartment.

ATMOSPHERIC PRESSURE

It is readily apparent on attempting to remove a femoral head from the ace-tabulum that atmospheric pressure plays an important role in providing stability for the hip joint. Semlak and Ferguson[10] demonstrated that atmospheric pressure also functions to stabilize the knee joint. They evaluated both normal knees and those with damage to the collateral ligaments by applying valgus forces to the distal tibial shaft (Fig. 2-7). They consistently demonstrated in the normal knees that no widening of the medial joint space was produced until a load of more than 4.5 kg was applied to the tibia. In the normal knees, if the load exceeded 4.5 kg, vaporization occurred in the medial compartment of the knee as the effect of atmospheric pressure was overcome. In knees with an effusion and torn medial collateral ligaments, the knee distracted immediately without vaporization occurring. They concluded that varus and valgus stresses are not realized within the collateral ligaments of the normal knee until the effect of atmospheric pres-sure is exceeded. They also noted that atmospheric pressure can provide its protective function only when there is no effusion or communication of the joint with the atmosphere. Although they did not demonstrate it, they implied that mild laxity of the collateral ligaments would not necessarily negate the function of atmospheric pressure as long as a large effusion was not present.

MENISCI

The effect of the menisci on knee joint stability is discussed in Chapter 1.

MUSCLE FUNCTION

All orthopaedic surgeons have been taught that muscle rehabilitation is an important portion of recovery from any knee injury. Common sense and practical experience have clearly demonstrated that normal muscle activity protects the knee from harm. The quadriceps mechanism has received the greatest attention in this regard. Its primary function is clearly to extend the knee, but just as important is the fact that it also controls flexion by antagonizing gravity and the hamstring muscles. Because of its massive size and anatomic configuration, the quadriceps is undoubtedly the most important dynamic stabilizer of the knee, but it also serves several other functions. Its insertion into the tibial tubercle and orientation anterior to the transverse axis of rotation of the distal femur allow it to assist in prevention of posterior subluxation of the tibia on the femur. Thus it functions synergistically with the posterior cruciate ligament. It assists in sta-bilizing the patella within the patellofemoral groove by means of both vertically and obliquely oriented fibers. Distinct fibrous bands connect the anterior horns of the menisci to the patella, thus allowing the quadriceps mechanism to pull the menisci forward as the knee is actively extended.[3,4] Through the retinaculum it tenses the anteromedial and anterolateral joint capsule.

White and Raphael[12] demonstrated the importance of the quadriceps in protecting the medial collateral ligament by placing a strain transducer on the anterior fibers of the ligament in cadaver specimens and then measuring the effects of various positions and loading configurations on strain within the ligament. In the unloaded knee they observed that strain is least when the knee is in full flexion and that strain decreases as load is applied to the quadriceps mechanism, regardless of the degree of flexion at the time of loading. Strain within the medial collateral ligament increases when a valgus stress is applied to the knee, but this increase is reduced by simultaneously loading the quadriceps. Using this experimental model, they documented the role of the quadriceps in dynamically protecting the medial collateral ligament from abduction stresses applied to the knee.

At this point it is necessary to inject a note of caution when considering the protective role of muscles about the knee. It is impossible for a particular muscle or group of muscles to protect all structures within the joint simultaneously. For example, a modification of the classic anterior drawer test in an individual with a dramatic absence of anterior cruciate function can readily demonstrate that the quadriceps mechanism is an antagonist to the anterior cruciate ligament. To do this, firmly secure the foot of the supine patient to the surface of the examining table with the knee flexed to 90°. Then ask the patient to tighten the quadriceps mechanism; at that point an obvious anterior drawer sign will occur.

A simplified vector analysis of what occurs is depicted in Fig. 2-8. When the force P is applied to the quadriceps mechanism, a strain is produced within the anterior cruciate, which must be resisted by the force C to prevent anterior

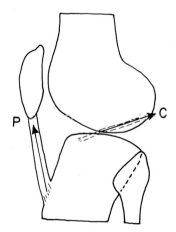

Fig. 2-8. Lateral view of knee. *P* represents load applied to the patellar tendon. *C* represents reaction force within anterior cruciate that must occur to prevent anterior subluxation of tibia on femur.

subluxation of the tibia on the femur. In resolution of this vector diagram, very large differences can be produced by slight variations in the angles between the long axis of the tibia and the direction of force representing the quadriceps loading and also in the exact position of the anterior cruciate ligament. For this reason the figures that will be given here can only be represented as reasonable estimates of what actually occurs. If 140 pounds of force (approximately that necessary to lift an unweighted adult leg) is applied to the quadriceps mechanism, then as much as 27 pounds may have to be resisted by the anterior cruciate ligament to prevent anterior subluxation of the tibia on the femur. Even more striking is the following example. If 422 pounds (a figure consistent with what occurs in climbing stairs) is applied to the quadriceps, up to 85 pounds is likely to be realized by the anterior cruciate ligament and any other structure that can resist the tendency to pull the tibia forward from beneath the femur. This evaluation of quadriceps function suggests that care must be taken in prescribing quadriceps exercises immediately after repair of an anterior cruciate ligament or reconstructive procedures that attempt to substitute for its loss. Likewise, this example stresses the importance of well-balanced rehabilitation of all muscles about the knee so that dynamic imbalance does not contribute to an increase in the static instability as time passes.

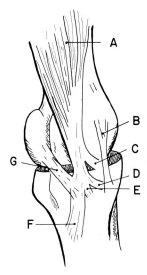

Fig. 2-9. Posteromedial view of knee. *A,* Semimembranosus muscle and its five insertions. *B,* Medial collateral ligament. *C,* Insertion of semimembranosus into posterior horn of medial meniscus. *D,* Anterior insertion of semimembranosus extending far forward parallel to joint line and deep to medial collateral ligament. *E,* Insertion of semimembranosus into posterior tubercle of tibia (direct insertion). *F,* Insertion of semimembranosus into gastrocnemius fascia. *G,* Insertion of semimembranosus into oblique popliteal ligament. (Modified from Kaplan, E. B.: Bull. Hosp. Joint Dis. **18:**53, 1957.)

The sartorius, gracilis, and semitendinosus tendons, which coalesce to form the pes anserinus, function primarily as flexors of the knee. One secondary function is to provide internal rotation of the tibia on the femur. Noyes and Sonstegard[9] demonstrated that as a unit the pes anserinus tendons are 4 to 10 times stronger in flexion than in internal rotation. Because of their anatomic configuration, they also can function to dynamically assist the medial capsule and medial collateral ligament. They protect the anterior cruciate by working in concert with it to prevent anterior subluxation of the tibia on the femur. Slocum and Larson[11] originated the principle of pes anserinus transplantation to assist in the control of anteromedial rotational instability. Noyes and Sonstegard[9] confirmed the efficacy of this procedure by demonstrating that pes anserinus transplantation reduces flexion power by approximately 30% in all positions of knee flexion between 0° and 90° and increases internal rotation power by as much as 50% at positions of 30° to 60° of knee flexion. Rotation power was increased, but to a lesser degree, at full extension and 90° of knee flexion.

Fig. 2-9 is a diagram of the posteromedial aspect of the knee.[4] It displays the five major insertions of the semimembranosus tendon. The complexity of this insertion indicates that this muscle provides several functional contributions to knee stability. Its primary purpose is its powerful ability to flex the knee and antagonistically resist the quadriceps to control extension of the joint. It dynamically bolsters the posterior and medial capsular structures. Although it has been classically stated to be a weak internal rotator of the tibia on the femur, its strong anterior tendon indicates the potential to be a powerful contributor to that function. It retracts the meniscus posteriorly and also augments the anterior cruciate by acting synergistically with it to prevent anterior subluxation of the tibia from beneath the femur.

Fig. 2-10 shows the lateral side of the knee with special reference to the iliotibial band. Kaplan[4,5] noted that, because of its attachment to Gerdy's tubercle inferiorly and to the supracondylar tubercle of the lateral femoral condyle and the intermuscular septum superiorly, the iliotibial band cannot be considered to be a true tendon of insertion. In fact, he believes that it acts as a static stabilizer of the knee and thus functions in reality as a ligament. He supported this contention by being unable to produce increased tension within the iliotibial band by stimulating the gluteus maximus or tensor fascia lata muscles in living patients and by noting no increase in varus instability of the knee caused by transecting the lateral collateral ligament and biceps tendon as long as the iliotibial band was left intact. Ellison[2] thinks that he may produce a dynamic stabilizer for the lateral side of the knee by freeing the inferior portion of the iliotibial band from its attachment to Gerdy's tubercle. Then, by isolating the major portion of its distal several inches, he also effectively detaches it from its distal femoral attachments. By passing it deep to the lateral collateral ligament and reattaching it distally just anteriorly to Gerdy's tubercle, he has not only been able to maintain the effectiveness of this structure as a static stabilizer but

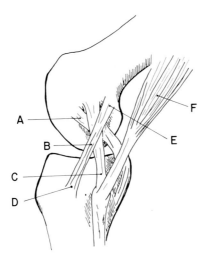

Fig. 2-10. Lateral aspect of knee with special reference to iliotibial band, *B. A*, Origin of popliteus tendon. *C*, Lateral collateral ligament. *D*, Gerdy's tubercle. *E*, Supracondylar tubercle of lateral femoral condyle. *F*, Biceps femoris. (Modified from Kaplan, E. B.: Bull. Hosp. Joint Dis. **18**:56, 1957.)

also has the advantage of dynamic support from the gluteus maximus and tensor fascia lata muscles from above. In this fashion his procedure has been able to eliminate the "pivot shift syndrome" first described by MacIntosh.[6]

The biceps femoris tendon inserts in three distinct layers into the fibular head, proximal tibia, fascia about the leg, posterior capsule of the knee joint, and even the lateral collateral ligament.[7] This indicates that the biceps serves to flex the knee, antagonistically control extension of the joint, externally rotate the tibia on the femur, tense the lateral and posterior capsule, and work synergistically with the anterior cruciate ligament.

The important anatomic features of the popliteus tendon of origin are depicted in Fig. 2-11. Approximately one half of the muscle originates from its tendon of origin from the femur, but the rest of it is attached to the posterior portion of the lateral meniscus medially and the arcuate ligament from the fibular head laterally. A direct extension of the meniscal attachment passes through the ligament of Wrisberg and then attaches to the medial femoral condyle.[1] This muscle thus serves to internally rotate the tibia on the femur and act, at least weakly, to flex the knee. It can forcefully draw the meniscus posteriorly and directly augments the function of the posterior cruciate ligament. It works antagonistically to the anterior cruciate ligament by tending to pull the tibia anteriorly beneath the femur.

Muscle stabilization of the knee is obviously very important, but one must consider the fact that muscles must be acting at the time loading is occurring to provide stability for the joint. It is doubtful that a relaxed muscle can contract

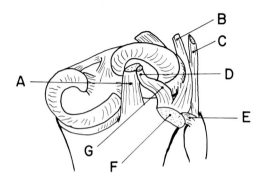

Fig. 2-11. Origin of popliteus muscle diagramatically depicted from posteriorly and slightly medially. *A*, Posterior cruciate ligament. *B*, Popliteus tendon from femur. *C*, Lateral collateral ligament. *D*, Ligament of Wrisberg. *E*, Origin of popliteus tendon from arcuate ligament. *F*, Major position of popliteus. *G*, Origin of popliteus tendon from posterior horn of lateral meniscus. (Modified from Kapandji, I. A.: The physiology of the joints. Vol. 2, lower limb, ed. 2, Edinburgh, 1970, Churchill Livingstone.)

rapidly enough to provide protection from forces instantaneously applied to the knee in such events as traffic accidents or athletic injuries. Thus ligaments may be torn before muscles have time to respond. Likewise, appropriate combinations of muscles must be functioning at the time of load application so that a coordinated effort can be made to resist the excessive loads encountered.

CONCLUSION

Knee joint stability obviously depends on many factors. Ligamentous function (which has not been a part of this discussion) is most important in stabilizing this inherently unstable joint. However, joint topography, atmospheric pressure, the menisci, and muscle function all contribute to stabilizing this large and complex joint.

References

1. Basmajian, J. V., and Lovejoy, J. F.: Functions of the popliteus muscle in man. A multi-factorial electromyographic study, J. Bone Joint Surg. **53-A**:557, 1971.
2. Ellison, A. E.: Personal communication, Williamstown, Mass., 1976.
3. Kapandji, I. A.: The physiology of the joints. Vol. 2, lower limb, ed. 2, Edinburgh, 1970, Churchill Livingstone.
4. Kaplan, E. B.: Factors responsible for the stability of the knee joint, Bull. Hosp. Joint Dis. **18**:51, 1957.
5. Kaplan, E. B.. The iliotibial tract: clinical and morphological significance, J. Bone Joint Surg. **40-A**:817, 1958.
6. MacIntosh, D. L.: Personal communication, Toronto, 1976.
7. Marshall, J. L., Girgis, F. G., and Zelko, R. R.: The biceps femoris tendon and its functional significance, J. Bone Joint Surg. **54-A**:1444, 1972.
8. McLeod, W. D.: Personal communication, Columbus, Ga., 1976.
9. Noyes, F. R., and Sonstegard, D. A.: Biomechanical function of the pes anserinus at the knee and the effect of its transplantation, J. Bone Joint Surg. **55-A**:1225, 1973.

10. Semlak, K., and Ferguson, A. B.: Joint stability maintained by atmospheric pressure, Clin. Orthop. **68**:294, 1970.
11. Slocum, D. B., and Larson, R. L.: Pes anserinus transplantation: a surgical procedure for control of rotatory instability of the knee, J. Bone Joint Surg. **50**-A:226, 1968.
12. White, A. A., and Raphael, I. G.: The effect of quadriceps loads and knee position on strain measurements of the tibial collateral ligament, Acta Orthop. Scand. **43**:176, 1972.

3. Contact areas and load transmission in the knee

Peter S. Walker

When two surfaces are touching, the apparent or nominal area of contact is the area within the common periphery. However, the real area of contact may be much smaller than the apparent area. For example, if two polished metal surfaces are pressed together, the real contact occurs at a number of small points, because of the hardness of the materials and the microirregularities on the surfaces. The contact stresses occurring at the contact points may be exceedingly high. As the materials become softer, the greater becomes the real area of contact, and the more even is the pressure distribution. A material is said to be compliant when it is sufficiently deformable to avoid localized peak stresses within a nominal area of contact; thus healthy cartilage is compliant, metal-on-polyethylene contact is a semicompliant combination, and metal-on-metal contact is noncompliant.

Two basic types of contact are "point contact," in which a sphere is pressed against a flat surface, and "line contact," in which a cylinder is pressed against a flat surface. For compliant materials that show a significant deformation of the bulk material in and around the contact zone, the real area of contact is a function of the initial conformity between the two surfaces and the elastic properties of the materials. In such a case the contact pressure is usually highest somewhere in the center of the contact area, reaching zero at the periphery. The maximum contact pressure for these types of contact is between 1.3 and 1.5 times the average pressure.

The effective compliance is reduced if the compliant materials are in the form of layers on a hard surface but is increased if the layers are viscoelastic and display creep.

In the articulations of the knee joint, the areas of contact and the contact pressures depend on the following:

1. Relative geometry between the articulating surfaces and any intervening structures such as the menisci
2. Loads and moments acting relatively between the articulating surfaces
3. Elastic properties of the materials at and below the surfaces
4. Viscoelastic, or time-dependent, properties of the materials

PATELLOFEMORAL ARTICULATION

For a given quadriceps force (Q), the resultant force on the patella (R) can be estimated by drawing a triangle of forces (Fig. 3-1). If there is minimal friction between the patellofemoral surfaces, the force in the patellar tendon is the same as the quadriceps force. Close to extension the patellar force is only about one third of the quadriceps force; at 60° of flexion and beyond the patellar force is about 1¼ times the quadriceps force.

Table 3-1 gives approximate values for the patellofemoral force, in units of body weight, for different activities.

As seen from the front, it appears that the resultant forces of the quadriceps and the patellar tendon are inclined such that there is a resultant force com-

Table 3-1. Patellofemoral forces in various activities

Activity	Angle of flexion	Maximum quadriceps force[*]	Patellofemoral force[*]
Level walking	0°-15°	1⅓	½
Walking up and down stairs	60°-75°	1½-2½	2-3
Rising from a chair	90°	1⅓	1⅔

[*]Given as multiples of body weight.

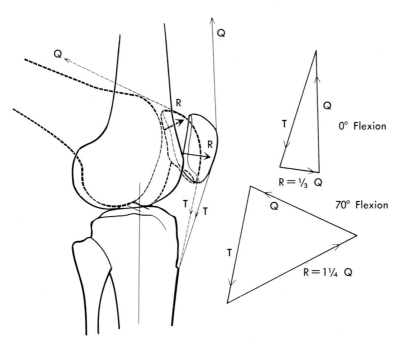

Fig. 3-1. Patellofemoral force in sagittal plane determined by triangle of forces. *Q,* Quadriceps force. *T,* Patellar tendon force. Q = T.

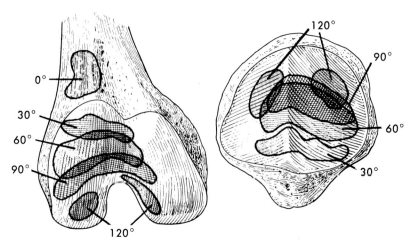

Fig. 3-2. Areas of contact on femur and patella for force of 1110 N at different flexion angles.

ponent of the patella laterally on the femur. This is reflected in the disposition of the contact area of the patella to the lateral side, the larger size of the lateral facet, and the greater prominence of the lateral femoral groove. The stability of the patella in the groove depends on the angle of the resultant force to the line of the femoral groove as seen in a sky view. If the angle is less than 90°, subluxation will occur.

In a transverse section the patella is seen to conform closely with the groove of the femur, but in sagittal sections there is only partial conformity. If a patella is fitted by hand into its femoral groove, there is felt to be a stable orientation for each position along the length of the groove. The implication is that areas of contact of reasonable size would be formed, elongated in the transverse direction. The size of the area depends on the direct force between the patella and the femur, which must not be confused with the force in the quadriceps.

Aglietti et al.[1] carried out experiments on cadaver knee specimens to determine the areas of contact for angles of flexion from 0° to 120° and a quadriceps force up to 1110 newtons (250 pounds force). The tibia was fixed, the femur was set at the required angle, and the force was applied in the quadriceps through a cable. Soft methyl methacrylate cement was used to obtain a casting of the area of contact.

At 0° of flexion the patella was just above the femoral articular surface; at 30° of flexion the inferior aspect of the patella contacted the femur; at 60° of flexion the contact was across the center; at 90° of flexion the contact was toward the superior patella; and beyond 90° the patella was astride the medial and lateral femoral condyles, forming two separate contacts (Fig. 3-2). With a quadriceps force of 1110 newtons, from 20° to 60° of flexion the average contact area increased linearly from 120 mm² to 480 mm². From 60° to 120° of flexion there

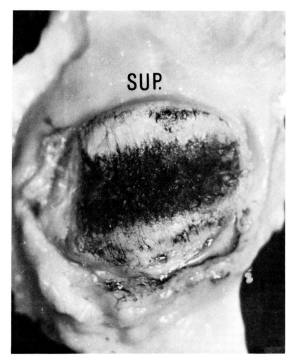

Fig. 3-3. Degenerate patella from 55-year-old man. India ink shows cartilage fibrillation. *SUP,* Superior.

was a linear fall to 360 mm². At any given angle of flexion the area of contact increased with load, but less than proportionately, a finding that was predicted by Goodfellow et al.[5] The explanation is that the larger portion of the contact area was accounted for by the initial conformity, whereas the curvatures of the femur and the patella diverged rapidly outside of that, especially in the sagittal plane.

The stresses on the articular surfaces can be calculated for different activities. For example, in walking upstairs, if the force is three times body weight and the contact area is 500 mm², the stress is about 4 newtons/mm². In level walking, for a force of half body weight and an area of 120 mm², the stress is 2.8 newtons/mm². In contrast, the stresses in the hip joint are approximately 1 newton/mm² for these activities, but in the ankle joint the stresses are at least as high as those in the patellofemoral joint, even in level walking.

There appears to be a correlation between the areas of the progressive degeneration in the patella and the areas that sustain the highest stresses.[2,3] These are not so much in the inferior half of the patella, which makes contact during level walking, but rather across the center and above, areas that are stressed when the knee is flexed to 60° and further (Fig. 3-3). Suggestions have been made that the areas of contact and the stresses imposed at these different areas could be correlated with certain stiffness and structural characteristics of the trabecular bone beneath.[9]

FEMOROTIBIAL ARTICULATION

If the menisci are removed, contact occurs between the femoral condyles, which are convex in two planes, and the tibial condyles; the medial tibial condyle is concave in two planes, with larger radii of curvature than the femur, and the lateral condyle is slightly concave or level in the frontal plane but convex in the sagittal plane. Consequently the contact areas under load are patches that

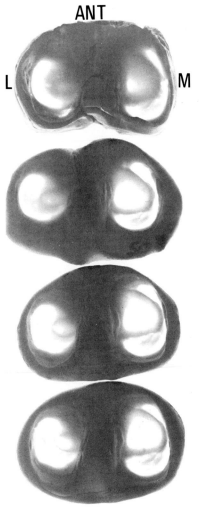

Fig. 3-4. Castings of areas of contact in normal 20-year-old knee at 30° of flexion. From top to bottom: Small load, 500 N, 1000 N, 1500 N (twice body weight).

are roughly elliptical in shape.[12] The average areas of contact under a total joint load of twice body weight were found to be 180 mm² and 140 mm² on the medial and lateral sides, respectively. Such a situation would apply to a knee after a meniscectomy.

At the time of the previous experiment there was no direct evidence available that the menisci carried much of the load across the knee. There is now strong evidence, however, that the menisci support a large fraction of the load.[7,8,10,11] The menisci are not simply space-filling washers but rather load-bearing structures with the important functions of distributing the load over a wider area than would otherwise be included, providing a measure of springiness to the knee, and giving a greater degree of stability. Also, Seedhom has demonstrated that although the joint surfaces themselves could be more conforming to spread the load, the range of motion and the capacity for transverse rotation would be greatly restricted.

Using a casting technique, Walker and Erkman[11] determined the areas of contact for knee specimens at different angles of flexion and under loads of as much as two times body weight (Fig. 3-4). At low loads, contact occurred primarily on the lateral and posterior borders of the menisci and often on a small area on the medial aspect of the tibial spine. As the load was increased, the contact areas on the menisci increased, as did the areas on the exposed cartilage

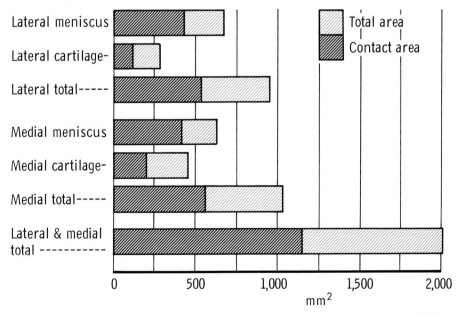

Fig. 3-5. Average areas of contact in knee at twice body weight, from 0° to 90° of flexion.

within the boundaries of the menisci. The latter were much more pronounced on the medial side than on the lateral. Whereas with a joint force of less than body weight a substantial fraction of the exposed cartilage on the medial side was in contact, it took a load of some one and one-half to two times body weight for the same to apply to the lateral side. The contact areas at 30° of flexion for a load of twice body weight, averaged for the 12 knees used in the experiments, are illustrated in Fig. 3-5. The average contact area was 1150 mm², of which more than half was on the menisci.

Care must be exercised in the distinction between contact area and contact stress, however. It is possible that the menisci were in contact but not experiencing much stress. This was tested by using a miniature pressure transducer placed at different locations in the intact knee specimens while a load was cycled on the joint. The highest pressure was on the exposed cartilage of the medial side; on the lateral side the highest pressure was on the meniscus. The pressures on the lateral and medial menisci were comparable. Calculating pressure times area shows that the exposed cartilage on the medial side carried about the same load as the meniscus; on the lateral side most of the load was carried by the meniscus. For the joint as a whole, the average contact stress across the joint was therefore approximately 1.2 newton/mm², which is comparable with that in the hip joint. With the menisci removed, as in the experiments of Walker and

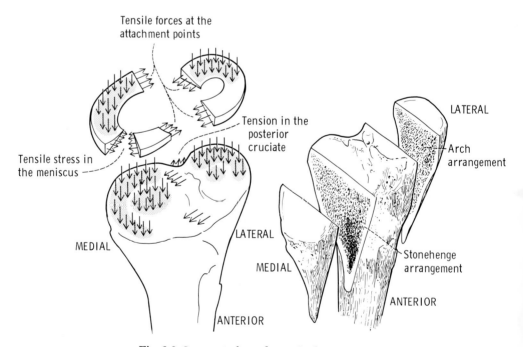

Fig. 3-6. Stresses in knee during load transmission.

Hajek, the average stress at twice body weight is nearly 5 newtons/mm². Thus the importance of the menisci in distributing the stresses, and the consequences of removing the menisci, are clearly demonstrated.

Fig. 3-6 gives a schematic representation of how the vertical loads are transmitted between the femur and the tibia at 30° of flexion. The stresses on the menisci are perpendicular to the angled surfaces, assuming very small frictional forces. These stresses have a radial component, expanding the menisci outward and causing a circumferential tension, which in turn produces tensile forces at the attachments with the bone at each end. Because most of the stress seems to be concentrated on the lateral and posterior surfaces of the menisci, there is an anteriorly directed horizontal component of force on the femur. This could be resisted by tension in the posterior cruciate ligament, although this has not been measured directly. Such a possibility, however, suggests that measurements of the ligamentous tensions of specimens in passive flexion and extension may not represent the situation in the more relevant load-bearing situations.

The vertical component of stress on the menisci reflects on the tibial surface beneath the menisci. Of course, there is the direct compressive stress acting on the cartilage not covered by the menisci.

These stresses on the upper tibia are transmitted to the cortex of the tibia through the subchondral plate, the trabeculae, and the bone around the periphery. The trabeculae are clearly oriented primarily in a vertical direction, in a slightly different way on the medial and lateral sides. On the medial side a large

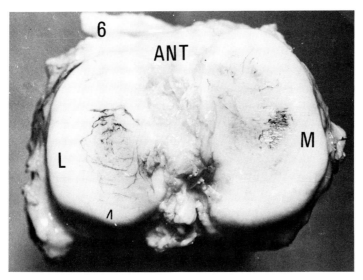

Fig. 3-7. Cracks on cartilage surface of 26-year-old upper tibia specimen. Cracks at posterolateral side are indicated by arrow. *ANT,* Anterior. *L,* Lateral. *M,* Medial.

fan of trabecular bone is present posteriorly, where most of the load-bearing occurs, and there is a smaller fan at the anterior to support the loads with the knee in extension. The high stresses acting on the exposed cartilage are borne on a substantial slab of bone supported across the aforementioned fans in a "Stonehenge" arrangement. On the lateral side the anterior and posterior fans intersect to produce an arch. The slab is much smaller on the lateral side than on the medial side, which may reflect the absence of high stresses on the exposed lateral cartilage.

In the contact area study described, it was found that as the angle of flexion was increased, the areas of contact shifted posteriorly. This was particularly true for the lateral side, because of the internal rotation of the tibia relative to the femur, with the pivot point on the medial tibial spine. One of the likely consequences of this phenomenon is the frequent cracking and ulceration that occur on the posterior lateral tibial condyle[2] (Fig. 3-7). This probably represents a materials failure, caused by high contact stresses between a posterior femoral condyle with diminished radii of curvature and the most posterior area of the tibial condyle, stresses something akin to those caused by standing on the edge of a sandbank. This condition occurs in rising from a low chair or rising from a squatting position.

COMBINATIONS OF FORCES AND MOMENTS

So far the only force that has been considered is one that is perpendicular to the upper tibia, but in many activities there are shearing forces and moments as well. In general these are resisted by the muscles, the ligaments, and the capsule, whereas in certain circumstances, the three-dimensional geometries of the femoral and tibial surfaces play an important role. The problem of stability of the knee is complex and is as yet incompletely understood, but a few basic comments will be made. It is useful to consider x, y, and z axes fixed in the tibia and to specify forces along and moments about each of the axes in turn.

1. Mediolateral forces are relatively small in level walking but higher in walking on slopes and on rough ground. The tibial eminence plays an important role here in forcing the knee to distract as movement takes place.

2. Anteroposterior forces are supported primarily by the cruciate ligaments,[4] with the menisci supplementary. The latter are only important if the cruciates are severed. When there is a compressive force across the joint, the curvatures of the condyles on the medial side provide a large fraction of the anteroposterior stability.[6]

3. A varus-valgus moment gradually applied to a loaded knee will increase the force on one condyle and decrease it on the other until tilting occurs. Beyond this stage there is tension in one of the collateral ligaments with some support from the iliotibial band, and in the cruciates. The menisci are important in providing as wide a base as possible in the frontal plane to maximize the moment at which tilting occurs.

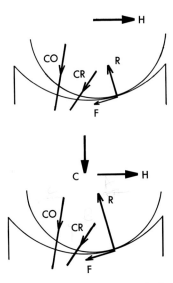

Fig. 3-8. Stability of knee when anterior force *H* is applied to femur relative to tibia. Top: No vertical compressive load. Bottom: Vertical compressive load *C* is applied.

4. An internal rotational moment on the tibia is resisted by a couple from the anterior cruciate and medial collateral ligament, with a raised area on the anterior of the inner medial side of the tibia giving additional support. External rotation is not so well resisted, the collaterals giving the main support. Again, when there is a compressive load acting, a large reduction in laxity occurs, indicating stability provided by the condylar surfaces.[13]

The principle by which support of forces and moments is provided by the shape of the condylar surfaces is explained with reference to Fig. 3-8, which depicts an anterior force applied to the femur relative to the tibia. When there is no vertical compressive load initially applied, the horizontal force H will move the femur forward to tense the posterior cruciate ligament (CR), the collateral ligaments (CO), and the capsule. The tension in the posterior cruciate is dominant. As a result of these ligamentous tensions there will be a pressing together of the joint surfaces, giving a resultant joint reaction force R, which is approximately equal to the sum of the ligament forces. The horizontal component of this reaction force on the concave medial side of the tibia provides some resistance to the horizontal force H. The frictional force F is unimportant here. When there is initially a vertical compressive force C, the reaction force R is increased by C. The horizontal component of R is now large and provides an important contribution to resisting H. Its contribution may be larger than that of the posterior cruciate if C is large enough.[6] The frictional force F will also provide a useful contribution.

Such stabilizing forces at the condylar surfaces, applicable to anteroposterior forces, mediolateral forces, and rotational moments, are an important factor in understanding the stability and load transmissions in the knee joint.

References

1. Aglietti, P., Insall, J. N., Walker, P. S., and Trent, P. S.: A new patella prosthesis— design and application, Clin. Orthop. **107**:175, 1975.
2. Bennett, G. A., Waine, H., and Bauer, W.: Changes in the knee joint at various ages, New York, 1942, The Commonwealth Fund.
3. Bullough, P. G., and Walker, P. S.: The distribution of load through the knee joint and its possible significance to the observed patterns of articular cartilage breakdown. Bull. Hosp. Joint Dis., New York, in the press, 1977.
4. Girgis, F. G., Marshall, J. L., and Monajem, A. R. S.: The cruciate ligaments of the knee joint, Clin. Orthop. **106**:216, 1975.
5. Goodfellow, J., Hungerford, D. S., and Zindel, M.: Patello-femoral joint mechanics and pathology, J. Bone Joint Surg. **58-B**:287, 1976.
6. Hsieh, H.-H., and Walker, P. S.: Stabilizing mechanics of the loaded and unloaded knee joint, J. Bone Joint Surg. **58-A**:87, 1976.
7. Kettelkamp, D. B., and Jacobs, A. W.: Tibiofemoral contact area, J. Bone Joint Surg. **54-A**:349, 1972.
8. Maquet, P. G., DeBerg, A. J., and Simonet, J. C.: Femorotibial weight-bearing areas, J. Bone Joint Surg. **57-A**:766, 1975.
9. Raux, R., Townsend, P. R., Miegel, R., Rose, R. M., Radin, E. L.: Trabecular architecture of the human patella, J. Biomech. **8**:1, 1975.
10. Seedhom B. B., Dowson, D., and Wright, V.: The load-bearing function of the menisci. In Proceedings of the international congress, Rotterdam, Sept. 1973, published New York, 1974, American Elsevier Publishing Co., Inc.
11. Walker, P. S., and Erkman, M. J.: The role of the menisci in force transmission across the knee, Clin. Orthop. **109**:184, 1975.
12. Walker, P. S., and Hajek, J. V.: The load-bearing areas in the knee joint, J. Biomech. **5**:581, 1972.
13. Wang, C. J., and Walker, P. S.: Rotatory laxity of the human knee joint, J. Bone Joint Surg. **56-A**:161, 1974.

4. Our current understanding of normal knee mechanics and implications for successful knee surgery

Eric L. Radin

The realization that the knee is a much more complicated joint than the hip finally appears to be entering the orthopaedic consciousness. The relatively high failure rate of total knee replacement as contrasted to total hip replacement,[5] the long-term problems created by meniscectomy[1] and patellectomy,[24] and the relative lack of success most surgeons have had with late knee ligament reconstruction have led to a significant amount of experimental work and clinical observations aimed at better understanding the mechanics and pathomechanics of the knee.

Although all the evidence does not yet exist, certain ideas have begun to emerge that help to clarify our thinking about this most important joint and that should alter our clinical approach to many common knee problems. This chapter will delineate some of these emerging concepts and point out their implications in the practice of orthopaedics about the knee.

ANTEROPOSTERIOR STABILITY AND REPAIR OF CRUCIATE LIGAMENTS

For the past 40 years arguments have flourished as to the role of the cruciate ligaments. Their function has been downgraded by many who find that section of the anterior cruciate ligaments seems to make no difference and who have ascribed the major anteroposterior stability to posterior capsular structures and the dynamic effects of the hamstrings and popliteus. Attempts continue to define the centers of rotation of the knee in the hope that some pattern of instantaneous centers will emerge that will make it possible to construct a joint replacement able to mimic knee motion. The assumption has been made that the irregular shapes of the distal femur and proximal tibia are the major contributory factors to knee stability and movement.

First of all, the knee not only moves in flexion but also in rotation.[4] The femoral condyles differ quite significantly in size, and thus an accurate plot of

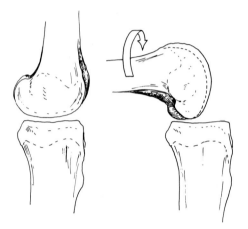

Fig. 4-1. Femoral condyles do not remain in single sagittal plane because of obligatory knee rotation throughout entire range of flexion.

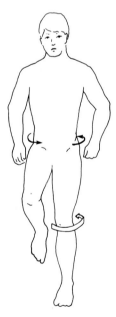

Fig. 4-2. Axial rotation takes place as one pivots over the stance leg in gait whether knee is fused or replaced. Normally knee rotation helps dissipate some of this torque.

the successive centers of rotation must be a complicated three-dimensional one. There can be no curve of reliable instantaneous centers of rotation for the knee as a whole, only one for the medial condyle and one for the lateral condyle. These will not remain in a single sagittal plane because of the obligatory knee rotation throughout the entire range of flexion[25] (Fig. 4-1). Even in the absence of different condylar sizes and shapes, as in a geometric prosthesis, axial rotation still takes place in pivoting over the stance leg in gait, with some of the torque relieved by the knee acting as the central linkage in the lower limb[12] (Fig. 4-2).

Second, the knee has a problem maintaining the collateral ligaments taut in all degrees of flexion. If this could not be accomplished, loading the knee in flexion, as in climbing stairs or pedaling a bicycle, would make the knee unstable and subject the articular cartilage to significant internal shear stresses that probably would be well above what it could sustain. The posterior capsular structures would be relaxed when the knee was flexed and would not be able to maintain anteroposterior stability (Fig. 4-3). Keeping the ligaments taut is accomplished by making the distal femur a cam and the collateral ligaments and their associated structure basically fan shaped so that some aspects of them keep taut as the knee is bent and the cam action goes to work[3] (Fig. 4-4). Furthermore, the cruciate ligaments twist as the knee is flexed and the femur rotates on the tibia.[3] In the flexed knee these ligaments can act to maintain anteroposterior stability.

In such a complicated articular arrangement it is essential that both rolling and sliding motions take place at the knee joint surfaces. As flexion commences, the femoral condyles begin to roll and then slide.[4] The proportion of sliding to rolling changes during flexion, but the combination is essential.[4,17-19] If the motion were just rolling, the femoral condyles would roll right off the back of the tibia[13] (Fig. 4-5). If the motion were just sliding, the femoral condyles would slide along one place in the tibial plateaus until motion would finally be blocked

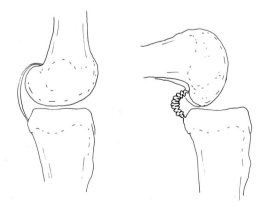

Fig. 4-3. When knee is flexed, posterior capsular structures will not participate in anteroposterior stability.

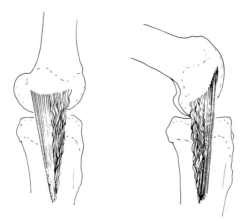

Fig. 4-4. Cam-shaped distal femur maintains tension in fan-shaped collateral ligaments throughout range of flexion.

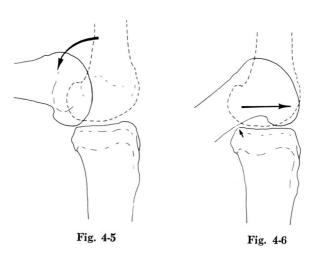

Fig. 4-5   **Fig. 4-6**

Fig. 4-5. If tibiofemoral motion were pure rolling, femoral condyles would roll right off tibia.
Fig. 4-6. If tibiofemoral motion were pure sliding, femoral condyles would slide over one point on tibial plateaus until flexion was blocked by posterior shaft of femur.

by the posterior shaft of the femur, perhaps at 110° or 120° of flexion[13] (Fig. 4-6). The relative amounts of tibiofemoral rolling and sliding are dictated by the cruciate ligaments, which act as parts of a four-bar linkage[11,17-19] (Fig. 4-7).

   This critical role of the cruciate ligaments has been so drastically misunderstood that some designers of total joint replacement would have us surgically extirpate these ligaments before inserting a joint prosthesis. Some, if the cruciate ligaments are absent, recommend the use of various sorts of hinges or ball and socket arrangements; however, none of these can adequately follow the pattern

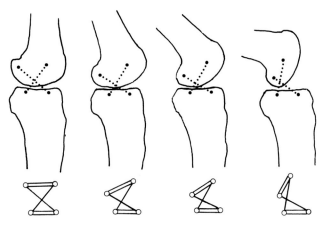

Fig. 4-7. Cruciate ligaments act as parts of four-bar linkage and dictate degree of rolling and sliding that occur during tibiofemoral motion.

of knee motion demanded by functional activity and, because of intolerable stresses, they either break or loosen at the bone-cement interface.

The problem of late repair or replacement of the cruciate ligaments remains a significant one. Although it is probably within the scope of our present technology to develop materials that would have mechanical properties similar to those of tendon (and polyethylene and Silastic are certainly not such materials), proper attachment of artificial ligaments still remains an almost unsolvable problem. What has been suggested is a porous interface that would allow bone to grow into it. This would, however, require a long period of postoperative immobilization, probably leading to a functional failure after successful surgery. Bolts, screws, staples, and other such devices would certainly cause surrounding osteolysis and loosening because of the high stress concentration, as does cement.

What we probably should do is stop ignoring isolated cruciate ligament tears, repair them with some piece of fascial material, and then put the knee in an external four-bar linkage brace for a long period to allow healing and revascularization to take place. Trying to replace these ligaments with various tendons as a dynamic transfer does not make much sense; these transfers are not dynamic at the appropriate time, and what we want is a static checkrein anyway.

ROTATIONAL FUNCTION AND MENISCECTOMY

Whether the knee is allowed to rotate or not, torsional stresses will pass through it, and the knee has to dissipate these stresses. As the body weight passes over the stance leg, an external rotation torsion is put on the lower extremity. The knee begins to bend and the femur externally rotates on the tibia, helping to dissipate this torsion[12] (Fig. 4-2). Any restraint at the knee that does not allow for this rotation is simply torqued loose. Stress has to be transmitted from the hip to the floor, and its transmission is directly through the knee joint. Allowing a flexion-extension joint a rotatory movement is the major function of the menisci, which act as washers to stabilize the joint in extension. They certainly bear load, and the degeneration that frequently follows meniscectomy has been experimentally related to the fact that the surgeon has not allowed the knee sufficient time to regrow a functional meniscal rim.[6] There is ample evidence now to support this view, and it has been shown that several weeks of non–weight bearing with motion almost doubles the rate of meniscal regeneration.[22] Fibrocartilage can form through metaplasia from the cut synovium; the source of cells is there. Encouraging early active motion helps change the clot that forms into fibrocartilage. One just has to be careful with weight bearing and weight lifting in the immediate postoperative period, and obviously a torn meniscus must be removed before it has a chance to create significant articular cartilage damage.

The recently renewed popularity of removing just the inner aspect of a bucket-handle tear and leaving the rim of the meniscus may have some rational basis. The older warnings that such a procedure invariably leads to severe degeneration might have been related to a failure to understand that the whole rim must be left. Partial peripheral meniscectomy represents a reliable model for the creation of osteoarthrosis of the knee[20] and clinically must be avoided. A recent study has pointed out that horizontal cleavage lesions are of little functional consequence and that we should leave such horizontally torn menisci alone.[21]

LATERAL STABILITY AND OSTEOTOMY

As seen in the frontal plane, the body weight in a single-leg stance acts medially to the knee and is balanced by the lateral structures of the knee, in particular the fascia lata and tensor fascia lata.[14] Their resultant is centered over the intercondylar notch and tibial spines. The so-called normal physiologic valgus alignment of the knee results from the fact that the femoral shaft begins at the end of the femoral neck, that is, quite laterally. For equilibrium the weight-bearing foot must be under the center of gravity. The femoral shaft curves back in, and if a physiologic valgus alignment did not exist at the knee, one would tend to stand with one foot on top of the other (Fig. 4-8). Obesity can overwhelm the power of the lateral muscles, displacing the resultant force medially, and force the knee into varus, or the stance can be widened as a compensatory mechanism. This increases the leverage of the body weight through the knee, tending to increase the physiologic valgus alignment. Inability to bring the thighs together because of increased girth might also play a role, as may hereditary predispositions to varus or valgus deformity. Degeneration of the knee is the only joint degeneration related to overweight.

There are several clinically important points that should be made on the basis of this information. First of all, x-ray films to determine if significant varus or valgus deformity exists at the knee must be made in single-leg stance (to fully appreciate the effect of lax collateral ligaments during weight bearing) and measured not on the basis of a few inches of the femoral and tibial shafts but

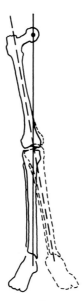

Fig. 4-8. Because optimal balance is achieved with foot directly under center of hip joint, femoral shaft curves medially, creating physiologic valgus deformity at the knee.

rather from the center of the hip joint to the center of the ankle.[14] Second, varus deformity associated with a lax lateral collateral ligament should not be considered a contraindication to osteotomy as long as the corrective osteotomy slightly overcorrects the deformity.[16] The reason is that the collateral ligaments are made of fibrous tissue that acts like scar tissue, and if the abnormal stress is removed from any scar, it will tighten.

There is evidence to show that patients with early degenerative joint disease and a tendency to varus deformity of the knee have weak abductors and that in some of these patients strengthening the abductors with weight lifting has relieved their symptoms.[2]

TREATMENT OF PAIN IN THE PATELLOFEMORAL JOINT

The term "chondromalacia" is used by most orthopaedic surgeons to mean cartilage damage on the underside of the patella, which can be symptomatic but more often is not. More controversy surrounds the treatment of this common condition than perhaps any other in orthopaedic practice. We are advised to ignore it, extirpate it (with a patellectomy), laterally release it, medially tighten it, inferiorly transpose it (with a Hauser procedure), curette and drill it, and replace it. Confusion reigns.

Population studies have indicated that fibrillation of the central medial facet articular cartilage is an age-related, almost physiologic change.[7] In my opinion, central medial facet fibrillation found at arthrotomy should be ignored and considered an incidental finding. Pain in the patellofemoral joint that is more than

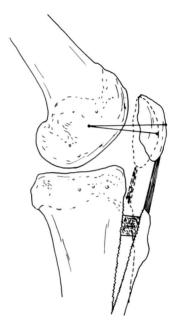

Fig. 4-9. Lever arm of quadriceps mechanism can be lengthened by anterior tibial tubercle transfer using iliac bone block. Increasing leverage of quadriceps decreases force required to straighten knee and thus lowers pressure on patellofemoral joint.

transient and does not fairly quickly respond to conservative measures should be considered as resulting from something other than "chondromalacia." The cause could be an odd facet lesion[9]; entrapped peripheral synovial folds; osteochondral damage resulting from subluxation, malposition, or trauma; or osteoarthrosic change that begins on the lateral facet. Unlike fibrillation on the medial facet, fibrillation on the lateral facet is osteoarthrosic and must not be ignored if found at surgery. Taken in this context, lateral release would be indicated where there is a slight tendency toward lateral subluxation.[8] Drilling and curetting may be indicated for lateral facet lesions. This procedure must then be followed by several months of non–weight bearing and passive motion. Active straight leg raising puts considerable stress across this joint; if healing is to be expected the stress in the joint must be diminished for a relatively long time.[23] Patellectomy, which has been shown to reduce the effect of quadriceps force by almost 50%, should rarely be carried out.[24] Severe or moderately severe osteoarthrosis of the patellofemoral joint should be treated by lowering the stress in the joint by moving the tibial tubercle forward (Fig. 4-9), increasing the leverage through which the quadriceps works.[14,15] Moving the anterior tibial tubercle distally only increases the stress across this joint and has been shown to be related to the development of late osteoarthrosic change.[10] Lateral release and medial reefing or lateral transplantation of the vastus medialis insertion frequently suffice. If the tibial tubercle has to be moved because of recurrent subluxation, then it should be moved only medially. If significant valgus deformity of the knee exists and is the cause of the subluxation, the surgeon is probably wiser to do a varus osteotomy. Valgus osteotomies can be carried out through the proximal tibia. Varus osteotomies of more than 15° must be carried out through the proximal femur, or considerable skewing of the tibial femoral joint line will be produced, with resultant stress concentration in the lateral compartment.[16]

It is of interest that many of the early failures of total knee joint replacement have come from persistent patellofemoral symptoms. No prosthetic replacement of the patella can duplicate its extremely deformable articular surface. The patellofemoral joint has a poor bony fit, and without deformable surfacing the joint rapidly develops areas of considerable stress concentration and degeneration. The answer in patellar replacement would seem to lie in designing a femoral intercondylar notch that allows a prosthetic patella an even ride and a wide contact area throughout the range of flexion.

Rotational stability such as is provided by the Lenox Hill brace will allow certain posterior capsular structures to tighten if the brace is worn on a full-time basis for 3 to 6 months. It makes perfect sense physiologically that all collateral ligamentous tears, particularly ones in which ligamentous ends are still intact, do not need to be operated on, or even immobilized for long, if the healing area is not under abnormal stress; one hopes that this idea will save a great number of patients a great deal of unnecessary surgery. In fact, it is a rare isolated tear of the medial collateral ligament that needs to be sewn together, and attenuation of this ligament, as long as the knee is not in valgus alignment, can be best treated by bracing for an appropriate period of time.

CONCLUSION

We were lucky with the hip. It is basically a ball-and-socket configuration, well controlled and stabilized by several surrounding muscles. The knee is a much more complicated joint, has need of many nondynamic constraints to its motion, and is in fact one of the more complicated joints in the body. The knee is a rotating cam whose oscillations in the sagittal plane are controlled by the cruciate ligaments acting as parts of a four-bar linkage: It is difficult to conceive of anything more complicated. However complicated it may be, if we clearly approach knee reconstruction and replacement in terms of function, we might fashion more realistic operative procedures and pursue more rational postoperative courses that would improve our therapeutic success rate.

References

1. Appel, H.: Late results after meniscectomy in the knee joint, Acta Orthop. Scand. Suppl. 133:1, 1970.
2. Blaimont, P., Burnotte, J., and Halleaux, P.: La préarthrose du genue: pathogenie, biomechanique et traitement prophylactique, Acta Orthop. Belg. 41:177, 1975.
3. Brantigan, O. C., and Voshell, A. F.: The mechanics of the ligaments and menisci of the knee joint, J. Bone Joint Surg. 23:44, 1941.
4. Braune, W., and Fischer, O.: Bewegungen des Kniegelenkes nach einer neuen Methode

an lebenden Menschen gemessen, Abh. Math. Phys. Sächs. Gesellsch. Wissensch. **17**:75, 1891.

5. Cracchiolo, A., III: Statistics of total knee replacement, Clin. Orthop. **120**:2, 1976.
6. Elmer, R. M., Moskowitz, R. M., and Frankel, V. H.: Meniscal regeneration: its relationship to postmeniscectomy degenerative joint disease, Clin. Orthop. **124**:304, 1977.
7. Emery, I. H., and Meachim, G.: Surface morphology and topography of patello-femoral cartilage fibrillation in Liverpool necropsies, J. Anat. **116**:103, 1973.
8. Ficat, P.: Pathologie féméro-patellaire, Paris, 1970, Masson & Cie Editeurs.
9. Goodfellow, J., Hungerford, D. S., and Woods, C.: Patello-femoral joint mechanics and pathology. 2. Chondromalacia patellae, J. Bone Joint Surg. **58-B**:291, 1976.
10. Hampson, W. G. J., and Hill, P.: Late results of transfer of the tibial tubercle for recurrent dislocation of the patella, J. Bone Joint Surg. **57-B**:209, 1975.
11. Husson, A.: The functional anatomy of the knee joint: the closed kinematic chain as a model of a knee joint. In Ingwersen, O. S., et al., editors: The knee joint, Amsterdam, 1973, Excerpta Medica.
12. Inman, V. T., and Mann, R. A.: Biomechanics of the foot and ankle. In Inman, V. T., editor: DuVries' surgery of the foot, ed. 3, St. Louis, 1973, The C. V. Mosby Co.
13. Kapandji, I. A.: The physiology of the joints. Vol. 2, lower limb, ed. 2, Edinburgh, 1970, Churchill Livingstone.
14. Maquet, P.: Biomechanics and osteoarthritis of the knee, Proc. SICOT, **11**:317, 1969.
15. Maquet, P.: Advancement of the tibial tuberosity, Clin. Orthop. **115**:225, 1976.
16. Maquet, P.: Valgus osteotomy for osteoarthritis of the knee, Clin. Orthop. **120**:143, 1976.
17. Menshik, A.: Mechanik des Kniegelenkes. 1, Z. Orthop. **112**:481, 1974.
18. Menshik, A.: Mechanik des Kniegelenkes. 2, Z. Orthop. **113**:388, 1975.
19. Menshik, A.: Mechanik des Kniegelenkes. 3, Vienna, 1976, F. Sailer.
20. Moskowitz, R. W., Davis, W., and Sammarco, J.: Experimentally induced degenerative joint lesions following partial meniscectomy in the rabbit, Arthritis Rheum. **16**:397, 1973.
21. Noble, J., and Hamblen, D. L.: The pathology of the degenerative meniscus lesion, J. Bone Joint Surg. **57-B**:180, 1975.
22. Radin, E. L., and Bryan, R. S.: The effect of weightbearing on regrowth of the medial meniscus after meniscectomy, J. Trauma **10**:164, 1970.
23. Radin, E. L., Ehrlich, M. G., Weiss, C. A., and Parker, H. G.: Osteoarthrosis as a state of altered physiology. In Buchanan, W. W., and Dick, W. C., editors: Recent advances in rheumatology, Edinburgh, 1976, Churchill Livingstone.
24. Sutton, F. S., Thompson, C. H., Lipke, J., and Kettelkamp, D. B.: The effect of patellectomy on knee function, J. Bone Joint Surg. **58-A**:537, 1976.
25. Walker, P. S., Shoji, H., and Erkman, M. J.: The rotational axis of the knee and its significance to prosthesis design, Clin. Orthop. **89**:160, 1972.

5. Gait characteristics of the knee: normal, abnormal, and postreconstruction

Donald B. Kettelkamp

Knee motion occurs in three planes during walking and the performance of daily activities. This motion is a characteristic of the knee as a diarthroidal joint. Motion during walking in the normal knee has been studied by a number of investigators using photometric and goniometric methods with close agreement as to the magnitude and sequence of motion.[2-4,8] Considerably less information is available for the normal knee during the activities of daily living[7] and for the abnormal and reconstructed knee.[*] The purpose of this chapter is to present the gait characteristics of normal, abnormal, and postreconstruction knees and to discuss the possible implications of these findings to total joint replacement.

MATERIALS AND METHODS

Knee motion for walking and for activities of daily living was measured with a three-plane electrogoniometer.[4] The goniometer was attached to the thigh and the calf using ECG straps. The flexion-extension pot of the goniometer was centered on the lateral side of the knee ½ inch proximal to the joint line and at the midpoint on the lateral femoral condyle from front to back. The extension along the tibia was parallel to the tibia in the frontal and sagittal planes. The degree of accuracy of this appliance has been previously described.[4]

In some of the earlier studies, cadence, stride length, and velocity were not determined. Where these determinations were made, cadence was obtained from the chart recorder, which moves at a fixed rate of speed, stride length was measured on the walkway, and velocity was a multiple of the two divided by 60 to give a measurement in centimeters per second. All patients were permitted to walk at their normal rate of speed.

Periods of weight bearing were determined from heel switches and had primary application to the activities of daily living with implants, particularly sitting and rising from a chair.

The gait characteristics of knee motion in 44 normal knees,[4] 41 rheumatoid

---

[*]References 1, 3, 5, 6, 9, 10.

knees,[5] 27 degenerative knees,[6] and 52 postmeniscectomy knees[3] will be presented in separate sections. Knee motion during walking will also be presented for 37 knees with MacIntosh prostheses,[10] 32 with proximal tibial osteotomies,[6] and a limited number with various types of total knee replacements.

Data for the activities of daily living, sitting and rising from a chair, and going up and down stairs, will be presented for 30 normal knees[7] and for a limited number of knees with total knee replacements.

MOTION IN NORMAL KNEES

Knee motion measurements in 22 normal persons—16 men and 6 women (44 knees)—are presented in Table 5-1. Cadence and stride length values were obtained from a publication by Murray et al.[8] It should be pointed out that these were average normal values from a relatively young group with an age range of 21 to 35 years and a mean of 28.7 years. The pattern of knee motion was consistent for each knee from stride to stride, although there were slight fluctuations in ranges of motion. Greater variation occurred from knee to knee and individual to individual; however, the overall patterns of motion were fairly consistent, particularly in the sagittal plane.

The pattern of normal motion in the sagittal plane was one of maximum extension occurring at or just before heel strike; flexion occurred during early stance phase to approximately the point of foot flat; secondary extension occurred between the time that the foot was flat and the time the heel was raised from the ground; the knee then flexed between heel off and toe off, continuing into swing phase (Fig. 5-1). Maximum extension occurred at or just before heel strike, and secondary extension only rarely reached the magnitude of the first extension (in a normal knee). Thus the so-called double screw-home mechanism probably does not occur during normal walking.

The normal pattern for abduction and adduction was somewhat less consistent, but in general maximum abduction occurred at approximately the same time as maximum extension. The knee adducted with stance-phase flexion and tended to abduct again as extension occurred. These findings were as anticipated on the basis of the anatomic characteristics of the knee; the maximum valgus femorotibial angle is present with the knee in a fully extended position. As the knee flexes, this angle decreases, so that at full flexion the tibia and femur are superimposed. Slight additional abduction and adduction can occur because of normal ligamentous laxity and because of compliance of the articular cartilage.

Rotation was the least consistent of the patterns of motion. Maximum external rotation occurred during swing phase, usually preceeding maximum extension. The tibia then internally rotated during early stance phase, externally rotated slightly as secondary extension occurred, and then internally rotated into swing phase.

Although there was some individual variation, these overall patterns were quite consistent.

Table 5-1. Knee motion (in degrees) during walking

| | Normal knees | | Abnormal knees | | | | Knees after reconstruction | | | Geometric | |
	Young	Old	Post-meniscectomy	Degenerative	Rheumatoid	Osteotomy	Mac-Intosh	Herbert	Shiers	IU	Mayo Clinic
Number of knees	44	32	52	27	41	32	37	12	9	9	50
Swing-phase flexion-extension	67.4	60.0	66.6	42.4	30.0	42.4	27.7	44.0	47.0	44.0	51.0
Stance-phase flexion-extension	20.6	—	19.6	7.4	6.0	8.7	4.6	2.0	2.0	5.4	13.0
Abduction-adduction	11.2	11.6	12.4	9.2	10.0	9.4	10.0	9.0	10.0	8.0	10.0
Rotation	13.3	15.0	12.9	12.1	8.0	8.1	8.0	13.0	10.0	7.0	12.6
Cadence (step/min)	117	95.5	—	56.0	72.5	64.5	47.6	39.0	29.0	57.2	88.5
Stride length (cm)	156.5	120.0	—	94.3	80.5	93.8	72.6	80.0	77.0	90.0	96.0
Velocity (cm/sec)	300	190	—	88.5	97.6	100.9	57.6	52	37	85.0	141.6

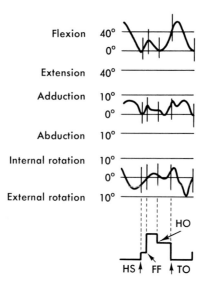

Fig. 5-1. Example of walking motion of normal knee. Maximum extension occurs at or just before heel strike (*HS*). Flexion rapidly occurs to foot flat (*FF*). Secondary extension then occurs, followed by flexion into swing phase. Stance-phase flexion and extension is from maximum extension to maximum flexion (approximately at or just after foot flat). Swing-phase flexion and extension is from maximum flexion during swing phase to maximum extension. (*HO*, Heel off. *TO*, Toe off.)

Normal data from an older group has been presented by DeWeerd et al.[1] Again, the patterns were fairly consistent, although the magnitude of motion was somewhat decreased in the sagittal plane and cadence and stride length were also somewhat decreased.

MOTION IN ABNORMAL KNEES
Postmeniscectomy

Johnson et al.[3] obtained goniometric studies for level walking in 52 postmeniscectomy knees using the unoperated opposite knee as a control (Table 5-1). The average values obtained showed no significant differences between the postmeniscectomy and unoperated knees for level walking. The postmeniscectomy knees had less stance-phase flexion (P = .05) than the previously mentioned 44 normal knees. Many of the postmeniscectomy knees had Fairbank's changes, including medial joint space narrowing, mild degrees of medial collateral laxity, and anteromedial rotatory instability.

This study implied that for level walking mild degrees of instability had very little effect on knee motion. It also suggested that the first alteration in the abnormal knee is decreased stance-phase flexion and extension.

Degenerative arthritis

A study of 27 knees with degenerative genu varum showed decreased motion in stance-phase and swing-phase flexion and extension[6] (Table 5-1). The mag-

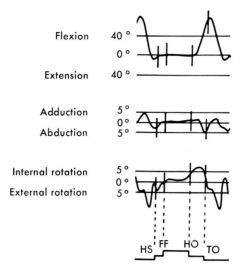

Fig. 5-2. This knee with degenerative varus deformity illustrates loss of stance-phase flexion and extension. This particular knee maintained a nearly normal range of swing-phase flexion and extension, which is more commonly decreased also.

nitude of abduction and adduction and of rotation were not significantly different from normal; however, fairly wide variations in patterns were observed. Complete loss of stance-phase flexion and extension was common in severely involved knees (Fig. 5-2). Cadence, stride length, and velocity were markedly decreased as compared to either the young or older normal knees.

Rheumatoid arthritis

The alterations in rheumatoid arthritis were more severe than those in degenerative arthritis.[5] The average values from 41 rheumatoid knees are presented in Table 5-1. The average stance-phase flexion and extension and average swing-phase flexion and extension were less in the rheumatoid knees than the degenerative varus knees. The average range of motion for abduction and adduction and for rotation were within normal limits. Cadence was a little greater in the rheumatoid knees than in those with degenerative arthritis. Stride length was less; however, the preponderance of patients with rheumatoid arthritis were women. Stride length is related to leg length; hence, one might expect a shorter stride length than in degenerative arthritis, in which the majority of patients were men.

Clinical findings and symptoms were related to decreased knee motion in the sagittal plane during walking in both the rheumatoid and degenerative knees. Those items that significantly decreased the amount of motion were pain with weight bearing, standing flexion, flexion contracture, severity of loss of articular surface, and varus or valgus angulation.

In arthritic knees, both degenerative and rheumatoid, the most significant alteration in knee motion during walking was a decrease in stance-phase flexion and extension. The postmeniscectomy knees seldom deviated from normal except for the decrease in stance-phase flexion and extension. These findings imply that stance-phase flexion and extension, one of the major determinants of gait,[9] is one of the earliest gait characteristics altered by arthritis of the knee.

Swing-phase flexion-extension also decreased in both rheumatoid and degenerative arthritis. It is interesting to note that the amount of swing-phase flexion and extension in normal young adults is about 49% of the available knee flexion and extension. A decreased use of the available passive flexion in the knee was characteristic of arthritic knees. Swing-phase flexion and extension was 39% of the available flexion in the degenerative knees and 25% of the available flexion in the rheumatoid knees. Thus in arthritic knees not only was there a decrease in stance-phase flexion and extension but also the relative amount of available motion used in swing phase was similarly decreased, to a greater degree in rheumatoid than in degenerative arthritis.

WALKING AFTER RECONSTRUCTIVE PROCEDURES

The clinical findings for which the patient seeks medical help and reconstructive procedures are pain, instability, flexion contracture, effusion, and synovitis. Since these factors were associated with decreased motion, the question that must be raised is, "Does motion during walking return toward normal after reconstructive procedures?" Data in this area are limited to studies of tibial osteotomy,[6] MacIntosh prostheses,[10] and, to a very minimal degree, total knee replacement arthroplasties.[1]

Proximal tibial osteotomy

We have recently reported the results of proximal tibial osteotomy performed for knees with degenerative varus deformity.[6] The mean values for the gait parameters for these patients are presented in Table 5-1. We found that a successful proximal tibial osteotomy (pain relief) improved knee motion during walking only in stance-phase flexion and extension. The stance-phase flexion and extension in the knees with good results increased an average of 3° (approximately 30%) compared to preoperative measurements but still was less than 50% of normal. The only other alteration in knee motion associated with a good result was a decrease in the magnitude of rotation. We are not able to explain this finding, but we suspect that it was related to a decrease in the translatory shift of the tibia on the femur so commonly seen in degenerative genu varus.

MacIntosh prosthesis

Stauffer et al.[10] reported the gait characteristics of 37 rheumatoid knees before and after MacIntosh prosthetic replacement arthroplasties. The mean values are presented in Table 5-1. Improvement in swing- and stance-phase flexion and extension was minimal and not significant. There was not a sigificant relationship between the postoperative gait characteristics and the clinical results. These findings indicate that in the rheumatoid patient the MacIntosh plateau prosthesis does not significantly improve the motion of the knee during walking, although most patients experienced significant pain relief and an improvement in ability to walk distances. One other clinical finding associated with decreased swing- and stance-phase flexion and extension, which may be related to the lack of improvement in this group of patients, was the presence of patellar widening and patellar osteophytes. Both significantly decreased swing- and stance-phase flexion and extension, and neither was corrected or improved by the operative procedure. The gait findings following MacIntosh implant arthroplasty correspond to the general clinical dissatisfaction with this procedure.

Total knee replacements

Gait studies of implant function in patients are in progress in a number of institutions, but few data are available. DeWeerd et al.[1] reported on 50 patients with geometric implants. We have similar data from study of nine geometric arthroplasties at Indiana University. Mean values from these two groups of patients are presented in Table 5-1. The values from the Mayo Clinic series show a definite improvement toward normal. The differences between their mean values and our findings may represent patient selection. Preoperatively our patients had tight knees with severe deformity. When less severe deformity was present, we used resurfacing implants other than the geometric. The data from Mayo Clinic may represent a less severely involved patient population. Clinical correlations with the gait findings are not available at this time. These findings, particularly those from Mayo Clinic, are encouraging and imply that knee replacement arthroplasty may return knee motion during walking toward normal. Perhaps the most

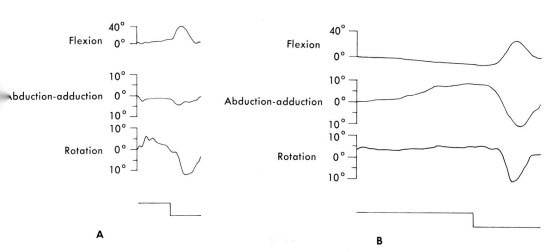

Fig. 5-3. Common patterns in knees with Herbert (**A**) and Shiers (**B**) prostheses. Knee with Herbert prosthesis shows gradual flexion throughout midstance, and knee with Shiers prosthesis show gradual extension throughout midstance.

significant finding was that the pattern of motion as well as amount of motion in the sagittal plane after geometric arthroplasty may return toward normal.

This differs from our findings in a limited number of Herbert and Shiers prostheses. Data from 12 Herbert prostheses show virtually no stance-phase flexion-extension. Two sagittal plane patterns were characteristic of this prostheses; one was gradual flexion throughout stance phase and the other gradual extension throughout stance phase (Fig. 5-3). This pattern, also seen with the Shiers prostheses, differs from those with the geometric and has no counterpart in either untreated degenerative or rheumatoid knees. It is possible, though unsubstantiated, that these abnormal patterns contribute to the breakage and loosening seen with both the Herbert and Shiers implants.

We have to date examined only three knees with variable axis implants. In

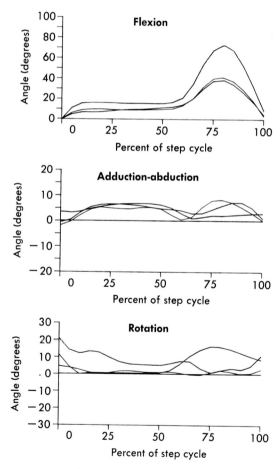

Fig. 5-4. Comparison of motion during walking for three knees with variable axis implants illustrates similarity of motion in sagittal and coronal planes (flexion and extension and abduction and adduction) given as percentage of gait cycle.

these three patients magnitudes of motion with this implant showed considerable improvement toward normal (Fig. 5-4). The sagittal plane pattern, though not the usual one seen in normal knees, does occur in a few normal knees. The differentiating point was lack of secondary extension during stance phase.

It is too early to make specific statements concerning the relationship between the patterns seen following total knee implant and either clinical results or subsequent evidence of mechanical failure. It is of interest that in some instances the pattern of motion seems to be implant specific, such as in the Herbert, the Shiers, and the variable axis implants. Certainly the sagittal plane pattern seen with the geometric knee and with the variable axis implant were patterns that can be seen in normal or untreated arthritic joints. The significance of these findings must await further studies.

ACTIVITIES OF DAILY LIVING

Activities of daily living consist of going up and down stairs, sitting and rising from a chair, and lifting an object from a lower level or from the floor. Laubenthal et al.[7] reported the knee motion used by normal subjects for these activities. They found that in going up stairs foot over foot, the subjects used an average of 83° of knee flexion. The average flexion for sitting and rising from a chair was 93°. The average flexion for tying a shoe was 106°. The average flexion for lifting an object from the floor was 71° when most of the flexion took place at the hip and back. After the subjects were instructed to squat to pick up the object, the average flexion increased to 117°. The patterns of knee flexion and extension were activity specific. The average tibial rotation that took place during these activities exceeded that found in walking. In going up and down stairs the average rotation was 16°; however, the consistency of pattern seen in walking was not present. This seemed to be related to foot placement in relation to the step. The closer the foot was to the step, the more rotation was required for going up stairs.

Similar information is not available for rheumatoid arthritic, degenerative arthritic, or postmeniscectomy knees, nor those that had tibial osteotomy or MacIntosh prosthesis arthroplasty. Stauffer et al.[10] did note, however, that the ability to go up and down stairs and get up and down from sitting was not significantly

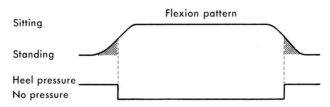

Fig. 5-5. Knee flexion with sitting down and knee extension with rising. Baseline represents standing. Cross-hatched areas represent time during which there was heel contact with floor. This pattern of limited weight bearing during sitting and rising was seen frequently in knees after implant surgery.

improved in patients with MacIntosh prostheses. Similar data from patients who have had total joint replacement are not available. Clinical reports indicate, however, that many of these patients go up and down stairs one step at a time. Our limited laboratory findings agree with this. It has been of interest to note sitting and rising from a chair. Using foot switches to demonstrate the period of foot contact and weight bearing, we have found that most patients with implants bear weight on the extremity only during the first degrees of flexion as they sit down and the last degrees of flexion as they rise from the chair (Fig. 5-5). This implies that many patients after total knee replacement are not bearing weight on their implant during the majority of the flexion that occurs with sitting and rising, thus tending to unload the joint.

Several of the current studies are making measurements of the knee motion that occurs with rising from and sitting on a chair and in going up and down stairs. This should provide more information as to the type of loads being placed on the implants during those activities.

DISCUSSION

Studies of arthritic knees and knees that have had various types of reconstruction have demonstrated alterations in knee motion. These studies show that the normal sagittal plane pattern of motion in an abnormal knee tends to decrease flexion and extension, with the most marked decrease occurring during stance phase. There is some evidence that satisfactory reconstruction, whether by osteotomy or implant, tends to restore stance-phase flexion and extension toward normal. It should be noted that the two hinged type of implants that we have studied, the Herbert and the Shiers, do not show improved stance-phase flexion and extension, even in relatively asymptomatic knees.

Motion in the transverse plane (rotation) and in the coronal plane (abduction and adduction) is more difficult to evaluate. The magnitude of motion was approximately the same in abnormal as in normal knees. The patterns of motion, however, appear to be altered by the knee abnormality. These altered patterns are not well understood at the present time. It has been found, however, that in knees with tibial osteotomy the better results showed a decreased amount of rotation when compared with the knees with poorer results, although the reasons are not known. It is of interest to note that irrespective of the amount of varus or valgus instability present, the magnitude of motion remains roughly within normal limits. I would interpret this finding to mean that weight bearing becomes impossible without some form of external support when those ranges of motion are exceeded. The patient may compensate for this by using thigh support as in the valgus rheumatoid knee, or by using crutches, a walker, or other form of external support.

Current data, although limited, imply that following total knee replacement most knees are not used in a normal manner for the activities of daily living. The majority of these patients are not bearing weight on the knee during the last part of flexion in sitting nor the early part of extension in rising. This tends to decrease the load on the joint during those activities. Many of these patients also are not stair climbers. They use the implanted knee as though it were arthrodesed, i.e., going up and down stairs a single step at a time with the implanted knee for the most part in an extended position or using only a few degrees of flexion. This, too, tends to decrease the load on the implant. This same manner of going up and down stairs was used by patients after patellectomy and may be related to residual patellofemoral arthritis.

At the present time on the basis of limited data it appears that there may be implant-specific patterns of flexion and extension during walking. Should additional studies bear out this finding, it may be possible to relate restricted motion or abnormalities of motion to the process of loosening.

References

1. DeWeerd, S. H., Jr., Stauffer, R. N., Chao, E. Y., and Axmear, F. E.: Functional evaluation of pre and postoperative total knee arthroplasty patients. In Transactions of the twenty-second annual meeting of the Orthopaedic Research Society, Vol. 1, 1976, p. 77.
2. Eberhart, H. D., Inman, V. T., Saunders, J. B. DeC. M., Levens, A. S., Bresler, B., and McCowen, T. D.: Fundamental studies of human locomotion and other information relating to the design of artificial limbs, vol. 1. A report to the National Research Council, Committee on Artificial Limbs, Berkeley, 1947, University of California.
3. Johnson, R. J., Kettelkamp, D. B., Clark, W., and Leaverton, P.: Factors affecting late meniscectomy results, J. Bone Joint Surg. 56-A:719, 1974.
4. Kettelkamp, D. B., Johnson, R. J., Smidt, G. L., Chao, E. Y. S., and Walker, M.: An electrogoniometric study of knee motion in normal gait, J. Bone Joint Surg. 52-A:775, 1970.
5. Kettelkamp, D. B., Leaverton, P. E., and Misol, S.: Gait characteristics of the rheumatoid knee, Arch. Surg. 104:30, 1972.
6. Kettelkamp, D. B., Wenger, D. R., Chao, E. Y. S., and Thompson, C.: Results of proximal tibial osteotomy. The effects of tibiofemoral angle, stance-phase flexion-extension, and medial plateau force, J. Bone Joint Surg. 58-A:952, 1976.
7. Laubenthal, K. N., Smidt, G. L., and Kettelkamp, D. B.: A quantitative analysis of knee motion during activities of daily living, Phys. Ther. 52:34, 1972.
8. Murray, M. P., Drought, A. B., and Kory, R. C.: Walking patterns of normal men, J. Bone Joint Surg. 46-A:335, 1964.
9. Saunders, J. B. DeC. M., Inman, V. T., and Eberhart, N. D.: The major determinants in normal and pathological gait, J. Bone Joint Surg. 35-A:543, 1953.
10. Stauffer, R., Kettelkamp, D. B., Thompson, C., and Wenger, D.: The MacIntosh prosthesis. Prospective clinical and gait evaluation, Arch. Surg. 110:717, 1975.

PART TWO

Diagnostic procedures

6. Value of arthrography for the problem knee

Martin W. Korn
Robert M. Spitzer
Harold E. Olsson

The purposes of the study described here have been (1) to determine the accuracy of arthrography in a clinical setting in which the clinical examination is performed by an orthopaedist and supervised by a radiologist and (2) to evaluate the benefits of arthrography in the evaluation and management of the problem knee.

Our study consisted of consecutively reviewed arthrograms of 100 knees (in 100 patients), all of which were operated on by the same surgeon. The arthrography and surgery were carried out between January, 1973, and December, 1975. The first 19 knees were studied by the single-contrast technique and the subsequent 81 by the double-contrast fluoroscopic technique.

The basic equipment for performing arthrograms at our hospital includes nitrous oxide, Conray 60 contrast medium, 1% solution of lidocaine, and the necessary tubing, syringes, and skin preparation materials. An angiographic head immobilizer was modified to make a snug cradle for holding the involved leg. Approximately 100 ml of nitrous oxide is injected after careful skin preparation and draping, followed by 3 to 4 ml of the contrast medium. Bubble formation is minimized by this order of injection and by not exercising the knee after injection. Fluoroscopic localization is then carried out and spot films are obtained. The knee is held in the cradle and the examiner holds the patient's ankle to obtain the desired position and stress.

Arthrograms were taken of the medial meniscus, lateral meniscus, and anterior cruciate ligament of each knee. The accuracy of results was as follows:

	Medial meniscus	Lateral meniscus	Cruciate ligament
Accurate	96%	95%	82%
False positive	2%	2%	9%
False negative	2%	3%	9%

The anterior cruciate ligament was analyzed as part of the overall study, but these results will not be discussed in this chapter.

As seen by the double-contrast technique, the normal medial meniscus has a triangular appearance, with the visible surfaces of the meniscus at a direct tangent to the central x-ray beam (Fig. 6-1). The surfaces are coated with contrast medium, which contrasts strongly with the nitrous oxide. The appearance of the medial meniscus varies from anterior to posterior. In the more *posterior* portion an important feature is the longer, thicker appearance of the meniscus and the tight attachment to the femoral condyle. Inconstant small recesses may

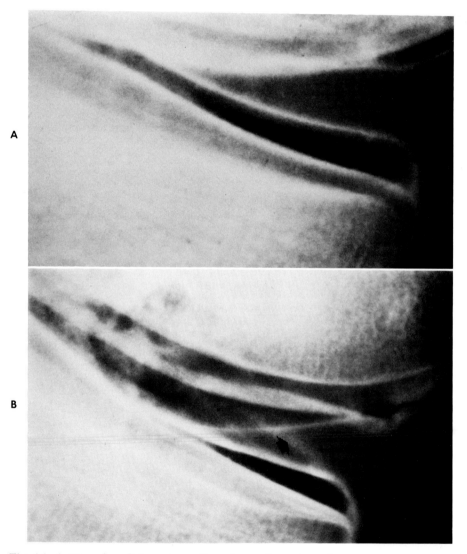

Fig. 6-1. A, Normal medial meniscus. Central x-ray beam is at direct tangent to meniscus. **B,** Normal medial meniscus with sharply defined triangular meniscus is directly tangential to central ray, and less sharply defined portion of meniscus is not tangential to central ray (arrow).

be present either superiorly or inferiorly. In the *midportion* of the meniscus the arthrographic appearance is similar to that of the more posterior segments but the meniscus is generally shorter and thinner. In the *anterior* segments the meniscus is tilted inferiorly and slightly displaced from the tibial surface by the distention of the joint with nitrous oxide, and the large infrapatellar joint space

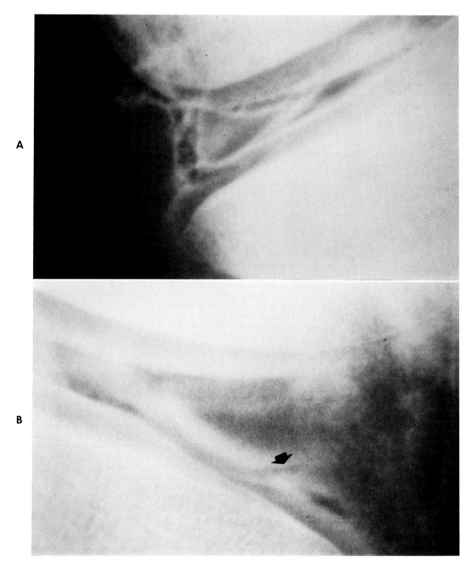

Fig. 6-2. A, Classic vertical tear. **B,** Inferior surface tear (arrow), with extension into body of meniscus with ill-defined margins and some increased absorption of contrast medium. Irregular, slightly bubbly appearance overlying peripheral half of this meniscus represents popliteal cyst containing contrast medium.

Continued.

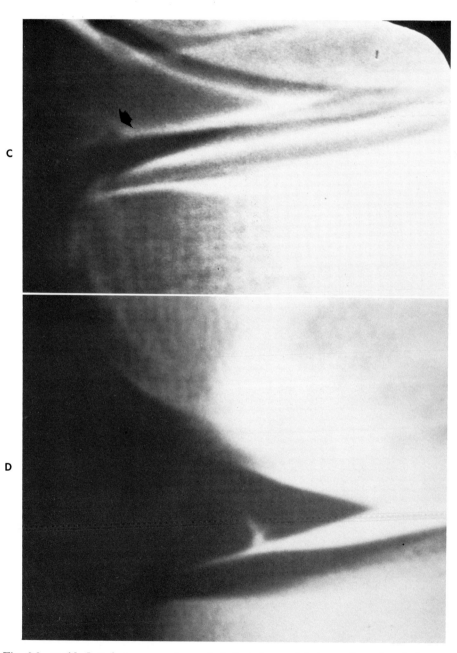

Fig. 6-2, cont'd. C, Inferior recess (arrow). Indentation on inferior surface of medial meniscus can be misinterpreted as a tear but instead represents overlap shadow from nontangential anterior recess. **D,** Inferior surface tear (arrow).

is readily apparent where the capsule is separated from the medial femoral condyle.

A classic vertical tear shows contrast medium crossing the body of the meniscus, with the inner and peripheral fragments each coated with contrast medium
and separated from one another by a region with an irregular appearance (Fig.
6-2). The appearance of a meniscal tear on the arthrogram may not correspond

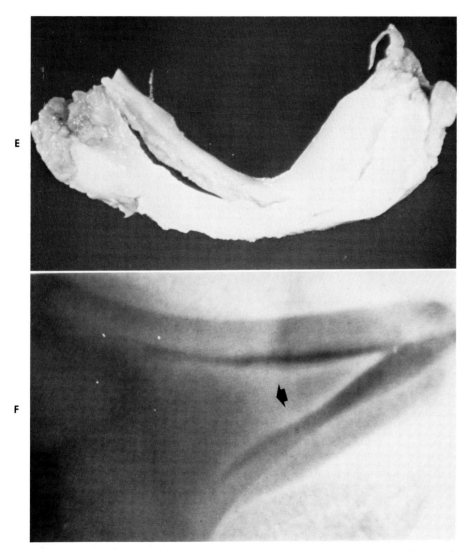

Fig. 6-2, cont'd. **E,** Gross specimen of knee shown in **D.** Note that arthrogram shows only an
inferior surface tear. **F,** Possible tear. Contrast medium absorption (arrow) arouses suspicion
of a tear.

Continued.

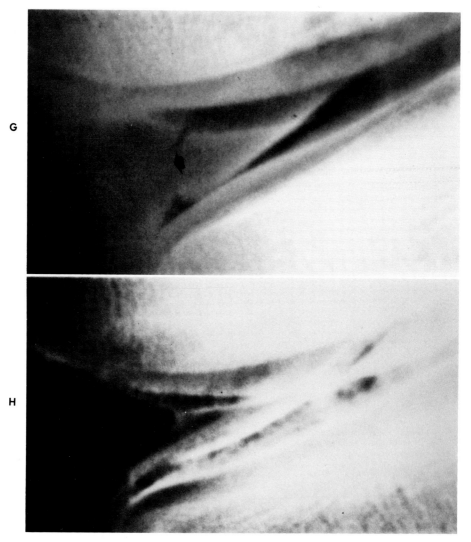

Fig. 6-2, cont'd. G, Confirmed tear. Additional views show vertical tear suspected in **F. H,** Peripheral recesses. In our experience, recess should extend no farther than 50% of thickness of meniscus. In this instance, first views of posterior aspect of this medial meniscus show a possible deep "recess" (arrow).

dependably to the gross anatomic tear. For instance, Fig. 6-2, *D*, shows a medial meniscus with what appears to be an inferior surface tear, but the gross specimen showed a typical bucket-handle tear.

In our study group two arthrograms of the medial meniscus gave false positive results. One occurred in a knee with a lateral meniscus tear and one was in a knee with an anterior cruciate ligament tear. The two false negative results in arthrograms of the medial meniscus were both in single-contrast studies.

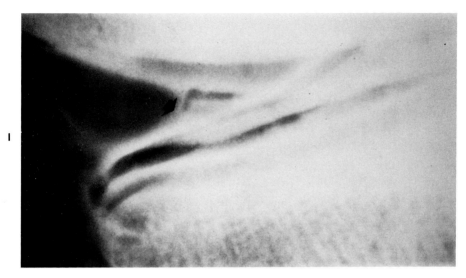

Fig. 6-2, cont'd. I, Confirmed tear (arrow). Additional views of knee shown in H with more stress reveal extensive tear of body of so-called "recess" representing most peripheral extent of tear. This illustrates value of fluoroscopic technique and additional positioning and stressing of knee in identifying pertinent view and obtaining spot films at the precise time that tear is best demonstrated.

The normal arthrographic anatomy of the posterior part of the lateral meniscus is reviewed in Fig. 6-3.

It is clear that knowledge of the precise location of the tangent of the lateral meniscus represented by a specific arthrogram is necessary if one is to interpret the significance of the superior and inferior attachments since presence or absence of either or both may be seen in a normal knee.

A classic peripheral tear of the lateral meniscus shows contrast medium extending across the body of the meniscus (Fig. 6-4).

There were two false positive results of arthrograms of the lateral meniscus; both of these were of knees with medial meniscal tears. There were three cases of false negative results in arthrograms of the lateral meniscus. One occurred in a remnant of a lateral meniscectomy and two in association with medial meniscal tears.

It is clear from the foregoing that bilateral tears require special attention in interpretation. There were 12 surgically proved bilateral tears in this study, only 1 of which was suspected clinically; 10 were thought to be medial tears only and 1 a lateral tear only. Arthrography, however, detected 10 of the 12 bilateral tears and gave two false negative results for the lateral meniscus.

Arthrography was found to be very safe. There were two minor, self-limited inflammations and no infections in the 100 knees. Arthrography has been highly accurate. It is certainly readily available and can be done as an outpatient procedure under local anesthesia. It has been a great help in decreasing procrastina-

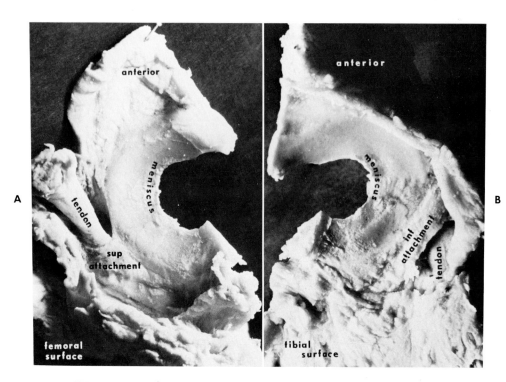

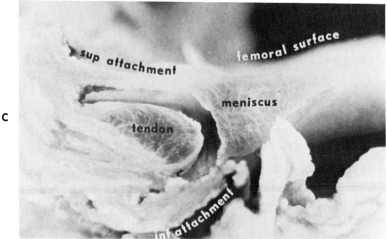

Fig. 6-3. **A,** Gross anatomic specimen of lateral meniscus seen from its femoral surface. **B,** Gross anatomic specimen of same meniscus seen from its tibial surface. Note oblique course of popliteal tendon traveling from below tibial margin posteriorly forward and upward to its attachment on lateral femoral epicondyle. That part of its oblique path contiguous to periphery of lateral meniscus represents popliteal portion of lateral meniscus, surrounded where possible by superior and inferior struts or attachments of lateral meniscus to lateral capsule. **C,** Cross section. Across midpart of popliteal portion of lateral meniscus, both superior and inferior attachments of lateral meniscus to lateral capsule are seen.

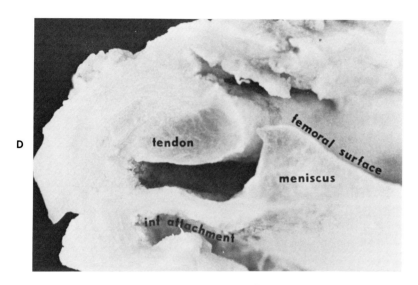

D

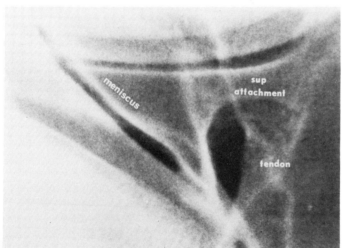

E

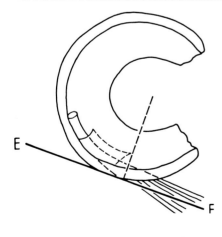

Fig. 6-3, cont'd. D, Cross section. Slightly more anterior cross section, where the popliteal tendon is more superior, reveals intact inferior attachment but no superior attachment, since tendon now occupies space where superior attachment normally would pass to lateral capsule. At this point, knee joint communicates with bursa surrounding popliteal tendon, thus permitting contrast medium to coat surfaces of popliteal bursa. E, Diagram showing tangent *EF* of central ray to lateral meniscus at posterior part of popliteal portion of meniscus; arthrographic cross section is of same tangent. Note that inferior attachment or strut is absent and superior attachment is present.

Continued.

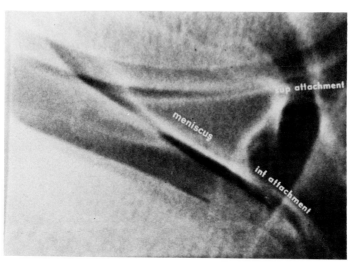

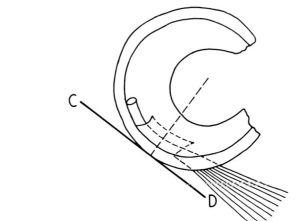

Fig. 6-3, cont'd. F, Diagram showing tangent *CO* through central part of popliteal portion of lateral meniscus. Arthrographic cross section shows intact superior and inferior attachments, and popliteal bursa itself is well seen and is lined with contrast medium.

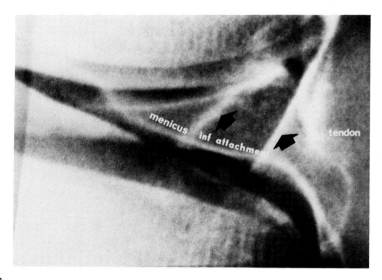

G

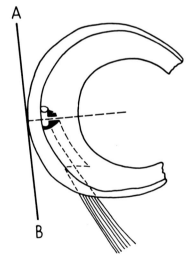

A

B

Fig. 6-3, cont'd. G, Diagram showing most anterior tangent *AB* of popliteal portion of lateral meniscus. Arthrographic cross section shows absence of superior attachment and intact inferior attachment. Contrast medium within popliteal bursa, especially just anterior to exit of popliteal tendon from its bursa, may be seen as vertical opaque line at periphery of lateral meniscus and can be mistaken for a tear of meniscus (arrow).

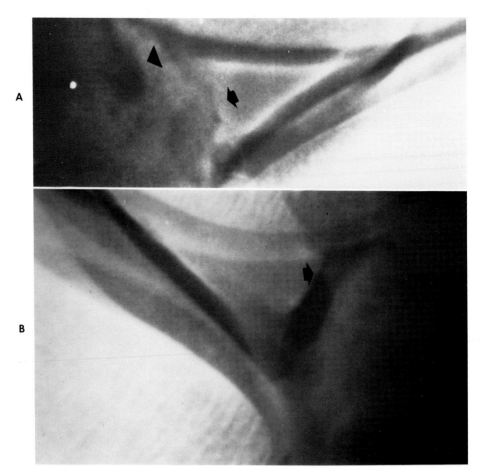

Fig. 6-4. A, Classic peripheral tear of lateral meniscus (arrow). Contrast medium extends across body of meniscus. Popliteal bursa is seen (◀) and its position superiorly clearly indicates that this is a tangent near anterior part of popliteal portion of lateral meniscus. **B,** Superior strut tear (arrow) showing lateral meniscus with central ray tangential to midpart of popliteal portion of meniscus. At this location there should be both superior and inferior attachments; there is no superior attachment.

tion in the decision to operate, and it caused us to change the site of incision in 6 of the 88 cases in which there was only one meniscus torn and in 1 of the 12 with bilateral meniscal tears. On the basis of this experience and the analysis of these cases, we recommend arthrography of the knee as a routine preoperative study, with the knowledge that positive findings can be confirmed in almost all cases by arthroscopy and by direct visualization at arthrotomy.

In summary, 100 knees were studied, with an accuracy of 96% for arthrograms of the medial meniscus and 95% for arthrograms of the lateral meniscus. Arthrography of the knee is considered an outpatient procedure and an extension of the clinical examination in patients for whom surgery is being considered.

7. Value of comprehensive arthroscopy in a patient being considered for reconstructive surgery

Lanny L. Johnson

A complete arthroscopic examination includes visualization through an anterior puncture into the medial and lateral compartments, intercondylar notch, and suprapatellar pouch (Fig. 7-1). More important, it is essential to visualize the posteromedial and posterolateral compartments in knees in which the view from anterior was either incomplete or normal. Experience has shown that it is not uncommon to identify a normal compartment in an anterior view and yet see a significant abnormality, i.e., a vertical tear of the meniscus or loose bodies, through a separate posteromedial or posterolateral puncture.

In addition, a complete arthroscopic examination assesses the articular surfaces of the patella, tibia, and femur. It is possible to document the menisci and their inner borders, bodies, attachments, and posteromedial and posterolateral moorings. Identification of the anterior cruciate ligament and its condition both by observation and by watching the ligament under stress of a drawer sign is possible. The posterior cruciate ligament can be seen through a posteromedial puncture in most patients because it is immediately beneath the synovium on the posterior septum as seen from the medial side. Observations include the popliteus tendon at its attachment, the posteromedial and posterior capsular structures, and the tibial collateral ligament. Last but not least, it is possible to identify morphologically the various characteristics of the synovium that can often classify the specific rheumatoid condition in an otherwise difficult case to diagnose.

It has been my contention that the history, physical examination, plain film x-rays, and air-contrast arthrogram, as important as they are, really represent circumstantial evidence. A complete arthroscopic examination of all chambers, front and back, provides direct evidence for a diagnosis. Arthroscopy should not be considered a substitute for the clinical assessment, but certainly it serves as adjunct in the surgical planning.

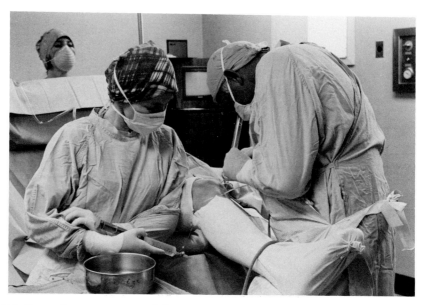

Fig. 7-1. Inspection into anteromedial compartment is facilitated by fulcrum placed against lateral distal femur by assistant and force applied to patient's leg by hip and thigh of arthroscopist. This allows two-handed manipulation of small-diameter endoscope to view medial compartment as well as under and above meniscus.

RETAINED POSTERIOR HORN OF MENISCUS

Of patients with a prearthroscopic diagnosis of meniscal disease, the ones who most commonly require reconstructive surgery are those who have had a previous meniscectomy through a single short anterior arthrotomy. Of the first 400 patients I reviewed who had undergone arthroscopy for diagnostic purposes, 28 were in this category.[1] The typical finding in such patients includes articular cartilage disease in addition to a retained posterior horn producing unresolved symptoms following surgery. Often the original injury included the anterior cruciate ligament. No amount of progressive quadriceps exercises alters this mechanical problem. A separate posteromedial or posterolateral arthroscopic entry can be used to identify the size of the retained posterior horn. With the patient under local anesthesia it is possible to palpate the posterior horn and pop it back and forth with the arthroscope and correlate that with the patient's symptoms. Questioning the patient at the time of manipulation of the retained posterior horn confirms the diagnosis. This further establishes a confidence in the diagnosis on the part of both the physician and the patient. The subsequent surgical excision relieves the patient's symptoms and interrupts the repeated articular injury and production of loose bodies that resulted in effusions, synovitis, and discomfort.

CONDYLAR CONDITIONS

In those patients who had a prearthroscopic diagnosis of condylar disease, there are several categories in which arthroscopy proved beneficial. One such group included individuals with meniscal symptoms with medial compartment loss demonstrated by a standing anteroposterior x-ray film of the knee. They had a history of effusions and pain but no clear-cut mechanical findings on physical examination. Arthroscopic examination can divide this group into two categories. The first includes patients with a bonafide mechanical tear of the meniscus that is injuring the articular cartilage. Such patients can profit symptomatically and biologically by meniscectomy. The second category is patients who have diffuse degenerative articular disease and diffuse degenerative meniscal disease without gross mechanical disruption of the meniscus. It is my opinion that such patients have a diffuse degenerative process and that meniscectomy has not been and would not prove to be beneficial. Such patients may be candidates for high tibial osteotomy.

ARTICULAR DEFECTS

Articular defects curetted to raw bone and drilling chondroplasties have also been studied. A lesion the size of a dime usually is revascularized and fibrotic within 6 weeks, and one the size of a nickle or a quarter with osteochondritis dissecans takes approximately 3 months to revascularize. Larger lesions, of course, pose a problem of considerably more magnitude and have a higher morbidity; revascularization of these can take 6 to 9 months. I think that at this early stage full weight bearing or physical activity should not be initiated until there is arthroscopic evidence of absence of vascularity and maturation of the fibro-cartilage surface.

OSTEOTOMY VERSUS RESURFACING

Arthroscopic examinations of patients whose clinical and x-ray examinations have been thought to show unicompartmental abnormalities have been performed. True unicompartmental disease has been a rare finding. Most patients have some degenerative meniscal and articular disease in the opposite compartment as well. Arthroscopy should be beneficial in any future studies of patients who are to undergo a high tibial osteotomy, unicompartmental condylar resurfacing, or bicompartmental condylar resurfacing. Arthroscopy should provide valuable data to be reviewed to improve patient selection for the various operative procedures.

LOOSE BODIES

Arthroscopy of patients with diffuse degenerative arthritis and mechanically stable knees has shown diffuse articular disease with multiple loose bodies of various sizes. These patients could be considered for condylar replacements or so-called total knee replacements. This condition may be managed by vacuuming the joint of all the small loose bodies and removing the larger loose bodies with a modified pituitary rongeur.[1] Surgery has not been necessary for these patients. Management with lavage, vacuuming, salicylates, and isometrics has successfully carried these patients for more than 2 years without symptoms. This certainly would be considered a good result for either tibial osteotomy or total knee replacement.

PATELLAR SUBLUXATION

Patients with patellar abnormalities have benefited considerably by arthroscopy. These patients are typically adolescent girls with meniscal symptoms and some patellar complaints sufficient to be unresponsive to conservative measures. They have a stable patella to manipulation, and arthroscopic evaluation is normal. I have learned that they can be advised to be alert for patellar subluxation, although the patella may be stable at the time of examination. It has been observed that within a year these patients develop a frank subluxating, if not dislocating, patella.

PATELLAR DISLOCATION

Patients with acute dislocation of the patella are excellent candidiates for arthroscopy. There may well be a torn meniscus or cruciate ligament that would not be identifiable because of pain and hemorrhage. These patients, if managed without arthroscopy, cast immobilization, and physiotherapy, obviously would do poorly. Therefore arthroscopic examination with removal of the blood, lavage of the joint, and complete inspection is imperative. Arthroscopy can rule out loose bodies and intra-articular lesions, i.e., a torn meniscus or anterior cruciate ligament. Then immobilization followed by rehabilitation results in a universally smooth course. Unfortunately it has not been routine to inspect the posteromedial and posterolateral compartments for loose bodies, which gravitate in these dependant areas. Therefore in reconstruction for recurrent dislocation of the patella the inspection of those compartments is essential in order that any loose articular debris can be either suctioned out through the arthroscope or washed out completely at the time of surgery.

CYSTIC MENISCI

The category of patients with extrasynovial abnormalities includes ligamentous injury, degenerative cysts of the meniscus, and Baker's cysts. Patients with degenerative cystic changes on a meniscus have been under study and have been examined arthroscopically under general anesthesia prior to surgical intervention. If no abnormality of the meniscus is seen and there is no degeneration of the meniscus or tear, then I have simply removed the cyst even though it goes down to the meniscus. If the degeneration is marked at the site of entry into the meniscus with cystic changes, a meniscectomy is performed. If it has not shown marked degeneration into the meniscus and has been a superficial attachment of capsule, then the meniscus has been saved. This study is not complete, but early observations indicate that about half of the patients with a cyst on a normal meniscus have a subsequent degenerative meniscal tear requiring surgery within 6 to 8 months. But in the half of these patients who have not had that injury yet, the meniscus and articular cartilage have been spared.

BAKER'S CYST

In a patient older than 16 years with Baker's cyst of unknown etiology, arthroscopy can be used to establish the etiology of the cyst. It often is a result of a posterior tear of the meniscus, but the cause may also be a rheumatoid condition. The latter may be identified by the synovial morphologic characteristics. A diffuse degenerative arthritis with loose bodies in the joint may be the cause. These can be removed at the time of arthroscopy, not only from the cyst, which can be penetrated with the arthroscope, but also from the joint, providing resolution of Baker's cyst by arthroscopic management.

JOINT INSTABILITY

In patients with old ligamentous injuries seeking reconstruction, we assess the medial, lateral, anterior, and posterior rotary instability of the joint. In patients who have had multiple operations an arthroscopic examination may be done with local anesthesia to discuss ahead of time the surgical planning and potential results. Patients in whom reconstruction is necessary are advised that the opposite compartment, which is not thought to be injured, should be inspected with the arthroscope. Any underlying tear of an existing meniscus or any loose bodies would be identified and removed, resulting in a smoother rehabilitation. Patients undergoing reconstructive surgery in whom the articular cartilage injury is identified ahead of time, can be better advised of their prognosis in spite of appropriate surgical reconstruction.

TIBIAL COLLATERAL LIGAMENT INJURY

Arthroscopy can be beneficial for patients with acute ligamentous injuries. A knee with a partial tear of a tibial collateral ligament, without palpable defect and gross instability, may have a torn cartilage or anterior cruciate ligament tear. In approximately half these patients there is a surgically corectable lesion, i.e., a torn meniscus, a loose body, or a cruciate ligament tear that would be amenable to repair or require débridement because it is catching in the joint.

ANTERIOR CRUCIATE LIGAMENT INJURY

Patients who have knee injuries that indicate a slight cruciate instability are candidates for arthroscopy. Valgus strain applied to the knee in 5° to 10° of flexion will move the tibia anteromedially on the femur.

An isolated tear of the anterior cruciate ligament is usually accompanied by hemorrhagic changes in either the posteromedial or the posterolateral capsule, even though no meniscal or ligament tear accompanies it. In such cases arthroscopy can be used in deciding whether the cruciate can be repaired or requires resection. More important, we have learned that in a so-called isolated tear of the cruciate in which no abnormality of the meniscus or loose bodies have been seen by *anterior inspection,* it is not uncommon to find a posterior abnormality. A tear of the medial or lateral meniscus may be seen only from the posteromedial or posterolateral puncture. There may be a loose body of significant size in either of those compartments; this would slow the rehabilitation following either surgical intervention or conservative management.

CONCLUSION

Comprehensive arthroscopy of the knee, including posteromedial and posterolateral inspection, has resulted in better diagnosis and smoother postoperative rehabilitation. No unknown abnormalities remain in the joint. In addition, it has improved physician-patient relationships because assessing the magnitude of the injury by the extent of the capsular hemorrhage and tear and/or degenerative changes of the joint has improved the ability to predict the course in each patient. Last, in the rheumatologic diseases it has been possible for us to identify morphologically the differences between the rheumatologic conditions. We have inspected arthroscopically some joints that, because of their heat and thickening, were thought to require synovectomy, only to find that the synovium was not proliferative or villous. The symptoms were the result of capsular edema secondary to acute inflammation of the synovium, and the patient would not be a candidate for synovectomy. In other situations it is clear that the patient would profit by synovectomy and/or condylar replacement, depending on the status of the articular surfaces. We have also had occasion to inspect patients with total knee replacements in rheumatologic conditions, finding that their symptoms are a result of the regrowth of synovium and the inability to control the condition medically.

Reference

1. Johnson, L. L.: Comprehensive arthroscopic examination of the knee, St. Louis, 1977, The C. V. Mosby Co.

8. Practical value of arthroscopy

Kenneth E. DeHaven

Arthroscopy of the knee has added another dimension to the evaluation of the knee by providing an alternative to arthrotomy for direct visualization of intra-articular structures. Arthroscopy has been and is currently being employed primarily as a diagnostic procedure, but new developments in instrumentation and technique[8] offer considerable promise of therapeutic applications in the future. An important question frequently raised is whether arthroscopy is of sufficient practical value in the clinical management of knee problems to justify the effort and commitment required to learn the procedure. This chapter focuses on these practical considerations in the following categories of knee problems: chronic internal derangements, acute injury, monoarticular arthritis, osteoarthritis, and popliteal cyst. Its use as a research tool is also discussed.

CHRONIC INTERNAL DERANGEMENTS

Meniscal lesions are the most common cause of chronic internal derangement, and we are all familiar with the typical case, with the history of a twisting injury followed by pain, swelling, giving way, and locking and the physical findings of effusion, joint line tenderness, limitation of motion, trapping with circumduction maneuvers, and normal appearance on x-ray films. The diagnosis is torn meniscus and the treatment meniscectomy—very simple.

Unfortunately it is not so simple: the meniscus may not be torn, the opposite meniscus may be torn in addition to or instead of the one in question, and there may be other additional pathologic conditions. In a prospective study correlating the preoperative clinical, arthrographic, and arthroscopic diagnoses with the findings at arthrotomy in 100 cases of internal derangement of the knee, we[3] found the clinical diagnosis to be completely correct in 72, correct but incomplete in 10, and incorrect in 18 cases.[3]

In the cases in which the clinical diagnosis was correct and there was full positive correlation between the various parameters studied (51 of 72), arthroscopy served only to confirm the diagnosis in 80%, but in the remaining 20% the arthroscopic findings directly influenced surgical treatment. Included were cases of retained posterior horn of the medial meniscus, posterior tears not readily visualized at arthrotomy, and lateral meniscal tears with equivocal arthrograms.

In other cases in which the clinical diagnosis was correct there was conflicting adjunctive information (21 of 72), most frequently involving falsely abnormal and falsely normal arthrograms for meniscal lesions and nondiagnostic arthrograms for anterior cruciate ligament tears or chondromalacia of the patella. Athroscopy was quite useful in demonstrating that the clinical diagnosis was indeed correct in these cases.

In the cases in which the clinical diagnosis was correct but incomplete (10% of the series) the opposite meniscus was found to be torn, in addition to the one clinically suspected, in eight cases. This was clinically unsuspected in all eight and missed on arthrography in seven. Even when it was known from arthroscopic visualization that additional lesions were present, they could not be seen at arthrotomy until the menisci were partially removed. The remaining cases in the correct but incomplete category were cases of "not so isolated" anterior cruciate ligament tears found to have vertical tears through the posterior horn of the lateral meniscus that had been missed by arthrography and also could not be seen at arthrotomy. The correct but incomplete category accounted for only 10% of our overall series, but the role of arthroscopy was critical in reaching the correct diagnosis in all of these cases.[3]

The clinical diagnosis was incorrect in the remaining 18% of cases in our study. Most were meniscal lesions, and particularly disturbing were four instances of "double-trouble" in which the incorrect clinical diagnosis of torn medial meniscus was supported by arthrograms that were falsely abnormal for the medial meniscus and falsely normal for the lateral. Without arthroscopic clarification of the correct diagnosis in these cases, one can readily imagine the disastrous possibility of removing a normal medial meniscus and leaving behind a torn lateral meniscus.

Other incorrect clinical diagnoses involved cases in which anterior cruciate ligament tears had appeared clinically to be meniscal lesions; there were supportive falsely abnormal arthrograms in some cases and nondiagnostic arthrograms in others. The same was true in cases of chondromalacia of the patella. Arthroscopic examination was also found to correctly clarify the diagnosis in the vast majority of these cases with incorrect clinical diagnoses.[3]

ACUTE INJURY

When there is a history of significant injury to the knee followed by immediate disability and the early onset of hemarthrosis, there are several potential diagnoses of surgical significance, including ligament tears, torn meniscus, intra-articular fracture, and extensor mechanism rupture. Although the definitive diagnosis, including the need for surgical intervention, can be made on the basis of clinical or x-ray examination in several of these categories (collateral and posterior cruciate ligament tears, intra-articular fractures, and extensor mechanism rupture), there remains a significant number of cases with acute injury and hemarthrosis that demonstrate no significant ligamentous laxity and have normal

x-ray films. My experience with arthroscopy in these cases has been most rewarding in demonstrating lesions that warrant prompt surgical intervention.

At one time hemarthrosis was thought to represent a contraindication, or at
least a relative contraindication, to arthroscopy because the blood obscured the
view of the joint.[1,5,6] By slightly modifying the normal technique to include
florid irrigation with a large-bore needle, and on occasion the use of a tourniquet,
it is possible to wash out the blood sufficiently to permit satisfactory arthroscopic
examination in nearly all of these cases.

In arthroscopy in acutely injured knees with hemarthrosis but no instability
and normal x-ray films (currently 75 cases), lesions warranting early surgical
intervention have been found in 90% of the cases. The most common finding is
torn anterior cruciate ligament (65%); most of these have associated meniscal
tears, but approximately one third are "isolated." Major meniscal tears (mostly
displaced bucket-handle tears) have been encountered in 23%, and osteochondral
fractures in 9%.[4]

Acute knee injury with hemarthrosis, rather than being a relative contraindication to arthroscopy, is in fact one of the best indications for this procedure,
which provides the opportunity to decide with a high degree of confidence
whether to operate or not.

MONARTICULAR ARTHRITIS

Persistent monarticular synovitis of the knee with an equivocal history of
trauma and nondiagnostic laboratory and radiographic studies frequently presents a diagnostic and therapeutic enigma. Arthroscopic examination is helpful
to exclude mechanical internal derangement, to obtain synovial biopsy under
direct vision for histologic and bacteriologic evaluation, and to document the
location and extent of any articular lesions that may be present. Approximately
half of our patients have subsequently developed seronegative polyarticular
rheumatoid arthritis, and another 20% continue to have nonspecific monarticular
synovitis. In the remaining 30% of cases, however, specific diagnoses have been
made by arthroscopy, including mechanical internal derangement, pigmented
villonodular synovitis, and crystalline synovitis.[4,7]

OSTEOARTHRITIS

Arthroscopic examination of patients with known osteoarthritis can be helpful
to document the extent of involvement, evaluate the status of the menisci, and
assist in selection of patients for tibial osteotomy or knee arthroplasty. In addition, the arthroscopic examination and irrigation frequently provide symptomatic relief in degenerative joints.[6]

Patients with mild or moderate osteoarthritis that does not respond to conservative management may have a degenerative meniscal tear that can be demonstrated by arthroscopy. Frequently these patients can be significantly helped by
meniscectomy, whereas other patients, clinically indistinguishable by other

means, may simply have osteoarthritis without associated meniscal lesions as the cause of their symptoms.

Also we are currently utilizing arthroscopy in patients with osteoarthritis to help refine selection for tibial osteotomy. In patients who are candidates for either osteotomy or total knee arthroplasty, osteotomy is performed if the arthroscopic examination confirms the involvement to be primarily unicompartmental, but arthroplasty is selected if significant degenerative changes are also encountered in the opposite compartment. It is hoped that this will lead to more reliable results following tibial osteotomy.

POPLITEAL CYST

In most instances popliteal collections of synovial fluid are secondary to some intra-articular lesion, and appropriate medical or surgical treatment of the intra-articular problem will allow the popliteal collection of synovial fluid to resolve. There are occasions, however, when popliteal swelling and pain are the presenting complaints and no intra-articular problem is apparent clinically or by arthrogram. Arthroscopy in these cases has usually demonstrated an intra-articular pathologic condition, establishing the need for arthrotomy, and surgical treatment of the popliteal cyst has been unnecessary. If no significant intra-articular disorder is found at arthroscopy, our approach has been to proceed with primary excision of the popliteal cyst.

RESEARCH TOOL

Because of the extremely low morbidity associated with arthroscopy[1,5,6] and the ease of photographic documentation, it is an ideal vehicle for follow-up studies to document the natural history of knee problems and to provide objective evaluation of surgical and nonsurgical treatment. Although there is limited information of this type available at the present, this may prove to be the area in which arthroscopy will make the greatest contribution.

SUMMARY

Various indications for diagnostic arthroscopy have been reviewed, with emphasis on the practical applications of the procedure. Arthroscopy has been found to be highly accurate (over 90%) and to influence the surgical treatment of knee problems in a meaningful way in more than 50% of cases.[2,3,5] Arthroscopy has been found to demonstrate unexpected pathologic conditions and to be critical for the totally correct diagnosis of knee problems in 15% to 25% of cases.[3] The procedure is not a panacea, however, and should not alter the time-honored approach to knee problems, which includes a careful history, thorough physical examination, and standard roentgenograms, and it must never be considered a substitute for sound clinical judgement. On the other hand, arthroscopy has proved to be an extremely valuable adjunct in the management of knees thought to have a lesion of surgical significance, and it should be included in the armamentarium of orthopaedic surgeons dealing with these problems.

References

1. Casscells, S. W.: Arthroscopy of the knee joint. A review of 150 cases, J. Bone Joint Surg. **53-A**:287, 1971.
2. Dandy, D. J., and Jackson, R. W.: The impact of arthroscopy on the management of disorders of the knee, J. Bone Joint Surg. **57-B**:346, 1975.
3. DeHaven, K. E., and Collins, H. R.: Diagnosis of internal derangements of the knee. The role of arthroscopy, J. Bone Joint Surg. **57-A**:802, 1975.
4. DeHaven, K. E.: Unpublished data.
5. Jackson, R. W., and Abe, I.: The role of arthroscopy in the management of disorders of the knee. An analysis of 200 consecutive examinations, J. Bone Joint Surg. **54-B**:310, 1972.
6. Jackson, R. W., and DeHaven, K. E.: Arthroscopy of the knee, Clin. Orthop. **107**:87, 1975.
7. O'Connor, R.: The arthroscope in the management of crystal-induced synovitis of the knee, J. Bone Joint Surg. **55-A**:1443, 1973.
8. O'Connor, R.: Arthroscopic surgery, Paper presented at American Academy of Orthopaedic Surgeons Postgraduate Course on Arthroscopy and Arthrography, Anaheim, Calif., 1976.

9. Arthroscopic surgery

Richard L. O'Connor

As a surgeon gains experience in diagnostic knee arthroscopy, his desire to use the arthroscope to improve his patient's clinical situation with as little morbidity as possible naturally increases. Obviously a history of injury and a complete knee examination with appropriate roentgenograms must be done prior to arthroscopy. Symptoms, physical findings, and the results of ancillary tests and arthroscopic examination must all be mentally synthesized to establish the appropriate diagnosis. Quite often the lesion encountered at arthroscopy may be dealt with using the arthroscope. It is my purpose to discuss, without being encyclopedic, a few conditions in which arthroscopic surgery has been useful in alleviating the patient's complaints with minimal morbidity. The indications and technique for partial meniscal excision are not included in this discussion.

The recent impetus for arthroscopic surgery was provided by Ikeuchi, Watanabe, and Takeda in Japan and Jackson, Casscells, and others in North America. However, examination of Burman's collection of arthroscopic instruments from the 1930s suggests that he had been performing arthroscopic intra-articular surgery much earlier.

Two important terms must be defined. The first of these is the *single-puncture technique*. With this method, only one port of entry into the joint is used during surgery. This technique is of limited usefulness, except in removing multiple small cartilaginous loose bodies and for minor use with an operating arthroscope. A large-diameter arthroscope is most appropriate for this application. In the *double-puncture technique,* the arthroscope is inserted through one portal and a second incision is made, usually on the other side of the patellar tendon but possibly posterior to the medial collateral ligament or in the quadriceps bursa. The operating instrument is inserted through a water sleeve introduced into the second incision (Figs. 9-1 and 9-2). A modification of the double-puncture technique involves the insertion of a retracting instrument through the second portal and a cutting instrument through the operating arthroscope. This technique is the most commonly used.

MULTIPLE CARTILAGINOUS LOOSE BODIES

Multiple cartilaginous loose bodies within the knee may be effectively dealt with using the single-puncture technique, as illustrated by the case of a 260-

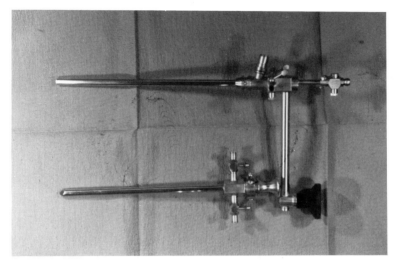

Fig. 9-1. Operating arthroscope (top) is introduced into joint through water sleeve after trocar has been removed.

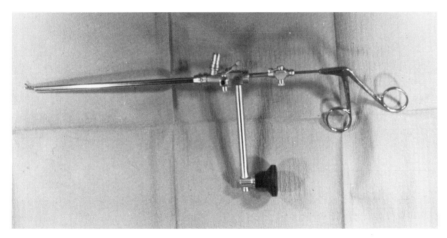

Fig. 9-2. Three-millimeter meniscal scissors has been introduced through operating channel. Instrument contains small telescope, light fiber bundles, and two irrigating channels in addition to operating channel.

pound, 22-year-old college offensive tackle. A 120 ml hemarthrosis was aspirated following a valgus injury that occurred during practice. Examination revealed tenderness but no instability of the medial capsule. The meniscal tests were equivocal, but the patellofemoral compression test was positive bilaterally. At arthroscopy, multiple cartilaginous loose bodies were found in all areas of the knee, and the retropatellar surface was quite fragmented (Fig. 9-3). No other pathologic condition was encountered. The telescope was removed from the water sleeve, an adapter was added, and a large-diameter irrigating syringe was

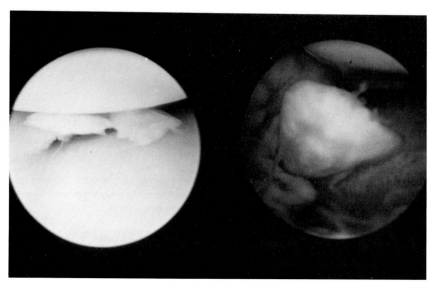

Fig. 9-3. Left, Two cartilaginous loose bodies lie beneath medial femoral condyle and medial meniscus. Right, Small cartilaginous loose body rests between anterior attachment of lateral meniscus and anterior cruciate ligament.

attached. Alternating positive and negative pressure was then used to remove the cartilaginous fragments. The sleeve was manipulated into all compartments and the irrigation was continued until the returning fluid was clear. The telescope was then reinserted and the joint inspected to ensure the adequacy of joint cleansing. The low morbidity of this technique is demonstrated by the patient's returning to play in his college game the following evening.

OSTEOCARTILAGINOUS LOOSE BODIES

Osteocartilaginous loose bodies are most often removed with a double-puncture or even triple-puncture technique. These loose bodies are most commonly located in the quadriceps bursa, in the intracondylar notch, in the lateral gutter, beneath the posterior third of the lateral meniscus, and in the posterior compartment. The relative ease or difficulty of removal of an osteocartilaginous loose body is determined not only by its location but also by its size, shape, and proportion of bone and cartilage. A loose body smaller than 6.5 mm may be removed using the irrigation single-puncture technique. In a young patient, however, the ossific nucleus may be small relative to its cartilaginous component, making the preoperative roentgenogram misleading and making retrieval at arthroscopy difficult because of the buoyancy of the fragment.

COMBINED INTRA-ARTICULAR PROBLEMS

Occasionally a combination of intra-articular problems can be solved using the arthroscope. Endoscopy was performed on the knee of a 35-year-old man

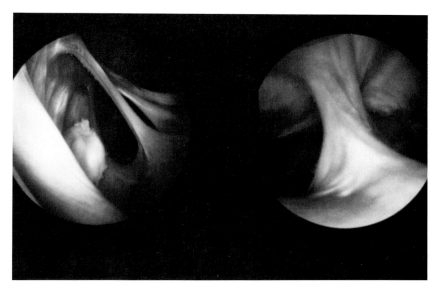

Fig. 9-4. Left, Small osteocartilaginous loose body is trapped in interstices of multiple adhesive bands. Right, Closeup of large fibrotic band. Lysis of these adhesive bands is easily accomplished with operating arthroscope.

after medial and lateral meniscectomy and patellectomy. The range of motion was limited, movement was jerky and quite painful, and occasionally he noted intermittent locking. Joint capacity, as determined by the saline distension of the joint, was markedly limited (40 ml—normal is 80 to 120 ml).

This is not an uncommon finding in patients with restriction of motion following patellectomy. Motion restriction is often caused by adhesions between the roof of the quadriceps bursa and the floor of the suprapatellar recess. These adhesions may be multiple strands of a thick fibrotic sheath.

In this instance multiple fibrotic adhesive bands were found with an osteocartilaginous loose body trapped within their interstitices (Fig. 9-4). The loose body, even though it contained an osseous core, was not seen on review of the preoperative roentgenograms. The loose body was removed and the adhesions were lysed with the operating arthroscope. The patient's range of motion has returned to normal, and his quadriceps strength is improving with appropriate physical therapy.

IMPROVEMENT OF KNEE ARTHROPLASTY RESULTS

Arthroscopy and arthroscopic surgery may also be useful in improving the results of knee arthroplasty. A 45-year-old man who had had a lateral compartmental replacement following severe fracture of the lateral tibial plateau had a full range of motion, a 10° genu varum, and medial joint line pain (Figs. 9-5 and 9-6). A spongy osteocartilaginous fragment was found in the medial compartment; its source was a crater in the medial femoral condyle. Roentgenograms

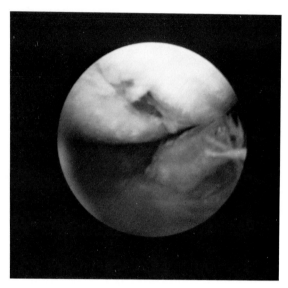

Fig. 9-5. Medial compartment of knee previously treated with lateral compartmental arthroplasty. Spongy osteocartilaginous loose body trapped in joint line arose from the overhanging medial femoral condyle.

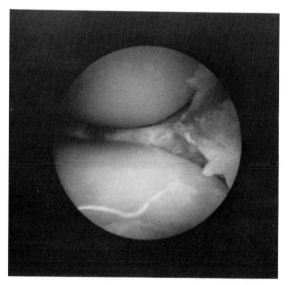

Fig. 9-6. Lateral compartment with metallic femoral component superiorly, polyethylene inferiorly, and ragged re-formed meniscus in center and to right.

identified a loose body in the lateral compartment. Extirpation was accomplished using the double-puncture technique.

RETAINED POSTERIOR HORN FOLLOWING MENISCECTOMY

A common problem following meniscectomy is a retained posterior horn. Assessment by conventional methods (arthrography) is apt to be misleading in predicting the presence and size of the retained fragment; it also gives little information regarding the fragment's propensity for interfering with joint motion. On the other hand, arthroscopy not only allows accurate determination of the presence of a retained fragment but also permits assessment of its size and estimation of the damage its presence has inflicted on the overlying articular cartilage. The fragment can be held with a grasping forceps and its mobility can be assessed visually. Although my experience with arthrotomy performed for the removal of retained posterior horns as an independent procedure is not great, the impression I have gained is that excision entails high mobility with unpredictable results. An ideal method for dealing with this common problem is to use the arthroscope to assess the situation and arthroscopic surgery to excise the fragment (Fig. 9-7, *left*).

Recurrent effusion and nonlocalizing discomfort were the indications for arthroscopy in a 45-year-old woman 1 year after a medial meniscectomy. In addition to a mobile 1 cm retained posterior horn of the medial meniscus, moder-

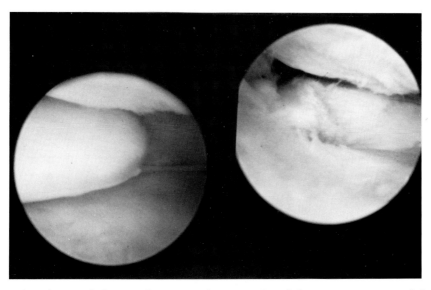

Fig. 9-7. Left, Rounded retained posterior fragment of medial meniscus is seen to left beneath medial condyle; re-formed rim is seen in background. Right, Postoperative appearance. Note area of excision and degeneration of femoral condyle and tibia.

ately severe degeneration of the retropatellar surface and of the posterior medial femoral condyle was found. The double-puncture technique was used, with a retractor introduced into the lateral portal and the operating arthroscope inserted medially to dissect the posterior horn. The preoperative and postoperative appearance of the medial compartment can be seen in Fig. 9-7. Although improvement in this patient's knee might have been a result of controlling the synovitis by joint lavage or removal of this fragment, the low morbidity associated with this technique represents an attractive alternative to arthrotomy.

SYNOVIAL CYSTS OR MASSES

Arthroscopic removal of synovial cysts or masses may also be quite rewarding. A 24-year-old man complained of lateral joint line pain with tenderness over the course of the popliteus tendon 3 years after surgery for a giant cell tumor of the lateral femoral condyle. Apley's compression test was positive in compression with internal rotation over the lateral joint line, but much more so in distraction. Roentgenograms showed no difference in the appearance of the lateral femoral condyle. Arthroscopy demonstrated an intact cartilaginous cover of the lateral femoral condyle, a normal lateral meniscus, and a cystic synovial mass surrounding the popliteus tendon (Fig. 9-8). Arthroscopic resection of this synovium alleviated the patient's symptoms. The specimen showed only nonspecific synovial changes.

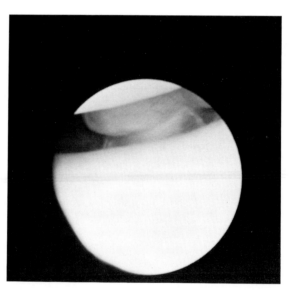

Fig. 9-8. Bulbous cyst of synovium overlying popliteus tendon is seen between lateral femoral condyle superiorly and lateral meniscus inferiorly. Excision of cyst relieved patient's symptoms.

INJURY TO MEDIAL INTRA-ARTICULAR BAND OR SHELF

A structure that can be injured by a variety of mechanisms and that can cause symptoms mimicking those caused by meniscal lesions is the shelf, or medial intra-articular band. This structure is most readily visualized arthroscopically, but it can also be seen by careful dissection during medial arthrotomy. The shelf runs along the medial sidewall of the quadriceps bursa and attaches distally to the fat pad. Its size and length vary from patient to patient. Synovial thickening is caused most often by blunt trauma to the anterior medial aspect of the flexed knee. Occasionally, however, a twisting injury tears the shelf from the medial sidewall, causing central displacement beneath the patella during flexion.

This was the case in a 22-year-old college lineman who had been kneeling following a play with his right knee resting on the ground and with his foot externally rotated. The ball carrier was forced into him, causing the knee to flex fully. He felt a sharp pain and a pop within the joint. An effusion developed, and examination revealed loss of the terminal 15° of extension and 20° of flexion. No ligamentous instability was noted, but there was a markedly positive Apley compression and distraction test in external rotation over the medial joint line. Arthroscopy demonstrated a completely normal medial joint line and a freely moving shelf, which had been torn from its peripheral attachment (Fig. 9-9). This was resected using the double-puncture technique. The patient returned to football practice the following day.

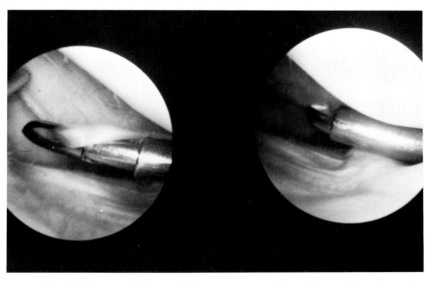

Fig. 9-9. Left, Shelf, retracted by small forceps, is seen through superolateral patellar approach. This structure was torn from its peripheral attachment, catching between patella and femur. Right, Orientation is easier when viewing patella and femur with operating instrument held in same position.

SUMMARY

Diagnostic arthroscopy will undoubtedly be further adapted to meet new problems and treatments, which will in turn necessitate a variety of new instruments. An ever-increasing number of orthopaedists are becoming proficient in diagnostic arthroscopy. Many will undoubtedly become interested in a subspecialty, and the incorporation of their observations, ideas, and suggestions for equipment modification will further advance the concepts of microscopic intraarticular surgery.

PART THREE

Fractures about the knee

10. Management of tibial condylar fractures

Mason Hohl

Over a period of 25 years 1,000 tibial condylar fractures have been studied.[8,11,12] Three hundred of these have been followed more than 2 years, and the findings have been analyzed for the purpose of identifying preferred treatment methods on the basis of results.[9,10] From the substantial literature of long-term results, it appears that some agreement on treatment indications is developing.[*] This chapter presents the highlights of personal study and draws on the written experience of others to discuss and develop an approach to the management of the different types of condylar fractures and their sequelae.

BACKGROUND

Historically tibial condylar fractures have been difficult to treat because of the uncertainty of outcome. Fifty years ago the general use of cast treatment was abandoned in favor of operative intervention utilizing screws, bolts, and bone grafts. Unfortunately the results were not sufficiently encouraging to justify continuation, largely as a result of the inadequacy of available internal fixative hardware and the necessity of using a supplementary cast to prevent loss of fracture reduction.[12] The common occurrence of permanently limited knee motion led to a revival of traction treatment.[1,18,22] Traction did result (as a rule) in good mobility of the knee, but late angular deformity and instability remained a problem in some patients. More recently the trend has been to tailor treatment to the patient and his fracture, utilizing whatever method will best assure an optimum result.[10,16]

The restoration of painless full function is the goal of fracture treatment about the knee. A good result, in general, is pain free and strong with full knee extension and flexion in excess of 120° without angular deformity or instability of more than 5°.

A number of problems may be encountered during treatment that tend to prevent a good result. Among these are failure to recognize soft tissue injuries or the extent and complexity of the fracture on x-ray examination, lack of apprecia-

---

*References 4, 9, 10, 16-18, 21, 22.

tion that certain fracture types tend to displace further with some forms of treatment, and failure to apply the general principle that when internal fixation is used, it should be sufficiently strong to obviate supplementary external cast support.

EVALUATION OF THE FRACTURE

Information derived both from clinical evaluation of the injured knee and from x-ray studies is necessary to plan appropriate treatment with the potential to achieve a good result.

Clinical stability testing of the knee is done basically to determine how much stability is present and whether significant angular deformity will require correction.[16,19] Stability is tested with the knee fully extended and with it flexed 20°. If the knee is stable in full extension, it is unlikely that open reduction will be necessary or helpful. If there is significant instability (10° or more), however, the cause (either fracture displacement or ligamentous instability or both) and extent should be determined by x-ray examination; in any event surgical management probably will be required. Instability occurring with the knee flexed 20° indicates ligament injury or a compression-type fracture in the midportion of the tibial condyle and also indicates the probable need for surgical management.

X-ray examination for tibial condylar fracture may require, in addition to the two routine views, oblique projections or laminagrams.[5] When depth in a compression fracture is critical to a decision about whether to operate, the tibial plateau view (10° caudal projection) or laminogram is most important.[14] Stress films are used all too seldom to document the cause and extent of instability.[7,11,22, 23,24] Local or general anesthesia is necessary to apply sufficient stress, and the injured knee is compared to the normal knee. Although temporary further fracture displacement may be seen with the stress, permanent loss of fracture position is rare. The stress views occasionally demonstrate some degree of capsular and ligamentous injury.

SOFT TISSUE INJURIES

Injuries to soft tissues (ligaments, capsule, and menisci) occur frequently in association with tibial condylar fractures.[7,11,22,24] Fortunately neurovascular damage is quite uncommon, but arterial laceration or compartment syndromes are seen. Prompt recognition of soft tissue injury is necessary so that proper and timely treatment can be rendered if permanent disability is to be minimized.

The diagnosis of ligament and capsular injuries is suggested by instability of the knee noted on clinical stress testing and documented by stress x-ray films (Fig. 10-1). At times, however, initial x-ray films show avulsive injuries at ligament attachments sites or widening of the joint space, which is also evidence of ligament injury, the significance of which can be determined by stress x-ray films.[11]

Although ligament injuries occur in nearly one half of tibial condylar frac-

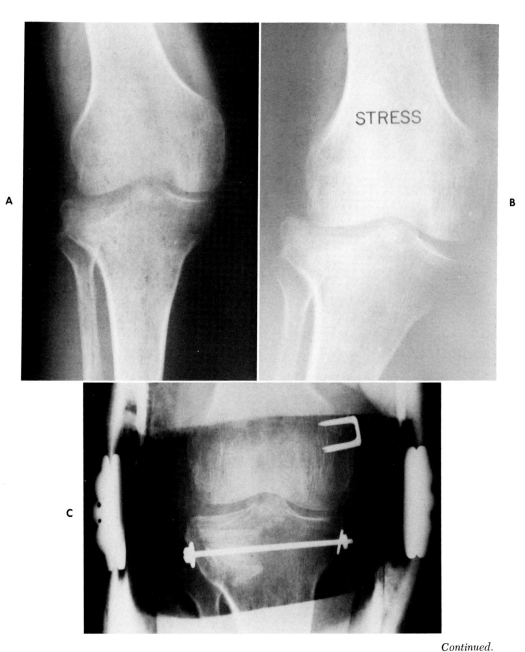

Continued.

Fig. 10-1. Forty-five–year–old man with family history of osteogenesis imperfecta sustained knee injury in a fall. **A,** Original film shows local compression fracture. **B,** Stress film without anesthesia demonstrates some medial cartilage space widening, which was more marked under anesthesia later. **C,** Film taken 2 months after iliac graft and placement of tibial bolt with staple to fix avulsed capsule and ligament to medial femoral condyle. **D,** Seventeen months later there is near-normal knee function and excellent clinical stability. **E,** Stress film at follow-up demonstrates excellent medial ligament stability.

D
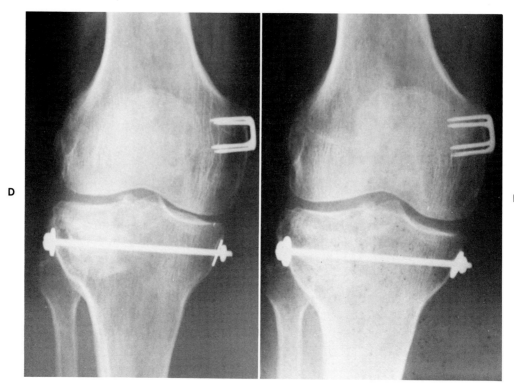
E

Fig. 10-1, cont'd. For legend see p. 97.

tures, most are of the avulsive type and tend to heal without surgery.[11] Ligament injuries are seen most commonly with undisplaced and compression fractures. The more dramatic injuries to ligaments, as determined by stress films, are much better treated by surgical repair.[11] Results after combined bone and ligament repair have been quite good.

Meniscal injuries usually occur as detachments along the periphery rather than intrinsic tears. These detachments can be repaired at the time of open reduction by simple resuture with little concern about future derangement.[19] It is seldom justifiable to remove a meniscus solely for better visualization of the upper tibial surface, but irreparably damaged menisci should be removed.

CLASSIFICATION AND MANAGEMENT

The following classification divides tibial condylar fractures into six types: undisplaced (less than 4 mm displacement), local compression, split compression, total condylar depression, split, and comminuted (Fig. 10-2).

Undisplaced fractures make up about one fourth of fractures seen.[9] These minimally displaced fractures are seen in a variety of configurations that may resemble one or more of the other types. These fractures rarely present a manage-

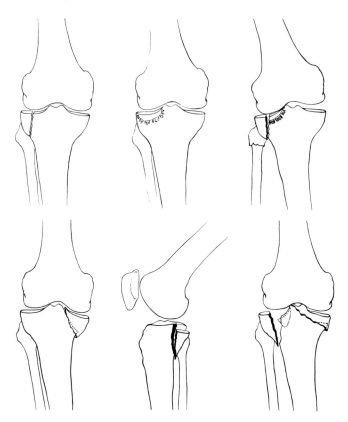

Fig. 10-2. Classification of tibial condylar fractures. (From Hohl, M.: J. Bone Joint Surg. 49-A:1455, 1967.)

ment problem and almost always have good end results seemingly independent of the treatment used. The major exceptions are those with associated ligament injury and the subtype with a fracture line extending from the intercondylar area obliquely to the medial cortex, similar to some total condylar depression fractures. This fracture tends to displace when treated in a long leg cast.[6,11,19] Potential loss of position must be considered in any treatment employed. Comparison of the fracture position by frequent x-ray films is indicated, and a change of treatment should be instituted if acceptable position is lost. The use of a cast brace as primary treatment may prevent loss of position, or its later use may prevent further change.[3] Traction may be used to retain position or to correct fracture alignment in the relatively early period, reserving open reduction for cases in which it is needed to restore reduction and provide internal fixation.

Local compression fractures are the most frequently encountered type, making up one third of fractures seen. Reduction of the depression is only possible by open surgical methods. Thus clinical stability, location of the depression from front to back on the condyle, and depth of the depression must be known for a proper treatment decision to be made. Clinical stress testing is helpful in determining stability of the knee and suggesting whether surgical treatment is necessary. Valgus deformity of the knee is dependent on the depth of the depression, especially if the defect is in the middle to anterior portion of the condyle. Also, since the functional position of the knee in walking is very near full extension, anterior to middle area depressions are much more significant than those located in the middle to posterior area. Ultimately the decision to operate and surgically elevate a local compression fracture is made on the same basis as with any other fracture—the requirements of the patient for appearance and function of the knee. In general, knees with a depression of 8 mm or more located anterior to the midportion of the lateral tibial condyle benefit from surgical elevation and bone grafting.[9,10,18]

In performing surgery for most lateral condylar fractures it is best to preserve the meniscus by approaching the tibial condyle between the meniscus and upper tibia, cutting the coronary ligaments, and resuturing them at the time of closure.[19]

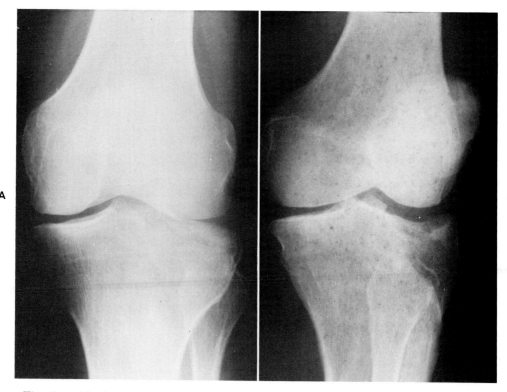

A

Fig. 10-3. Fifty-four–year–old bracemaker was struck by automobile and sustained local compression fracture. **A,** Anteroposterior view. Note that depth of depression cannot be defined. **B,** Oblique view shows depression in anterior portion of lateral condyle. **C,** One month after surgery patient is fully ambulatory in cast brace. Note iliac graft in place. **D,** Two years after injury there is near-normal knee function.

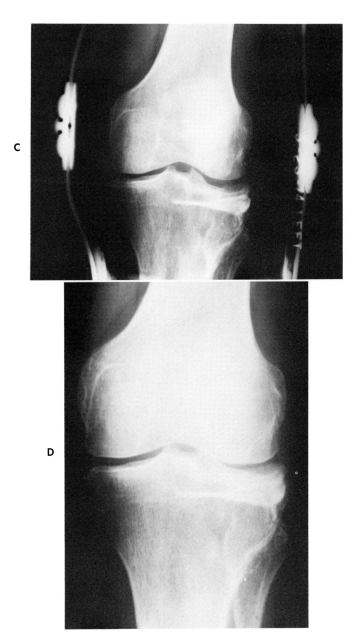

Fig. 10-3, cont'd. For legend see opposite page.

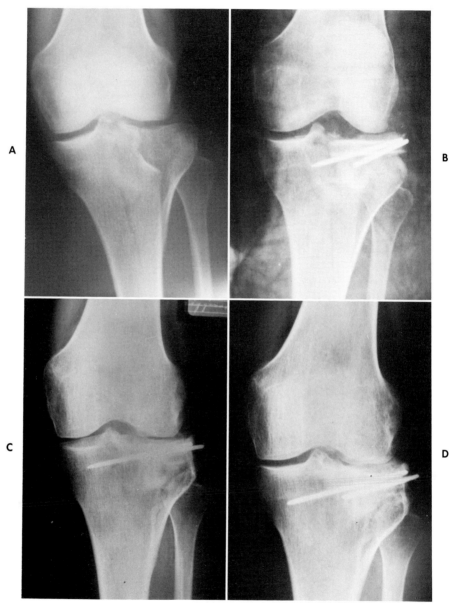

Fig. 10-4. Thirty-five–year–old secretary injured in automobile collision and treated by iliac replacement. **A,** Original film demonstrates marked local compression fracture. **B,** Postoperative view with leg in cast after iliac replacement of entire lateral condyle. **C,** Good functional recovery 5 years after surgery. Patient is working regularly. **D,** Ten years after surgery there are some degenerative changes, but they are accompanied by minimal symptoms.

This approach gives sufficient visualization for accurate elevation and fracture reduction. Despite this, it is important to check the reduction by intraoperative x-ray examination. Of necessity, raising the depressed fragments to position leaves the fragments avascular and subject to possible resorption. Redepression from femoral condylar pressure is also a real probability unless good support of fragments from below is provided. An iliac crest, tibial, or bone-bank cortical graft thrust immediately under the elevated fragments has proved best, but tight packing of the defect with cancellous bone does succeed at times (Fig. 10-3). When the articular surface is irreparably damaged, replacement of the surface by iliac graft is the best approach (Fig. 10-4).

Split compression fractures occur in 17% of condylar fractures and share some common features with the local compression type, but they are more easily and predictably treated by surgical means. The reason for this is that a portion of articular surface is split off and can be replaced anatomically and fixed to provide strong support for the femoral condyle, thus preventing redepression or displacement (Fig. 10-5). It is most likely that sufficient strength of internal fixation can be provided to eliminate the need for postoperative cast immobilization in many patients.

Open reduction is indicated if there is depression of 8 mm or more or widening or spreading of the condyles more than 3 mm if support for the femoral condyle is lacking. Surgical exposure of this fracture is carried out through the split fracture line, severing the meniscus from the tibia as in the approach for local compression fractures. The compressed area should be elevated before the split fragment is repositioned and fixed. Bone grafting is seldom required. Closed reduction utilizing traction and impaction may be successful in less displaced fractures.[8,19] Following successful manipulative reduction it is best to maintain the reduction in traction, although there are some reports of successful use of cast bracing.

Total condylar depression fractures make up only 8% of the total but are important since there is significant potential for the development of late angular deformity and its associated sequelae.[6,9] Some fractures of this type tend to displace, especially those in which the fracture extends from the intercondylar region medially to the medial cortex. A long leg cast does not seem to prevent gradual displacement. Although relatively easy reduction of this fracture is often accomplished at the scene of injury by the application of splints or is obtained later with the patient under anesthesia, it tends to be lost during the process of healing. For this reason, even for minimally displaced fractures, the use of a cast brace appropriately stressed to prevent further displacement is indicated; for more displaced fractures, open reduction with sufficient fixation to prevent loss of reduction may be required (Fig. 10-6). This generally means the use of a bolt or bolts together with a contoured side plate.[21]

Indications for manipulative or open reduction depend on the degree of displacement of the fracture. Experience has shown that if late angular deformity

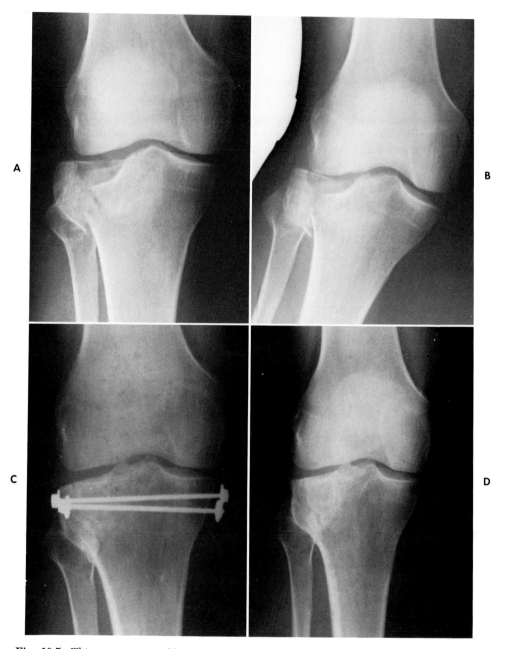

Fig. 10-5. Thirty-seven–year–old man injured in motorcycle accident. **A,** Split compression fracture shown. **B,** Stress film at surgery demonstrates minimal medial opening. **C,** Five months after open reduction without bone grafting. **D,** Two years after surgery there are excellent stability and function.

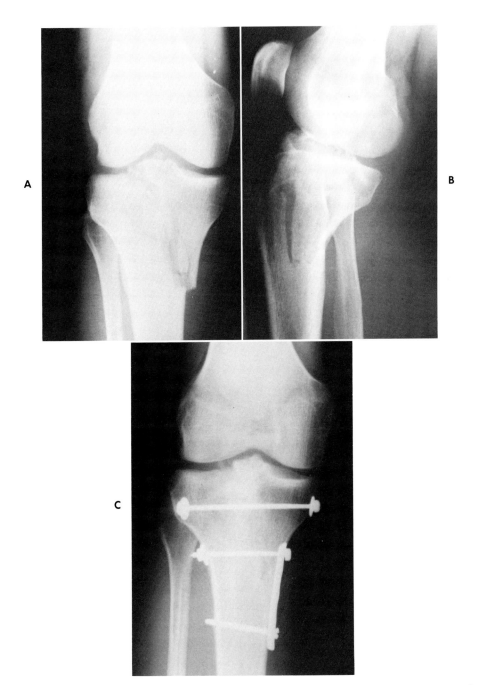

Fig. 10-6. Twenty-five–year–old climber who fell from height. **A** and **B,** Anteroposterior and lateral postinjury films demonstrating medial total condyle depression fracture. **C,** One year after open reduction and fixation. No postoperative cast was used. Excellent function was achieved.

of the knee is to be avoided, the proper height of tibial condyles must be maintained. It is generally recognized that the knee tolerates valgus deformity far better than varus deformity in terms of knee function and late arthritic changes are far more common with varus angulation.[6]

Split fractures are fortunately uncommon, but they are difficult to manage since they are commonly associated with a more serious injury to the knee such as a partially reduced knee dislocation or at least a ligament injury. The fracture line usually presents in a coronal plane so that the degree of displacement is not well appreciated on the anteroposterior x-ray view. At times the fracture tends to displace further with the knee in flexion, so that the femoral condyle articulates with the split fragment and reduces, or nearly so, in full extension. It is important to reduce and hold these fragments in good position if a good result is to be realized; this often means accurate open reduction. Long-term results in this series have been disappointing, regardless of treatment.[9]

Comminuted fractures make up 15% of the total and include a wide variety of fracture configurations involving both compartments of the proximal tibia and often an associated subcondylar fracture. The degree of comminution and the displacement seems too much to permit any reasonable reconstruction. Cast treatment frequently leads to fracture healing in some degree of displacement, but a cast brace has recently been shown effective in maintaining alignment and reduction.[3] Actually many of these fractures reduce satisfactorily in traction, and traction can be continued for several weeks, during which time passive and then active motion is used.[12] Others may require closed reduction with aftercare in traction. Selected fractures benefit from limited open reduction to solve particular displacement problems in one compartment of the knee, with traction in the postoperative period. A few lend themselves to an extensive open reduction and internal fixation utilizing side plates, bolts, and screws as necessary.[21] An extensive exposure is required to do this with an incision on either side of the knee or a Y-shaped incision centered on the tibial tubercle. Most important is to regain good alignment and utilize side plates and bolts for solid fixation. If knee motion can be started within a few weeks, the prognosis is good for restoration of function.

POSTFRACTURE MANAGEMENT

It is in the postreduction or postoperative care period that the ultimate functional result will be determined. For instance, open reduction of a fracture followed by immobilization in a long leg cast with the knee bent 15° for 10 weeks or more will likely doom the patient to live with a knee that does not fully extend or flex. In some cases this type of result may be inevitable, but it should be prevented whenever possible.

Ideal postoperative management includes the use of a soft dressing for a few days and encouraging early and continuing active motion. However, practical considerations often dictate the use of a splint or cast for a few days after surgery.

In such a cast it is important to keep the knee in the extended position and then begin motion as soon as possible.[6,19] Traction can be used in the postoperative period as a means of stabilizing the knee, yet allowing at least 90° of motion. A cast brace permits early motion, supplies considerable support to the knee, and decreases the forces across the elevated condyle.[3,6,13,20]

The presence of a repaired ligament injury necessarily modifies the post-operative regime to the extent that a minimum of at least 5 to 6 weeks of immobilization is suggested to permit ligament healing.[11] Unfortunately the best position for the repaired ligament may be flexion, and thus recovery of extension and motion will be slow and at times difficult.

During the period of convalescence from fracture, and after external support has been discontinued, active exercises to increase leg muscle strength and increase range of motion are encouraged.

MANAGEMENT OF FRACTURE SEQUELAE

The more serious long-term problems resulting from tibial condylar fractures are limited range of knee motion, lack of extension, angular deformity, instability, and traumatic arthritis.* Delayed union or nonunion is an uncommon occurrence, but malunion requiring corrective osteotomy or joint replacement is seen more frequently.

Follow-up studies have shown that the knee motion does improve for at least 2 years after fracture; however, it appears that if 90° of movement has not been achieved by the end of the first year, it is unlikely that the patient will ever achieve 120°. The key to recovery of motion is to start active movement as early as possible, preferably by 5 or 6 weeks after fracture. When this cannot be achieved because of associated injuries or other problems, it is important to start the patient working on a regular exercise program as soon as possible.

Surgical lysis of adhesions to increase range of motion may be helpful in well-motivated patients, but the gain in motion is never as much as hoped. Closed manipulation of the knee to recover motion is not productive and may cause other intra- or extra-articular injury.

Failure to achieve full extension is a result of immobilization in flexion with resultant scarring and pannus involving the anterior soft tissues and fat pad or a result of residual fracture deformity.[6] The key to retaining extension, of course, is to reduce the fracture and, if traction or cast is used, to make certain that the knee is extended, at least at rest. Late arthrotomy to excise the fat pad and lyse adhesions has helped an occasional patient to achieve full extension.

Angular deformity is a common sequel to tibial condylar fracture, but fortunately it mostly occurs as a few degrees of valgus or varus deformity. However, 36% of 300 followed patients had deformity of 10° or more, and some of these required subcondylar osteotomy for late correction.[9] Deformity is a result of fail-

---

*References 4, 6, 8, 9, 17, 18, 22.

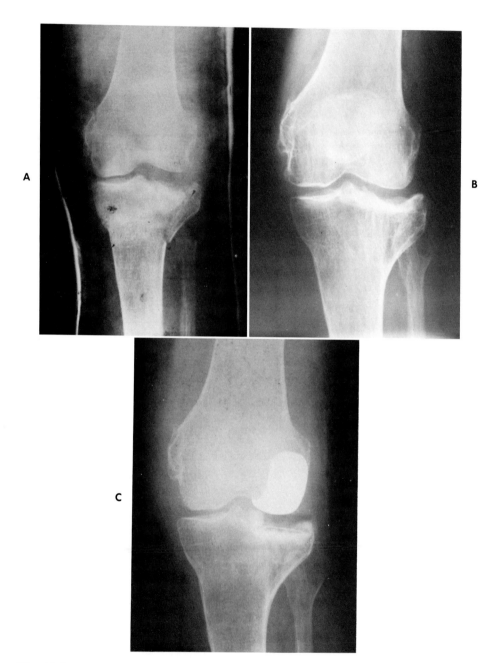

Fig. 10-7. Seventy-two–year–old woman who fell sustaining local compression fracture. **A,** View in long leg cast with knee flexed 20° 3 weeks after injury. **B,** Two years later walking is almost impossible because of flexion contracture of 20° and valgus deformity of 25°. **C,** Unicompartmental knee replacement corrected alignment and contracture.

ure to reduce or maintain condylar height at the correct level or later from loss of articular cartilage (Fig. 10-7). Angular deformity that interferes with function or that will surely result in the development of premature degenerative changes is an indication for subcondylar osteotomy or possibly knee replacement.

Instability of the knee is a difficult problem to treat late and thus is best anticipated and treated early. The causes are failure to restore normal condylar height, residual ligament instability, and loss of articular cartilage. Late ligament reconstruction is helpful in improving stability and is suggested if disabling instability is present. Most published follow-up series have indicated residual instability ranging from 10% to 36%.*

Traumatic arthritis has been shown to follow intra-articular fractures frequently. Sixty-three percent of patients in my series, who were followed an average of 5 years, had some degree of traumatic arthritis. Varus angulation led inevitably to traumatic arthritis.

SUMMARY

Treatment of the patient with tibial condylar fractures must be selected on an individual basis, taking into account the future requirements of the patient for knee function, stability, and alignment; the type and displacement of the fracture; and the treatment pitfalls and potentials. When treatment has been carried out with full awareness of all the involved factors the result can be gratifying, but these fractures are a continuing challenge.

---

*References 2, 4, 9, 11, 15-18, 22, 24.

References

1. Apley, A. G.: Fractures of the lateral tibial condyle treated by skeletal traction and early mobilization, J. Bone Joint Surg. **38-B**:699, 1956.
2. Bakalim, G., and Wilppula, E.: Fractures of the tibial condyles, Acta Orthop. Scand. **42**:429, 1971.
3. Brown, G. A., and Sprague, B. L.: Cast brace treatment of plateau and bicondylar fractures of the proximal tibia, Clin. Orthop. **119**:184, 1976.
4. Dovey, H., and Heerfordt, J.: Tibial condyle fractures. A follow-up of 200 cases, Acta Chir. Scand. **137**:521, 1971.
5. Elstrom, J., Pankovich, A. M., Sasson, H., and Rodriguez, J.: The use of tomography in the assessment of tibial plateau fracture, J. Bone Joint Surg. **58-A**:551, 1976.
6. Epps, C. H., Jr.: Complications in orthopedic surgery, J. B. Lippincott Co. (In press.)
7. Forster, E., Mole, L., and Coblentz, J.: Etude des lesions ligamentomes dans les fractures du plateau tibiale, Ned. Tijdschr. Geneeskd. **105**:2173, 1961.
8. Hohl, M.: Tibial condylar fractures, J. Bone Joint Surg. **49-A**:1455, 1967.
9. Hohl, M.: Tibial condylar fractures: long term follow-up, Tex. Med. **70**:46, 1974.
10. Hohl, M.: Treatment methods of tibial condylar fractures, South. Med. J. **68**:985, 1975.
11. Hohl, M., and Hopp, E.: Ligament injuries in tibial condylar fractures, J. Bone Joint Surg. **58-A**:279, 1976. (Abstract.)
12. Hohl, M., and Luck, J. V.: Fractures of tibial condyles. A clinical and experimental study, J. Bone Joint Surg. **38-A**:1001, 1956.
13. Mooney, V.: Cast bracing, Clin. Orthop. **102**:159, 1974.

14. Moore, T. M., and Harvey, J. P.: Roentgenographic measurement of tibial plateau depression due to fracture, J. Bone Joint Surg. **56-A**:155, 1974.
15. Moore, T. M., Meyers, M. H., and Harvey, J. P.: Collateral ligamentous laxity of the knee—long term comparison between plateau fractures and normal, J. Bone Joint Surg. **58-A**:594, 1976. (Reprint.)
16. Rasmussen, P. S.: Tibial condylar fractures, J. Bone Joint Surg. **55-A**:1331, 1973.
17. Reibel, D. B., and Wade, P. A.: Fractures of the tibial plateau, J. Trauma **2**:337, 1962.
18. Roberts, J. M.: Fractures of the condyles of the tibia, J. Bone Joint Surg. **50-A**:1505, 1968.
19. Rockwood, C. A., and Green, D. P.: Fractures (vol. 2). Philadelphia, 1975, J. B. Lippincott Co.
20. Rockwood, C. A., Ryan, V. L., and Richards, J. A.: Experience with quadrilateral cast brace, J. Bone Joint Surg. **55-A**:421, 1973. (Abstract.)
21. Rombold, C.: Depressed fractures of the tibial plateau, J. Bone Joint Surg. **42-A**:783, 1960.
22. Schulak, D. F., and Gunne, D.: Fractures of tibial plateau. A review of the literature, Clin. Orthop. **109**:166, 1975.
23. Shelton, M. E., Neer, C. S., II, and Grantham, S. A.: Occult knee ligament ruptures associated with fractures, J. Trauma **11**:852, 1971.
24. Wilppula, E., and Bakalim, G.: Ligamentous tear concomitant with tibial condylar fracture, Acta. Orthop. Scand. **43**:292, 1972.

11. Epidemiology, treatment, and prevention of patellar fractures

Stephen C. Robinson
John D. States

Patellar fractures comprise approximately 1% of all fractures and have increased in frequency because of motor vehicle trauma.[2] Direct trauma such as a knee striking a dashboard is a common method of injury, but indirect trauma such as stumbling with sudden flexion of the knee against a tightened quadriceps may also cause the patella to fracture. Patellar fractures are rare in the young and the old, occurring most often in patients in the 20- to 60-year range.[2] They are more common in men than women by almost two to one. The importance of understanding patellar fractures lies in the fact that they are intra-articular fractures involving the largest and one of the most stressed synovial joints in the human body.

ANATOMY

The patella is a unique bone in several ways. It is the only major bone that is an integral part of a joint capsule. Circumferential removal of the patella from a knee creates a large window in the anterior knee. It has been called a sesamoid bone, but a true sesamoid bone is embedded in the substance of a tendon, and according to some anatomists the patella actually lies behind the quadriceps tendon and the superior and inferior poles are covered by fat and synovium.[3,13] Embryologic studies have supported this and have shown that the nucleus of cells that form the patella is located well behind the strata of cells that form the quadriceps tendon and ligamentum patellae; embryologically the patella appears not to originate as a part of the quadriceps expansion.[3] However, Bruce and Walmsley's observations[4] suggest that the patella is an integral part of the quadriceps expansion, both embryologically and anatomically. Comparative anatomic studies suggest that animals with the most efficient quadriceps mechanisms in terms of speed or strength have the smallest patellae or none at all. The sloth has a patella that is relatively large for its body. The fox and deer have patellae that are relatively small. The kangaroo, the animal with perhaps the largest and most well-developed quadriceps system for its size, has no patella

111

at all. With growth, the human patella becomes relatively smaller in reation to the quadriceps muscles rather than larger as one might expect from the greater functional demands of the adult knee compared to the knee of a young child.[3]

CLINICAL STUDIES OF PATELLECTOMY

These embryologic and anatomic studies raised in Brooke's mind the question of whether the patella is a functionally important bone. In 1937 he reported 10 cases of patellectomy for patellar fractures in which the knees were tested for strength postoperatively.[3] In 9 of the 10 cases the injured leg was found to be actually stronger than the well leg. Also, in cadaver studies he demonstrated that the speed of knee extension was increased after removal of the patella. Ernest Hey-Groves noted that when he first read of Brooke's work, he was incredulous. He then personally reviewed many of Brooke's patients and confirmed his results.[13] Later Watson-Jones[31] stated that the knee operated more efficiently without a patella. Brooke's study, along with the endorsement of these famous orthopaedists, led to a marked increase in the number of patellectomies for fractures and for other problems of the patellofemoral joint.

Enthusiam for patellectomy waned somewhat when animal studies in the 1940s demonstrated what appeared to be a higher incidence of osteoarthritis of the femoral condyles after patellectomy.[4,5,9] These studies and the poorer clinical results from other series raised doubts of the wisdom of removing the patella.[30] More attention was turned to the study of the function of the patella, and one of the first good experimental studies was by Haxton[11] in 1945.[12] He determined the amount of force on the quadriceps tendon necessary to extend fresh cadaver limbs mounted on an experimental device. He then removed the patella from each limb, leaving the transversely cut quadriceps expansion unappoximated. By then suturing the quadriceps mechanism he obtained an average of 13° more extension but still was left with an extensor lag averaging 17°. He concluded that the patella was responsible for increasing the power of extension as the quadriceps muscle shortened.

O'Donoghue et al.[19] in 1952 supported Haxton's findings by comparing postoperative quadriceps strength in 10 patients with total patellectomies and 10 patients with partial patellectomies. In the patients with total patellectomies strength was 61% of that of the normal knee at full extension and 75% of normal at 90° of flexion. These figures compare with strengths of 98% of normal at 90° of flexion and at full extension in the patients with partial patellectomies.

In 1971 Kaufer[14] further confirmed these results by his work on fresh human amputation specimens and described the mechanical function of the patella. He analyzed knees in terms of their extension moment arms around an average of the instant centers of rotation. He found that the patella served a linkage function to transmit quadriceps pull directly to the patellar ligament. If the patella was absent and the extensor expansion over the patella was left open, the pull of the quadriceps tendon was diverted to the medial and lateral patellar retinacula. This shifted the extensor pull closer to the axis of knee flexion, resulting in a shorter moment arm and less extensor power. The linkage function could be partially restored by suturing the quadriceps tendon to the patellar ligament, but this restored only a small amount of the moment arm present with the intact patella. He found that after patellectomy with longitudinal closure 30% more force was needed to achieve full extension and that after patellectomy with transverse closure 15% more force was needed to achieve full extension. He showed experimentally that if the tibial tubercle was elevated anteriorly 1.5 cm, the mechanical disadvantage of patellectomy could be overcome by restoring a satisfactory moment arm. He did this in eight patients who had had patellectomies and who lacked full active extension, and all eight regained full active extension postoperatively.

A recent study by Sutton et al.[25] further suggests that the patella is a functionally important bone. In 20 cases of total patellectomy they found an average reduction of quadriceps strength at follow-up of 49% and an average measured quadriceps atrophy of 2.2 cm compared to the contralateral normal knee. In addition they found greater instability and a decrease in stance-phase flexion excursion in knees with total patellectomy as compared to normal knees and to those with partial patellectomies.

HISTORICAL TREATMENT OF FRACTURED PATELLA

These clinical and experimental studies on the mechanics of patellar function seem to refute Brooke's hypothesis that patellectomy is a functionally benign procedure. The history of patellar function thus returns to the position of Heineck,[12] who in 1909, on the basis of a review of more than 1100 patellar fractures, concluded that the patella was a functionally important bone. He cautioned about the generally poor results of patellectomy, and mentioned that patellectomy should be a procedure of necessity rather than choice.

The history of the treatment of patellar fractures roughly parallels the development of knowledge concerning the function of the patella. Prior to 1877 when the first reported surgical repair of a patellar fracture was done by Cameron in Glasgow, it was generally accepted that anyone unfortunate enough to have a serious patellar fracture would be left with some residual functional deficit. Sir Astley Cooper[7] in 1836 described an Army captain who sustained an open fracture of the patella when he struck a wagon with his knee while riding a horse. The bone fragments were placed together, a compressive dressing applied, and the leg was elevated. After 5 weeks the dressing was removed. The wound was healed, and at 3 months the patient was walking "without much lameness." Later the patient died of other causes and Cooper examined the knee postmortem. He found that fragments of the patella had united by fibrous union and gross motion was present.

About this time Malgaigne[15] used percutaneous hooks to hold patellar fragments together, but these were abandoned because of a high incidence of sepsis.

Surgeons of the late nineteenth and early twentieth centuries made every effort to save the patella after fracture, and techniques such as cerclage, hemi-cerclage, and screw fixation were developed. A wide variety of suture materials was used for cerclage techniques, and for a while the great controversies were over which were the best materials to use: silk, catgut, wire, or tendon.

Partial patellectomy

After publication of Brooke's article in the 1930s many patellectomies were performed for all types of patellar fractures, but after Haxton's work on patellectomized cadavers more physicians began to follow the approach of Thomson,[26] who advocated partial patellectomies when possible. Thomson maintained that the patella has a poor osteogenic potential since it has only one periosteal surface and that more rapid healing and faster return to function would be made possible by allowing tendon-to-bone healing with partial patellectomy.

TREATMENT OF PATELLAR FRACTURES
Rochester series

Compared to some fractures, the fractured patella is relatively easy to treat. In spite of this, there is no universally accepted method of treating the displaced fractured patella. A review of the experience of a Rochester, New York, hospital orthopaedic group illustrates this statement. Seventy patients treated over an 18-month period were studied (Table 11-1).

Undisplaced linear or comminuted fractures (20) and minimally displaced fractures (15) presented relatively few problems in treatment. Most of these cases were treated with cylinder casts and immobilization for 4 to 6 weeks. Long-term follow-up data for this group are not available, but previous experience indicates that a significant group develop traumatic arthritis and eventually require patellectomy.

Table 11-1. Method of treatment of patellar fractures

Type of fracture	Treatment							
	None	Soft dressing	Splint	Cast	Patellectomy	Partial patellectomy	Fragment removal	Open reduction
Transverse								
Undisplaced	4	1	3	8	0	0	0	0
Displaced	2	0	1	6	2	6	0	3
Vertical								
Undisplaced	0	0	0	0	0	0	0	0
Displaced	2	3	0	1	0	0	0	0
Comminuted								
Undisplaced	0	0	0	4	0	0	0	0
Displaced	0	0	0	0	13	2	0	3
Osteochondral	0	0	0	0	0	0	6	0

The remaining 35 fractures were more difficult and were treated by a variety of methods. Eleven of the fractures were displaced; 18 were displaced and comminuted and were treated by patellectomy, partial patellectomy, or open reduction. The remainder were osteochondral fractures and were treated by fragment removal.

The numbers in this series are too small to provide conclusions concerning desirable or undesirable treatment methods. The final determination of the method of treatment for specific clinical situations is left to the reader, based on the interpretation of the data presented, the literature reviewed, and his own experience.

Each type of fracture required different treatment, and no consensus existed locally regarding the treatment of choice for some types.

Until several years ago displaced transverse fractures were treated by excision of the minor fragment. Duthie and Hutchinson[10] in 1958 compared this treatment with total patellectomy and found that both were far from uniformly satisfactory. Total patellectomy was as successful as partial patellectomy.

Currently open reductions are being performed by many orthopaedists in an effort to preserve the patella. Techniques devised by the Swiss AOI group and occasionally other internal fixation methods are being employed. Wire fixation and screw fixation are being used, either separately or in combination. Open reduction with internal fixation has been performed in our series. One failed and required patellectomy. The other patients are doing well, but long-term results are not known.

Current status of patellectomy

To this day the question of how best to treat the displaced or comminuted patellar fracture remains controversial, and strong proponents of each type of treatment can be found. There is, however, general agreement on the seriousness of these fractures, and several studies have emphasized this specifically in terms of time for recovery, subjective complaints, and development of osteoarthritis after patellar fracture.

Recovery time. Nummi[18] reported that the median length of sick leave after patellar fractures treated by open reduction and internal fixation was 4 months; after partial patellectomy, slightly less than 4 months; and after total patellectomy, 5 months. Bostrom[2] found the median sick leave period after surgical treatment to be twice that required for those fractures that could be treated conservatively. Crenshaw and Wilson[8] stated that it took up to a year to fully recover from a patella fracture. Wass and Davies[30] found that the average time off from work for fractures treated by open reduction and internal fixation was 5 months. The time after total patellectomy was even longer.

Subjective complaints. Nummi[18] reported on 155 patients treated surgically, of whom 86% had subjective complaints referable to the knee; 52% of 236 patients with conservative treatment had complaints. Crenshaw and Wilson[8] reported that 15 of 25 patients complained of weakness and instability after patellectomy for fracture. Bond[1] noted that aching and discomfort were common complaints after patellectomy. Scott[20] found that 90% of 101 patients with total patellectomies had constant aching and 60% had giving way of the operated knee. Todd[27] observed that quadriceps power was less after total patellectomy than after repair of fractures. Bostrom[2] reviewed 300 cases of patellar fractures followed up for a mean of 8.9 years. Of the 108 surgically treated patients, only 30% had no pain and 39% had no functional limitations. West[32] noted that weakness and quadriceps atrophy were common after total patellectomy.

Osteoarthritis. In his series of 391 fractures Nummi[18] found that 76% of patients surgically treated developed osteoarthritis after injury, as compared to 41% of those treated conservatively. Crenshaw and Wilson[8] found a definite tendency toward development of osteoarthritis after partial patellectomy and after open reduction and internal fixation but not after total patellectomy. These data suggest that disability from the more severe patellar fractures can be significant and that consistently good results are difficult to obtain with currently available treatment.

Surgical technique of patellectomy

Total patellectomy continues to be an acceptable treatment for most displaced transverse fractures and for all severely comminuted fractures. Open reductions may be justified in younger patients, but total patellectomy appears preferable for an older patient.

The surgical technique of patellectomy in part depends on the experience and choice of the surgeon. However, shortening of the extensor mechanism is essential to ensure full active extension.

Our surgical technique consists of patellectomy through a transverse incision in the extensor retinaculum, centered over the apex of the patella. The patellar fragments are removed by sharp dissection, preserving as much of the soft tissue as possible. The cut ends of the extensor reticulum are overlapped 1 to 1.5 cm and sutured with a double row of interrupted sutures of No. 1 silk, chromic catgut, or similar material. Postoperative immobilization in a walking cylinder cast for 6 weeks is necessary to obtain satisfactory healing. Quadriceps exercises are initiated immediately postoperatively in the cast, and range of motion exercise is begun after cast removal. Progressive resistive exercises are begun 2½ months postoperatively. Six months is usually sufficient for full rehabilitation, although elderly patients may require more time.

Two problems remain with total patellectomy. Extensor lag may occur in spite of shortening the extensor mechanism in the repair. Kauffer[14] reported a 15% incidence of extensor lag in cases in which the extensor mechanism had been shortened. Various figures are reported for the incidence of femorotibial osteoarthritis, but up to 50% has been reported in some long-term follow-ups. Total joint replacement appears to be the treatment of choice in this group when seriously disabling osteoarthritis occurs.

Table 11-2. Causes of injury

Cause	Age of patients (years)				
	0-15	16-25	26-65	Over 65	All ages
Fall	2	5	33	12	52
Auto accident	1	2	10	1	14
Cycle	0	3	0	0	3
Sports	4	5	0	0	9
Other	0	0	1	0	1
TOTAL	7	15	44	13	79

EPIDEMIOLOGY AND PREVENTION OF PATELLAR FRACTURES

The prevention of patellar fractures is a logical way to decrease the morbidity of these injuries, and one common cause of patellar fractures that is subject to some control is motor vehicle trauma. Smillie[22] refers to the frequency of automobile injuries in the etiology of patellar fractures by describing the "dashboard fracture." Nagel et al.[18] describe the "dashboard knee." McMaster[16] noted that patellar fractures were common from dashboard injuries. Bostrom emphasized the frequency of this injury in motor vehicle accidents, reporting that 28% of 422 patellar fractures were caused by automobile, cycle, or pedestrian accidents. Of these 12% were from automobile accidents involving the driver or front seat passenger. In 156 males younger than 50 years old 45% of the fractured patellae occurred in automobile accidents. Sorenson[23] reported that 36 of 64 patients had fractures caused by traffic accidents, with 14 of these from automobile injuries. Crenshaw and Wilson[8] found that 27 of 62 patellar fractures were from dashboard injuries.

Of the fractured patellas studied in an extended Rochester series, falls accounted for the majority of fractures. Fourteen of the 79 (18%) patellar fractures occurred in automobile accidents (Table 11-2).

Prevention

Safety belt use reduces or eliminates dashboard impact injury in automobile accidents, but use rates remain discouragingly low. A statement issued June 9, 1976, by Secretary of Transportation William Coleman reported that use rates of all types of safety belts were less than 20%.[6] All efforts to induce safety belt usage short of mandatory usage laws have been ineffective.[24] In spite of repeated efforts in many states to enact usage laws in the past 4 years, no effective law has been passed in the United States.

This dilemma has been recognized by the Department of Transportation and by several manufacturers. Beginning in 1968 the Department of Transportation initiated a program to develop and introduce the airbag system of passive restraints. The program has required much more time, effort, and expense than anticipated, and airbags will not be available as an option until 1979.[28] Airbag

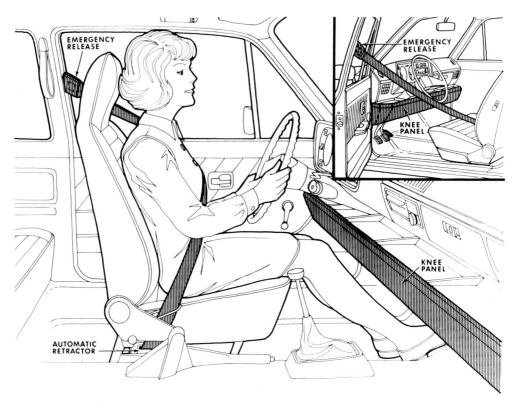

Fig. 11-1. Volkswagen Rabbit automatic (VWRA) belt consists of diagonal shoulder belt anchored to inertial reel below seat cushion and to door frame at shoulder level. Only kneebar is used to restrain lower extremities and lower torso; lap belt is not used. Kneebar is made of dense molded foam plastic mounted on deformable steel backing plate. Seat cushion is designed to take some of load in head-on collision by preventing forward motion of buttocks and pelvis. (Courtesy Volkswagen of America, Inc.)

systems promise improved knee protection, but development and ultimate application remain uncertain at this time.

Volkswagen Rabbit automatic (VWRA) belt system. Beginning in 1970 Volkswagen developed an experimental safety vehicle to provide protection against a serious injury in barrier impacts of up to 50 miles per hour. Combined airbag, belt, and dashboard kneebar restraints were used. The kneebar design proved so successful that it was introduced as a production option with an automatic door-mounted shoulder belt in 1975 models[21] (Fig. 11-1). In 1975, 30,000 vehicles equipped with the automatic belt system and kneebar were sold. The system became standard equipment in some models in 1976, and an additional 30,000 were sold.

The Volkswagen Rabbit system utilizes the knees as the principal target for energy in a head-on impact. The kneebar is a molded dense foam plastic structure with a steel back plate approximately 5 inches (13 cm) wide and 4 inches

(10 cm) deep. The bar extends across the lower edge of the dashboard and is positioned so that it contacts the legs over the patella or proximal tibia. The shoulder belt is anchored at shoulder level on the rear edge of the window frame. An interlock transfers load to the door pillar if the belt is loaded heavily enough to deform the door. The shoulder belt extends medially across the occupant's outboard shoulder, chest, abdomen and pelvis, and inboard hip to an inboard anchor mounted below the seat cushion. The anchor is an inertia reel, which automatically provides the proper tension on the belt and locks if the vehicle is decelerated by locked-wheel braking or an impact.

The seat is especially designed to complement the kneebar and shoulder belt. The lower cushion is firm plastic foam and rests on a metal pan, the front half of which rises at a 45° angle. The rise provides a stop for the forward motion of the pelvis that would occur in a head-on impact. This reduces kneebar and shoulder belt loading. The seat back and cushion are contoured to provide side support for positioning in rollover and side-impact accidents and for fatigue reduction during ordinary usage.

Volkswagen has investigated 39 accidents (with 46 occupants) involving Rabbits equipped with the automatic restraints system in which the amount of damage to the vehicle was $750 or more. In this series there have been no knee injuries. In 13 accidents the amount of damage was in excess of $2000. The kneebars appear to be particularly effective for protecting the knee.

Early dashboard safety designs. Beginning in 1963 dashboard designs have been modified to reduce the frequency and severity of knee injuries. Dense molded foam plastics over sheet metal are now universally used in passenger cars for knee impact protection. Controls, such as ignition keys, have been moved away from the target area in the lower dash or are made to break away. The 1963 English Rover 2000 was the first model marketed in the United States to provide knee protection.

In summary, dashboard design has significantly improved in the past 14 years so that fractured patellas occurring in automobile accidents should become less common. Lap belts are helpful in reducing the severity of knee impact, but usage rates are less than 20%. A highly effective kneebar has been introduced on production Volkswagen Rabbits; on the basis of limited accident studies, this bar promises to virtually eliminate fractured patellae occurring in automobile accidents.

References

1. Bond, J. A.: Excision of the patella. In Proceedings of the Joint Meeting of the Orthopaedic Association of the English Speaking World, J. Bone Joint Surg. 34-B:516, 1952.
2. Bostrom, A.: Fractures of the patella. Acta Orth. Scand. Suppl. 143:1, 1972.
3. Brooke, R.: The treatment of fractured patellae by excision, Br. J. Surg. 24:733, 1937.
4. Bruce, J., and Walmsley, R.: Excision of the patella. Some experimental and anatomical observations, J. Bone Joint Surg. 24:311, 1942.
5. Cohn, B. N. E.: Total and partial patellectomy. An experimental study, Surg. Gynecol. Obstet. 79:526, 1944.

6. Coleman, W. T.: Public notice concerning motor vehicle occupant crash protection, Washington, D.C., June 9, 1976, Office of the Secretary of Transportation.
7. Cooper, A.: Compound fracture of the patella, Guys Hosp. Rep. 1:241, 1836.
8. Crenshaw, A. M., and Wilson, F. D.: The surgical treatment of fractures of the patella, South. Med. J. 47:716, 1954.
9. DePalma, A. F., and Flynn, J. J.: Joint change following experimental partial and total patellectomy. J. Bone Joint Surg. 40-A:395, 1958.
10. Duthie, H. L., and Hutchinson, J. R.: The results of partial and total excision of the patella, J. Bone Joint Surg. 40-B:75, 1958.
11. Haxton, H.: The function of the patella and effects of its excision, Surg. Gynecol. Obstet. 80:389, 1945.
12. Heineck, A. P.: The modern operative treatment of fractures of the patella, Surg. Gynecol. Obstet. 9:177, 1909.
13. Hey-Groves, E.: A note on the extension apparatus of the knee joint, Br. J. Surg. 24:747, 1937.
14. Kaufer, H.: Mechanical function of the patella, J. Bone Joint Surg. 53-A:1551, 1971.
15. Malgaigne, J. F.: Dennis system of surgery, vol. 1, Philadelphia, 1895, Lea Brothers & Co.
16. McMaster, P. E.: Fractures of the patella, Clin. Orthop. 4:24, 1954.
17. Nagel, D. A., Burton, D. S., and Manning, J.: The dashboard knee, Clin. Orthop. (In press.)
18. Nummi, J.: Fractures of the patella. A clinical study of 707 patellar fractures, Ann. Chir. Gynaecol. Fenn. Suppl. 179:1, 1971.
19. O'Donoghue, D. M., Tompkins, F., and Hays, M. B.: Strength of quadriceps function after patellectomy, West. J. Surg. Gyn. Obstet. 60:159, 1952.
20. Scott, J. C.: Fractures of the patella, J. Bone Joint Surg. 31-B:76, 1949.
21. Seiffert, U., Oehm, K., and Paitula, H.: Description of the Volkswagen Restraint Automatic (VW-RA) used in a fleet test program, Society of Automotive Engineers No. 740046, Feb. 1974.
22. Smillie, I.: Injuries of the knee joint, ed. 4, Baltimore, 1971, The Williams & Wilkins Co.
23. Sorenson, K. M.: The late prognosis after fracture of the patella, Acta Orthop. Scand. 34:198, 1964.
24. States, J. D.: Restraint system usage—education electronic inducement systems or mandatory usage legislation? Proceedings of the seventeenth conference of the American Association for Automotive Medicine, Ann Arbor, 1973, University of Michigan Press.
25. Sutton, F. S., Thompson, C. M., Lipke, J., and Kefflekamp, D. B.: The effect of patellectomy on knee function, J. Bone Joint Surg. 58-A:537, 1976.
26. Thompson, J. E. M.: Fractures of the patella treated by removal of loose fragments and plastic repair of the tendon. A study of 554 cases, Surg. Gynecol. Obstet. 74:860, 1942.
27. Todd, J.: The end results of fracture of the patella. In Proceedings of the British Orthopaedic Association, J. Bone Joint Surg. 32-B:281, 1950.
28. U.S. Department of Transportation News—Office of the Secretary, DOT 16-17, Jan. 18, 1977.
29. VW study shows fatalities cut with passive restraints, Automotive News, Oct. 4, 1976.
30. Wass, S. H., and Davies, E. R.: Excision of the patella for fracture, Guys Hosp. Rep. 91:35, 1942.
31. Watson-Jones, R.: Excision of the patella correspondence, Br. Med. J. 2:195, 1945.
32. West, F. E.: End results of patellectomy, J. Bone Joint Surg. 44-A:1089, 1962.

PART FOUR

Management of knee joint disorders

12. Effects of patellectomy

Herbert Kaufer

Patellectomy is a common operation frequently performed for fracture, patellofemoral arthritis, and chondromalacia patellae.* Less common indications for patellectomy include chronic infection, tumor, and habitual patellar dislocation.[11,22] In cases of markedly comminuted displaced fractures, certain neoplasms, and some chronic infections, patellectomy is clearly indicated because there is no reasonable alternative. However, in most other situations in which patellectomy is performed there are other treatment alternatives and the patellectomy is highly elective. It is important therefore that the orthopaedist be fully aware of the effects of patellectomy so that the decision to perform an elective patellectomy can be made on a rational basis.

Clinical experience and laboratory studies have shown that patellectomy is associated with definite alterations in appearance, stability, motion, and extensor power.

APPEARANCE

The patellectomized limb's appearance is altered by the cutaneous scar, absence of the patella's subcutaneous prominence, and thigh atrophy (Fig. 12-1). Theoretically thigh atrophy ought to be reversible with a rigorous postoperative quadriceps strengthening program. Physical therapy can certainly minimize the degree of thigh atrophy. However, clinical experience has shown that some degree of thigh atrophy is a permanent feature of nearly all patellectomized limbs, regardless of operative technique or postoperative rehabilitation regimen.[2,4,11,18,21] Since neither patellectomy nor most prepatellectomy pathologic conditions subject the quadriceps muscle fibers to direct trauma, the evidence suggests that alteration of a muscle fiber's resting length may result in irreversible atrophy of that fiber.

Perhaps the most distressing cosmetic effect of patellectomy is loss of the subcutaneous patellar prominence. This is most apparent with the knee in acute flexion and becomes less apparent with the knee fully extended (Fig. 12-1). Some

---

*References 6, 8, 15, 19, 20, 23.

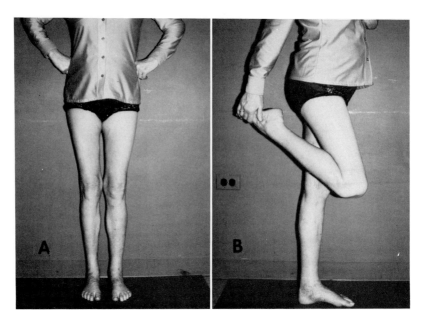

Fig. 12-1. Forty years after right total patellectomy. **A,** Frontal view. There is minimal but definite atrophy of right thigh. Absence of patella is not obvious. **B,** Side view. Minimal limitation of flexion; patellar absence is most apparent when acutely flexed knee is viewed from side.

techniques of patellectomy defect repair such as pursestring closure[9] or overlapping flaps[12,22] can decrease but cannot eliminate the postpatellectomy loss of subcutaneous patellar prominence.

Although a cutaneous scar is a feature of almost all operative procedures, a longitudinal scar over the anterior aspect of the knee is notoriously prominent and unsightly. Longitudinal incisions offer optimal exposure of longitudinal structures such as the extensor mechanism and are the incision of choice if one needs extensive exposure of these structures. Transverse incisions in this region are cosmetically much more acceptable and should be used in situations in which less than optimal exposure is adequate.

POWER

Active knee extension power is the result of extensor moment or torque and is the product of quadriceps force multiplied by the extensor moment arm[7] (Fig. 12-2). Patellectomy has a deleterious effect on both quadriceps force and extensor moment arm.[10]

Decreased quadriceps force is the result of muscle atrophy and alteration of the muscle fiber's resting length.[2] As discussed in the section on appearance, patellectomy seems to be associated with a nearly universal measurable degree of atrophy. Since there is a definite positive relationship between a muscle's active

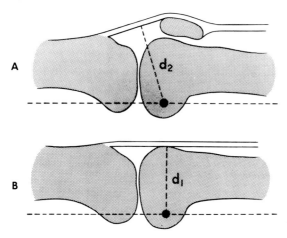

Fig. 12-2. Length of knee's extensor moment arm is perpendicular or shortest distance from line of extensor pull to flexion axis. Extension moment arm is significantly shortened by total patellectomy.

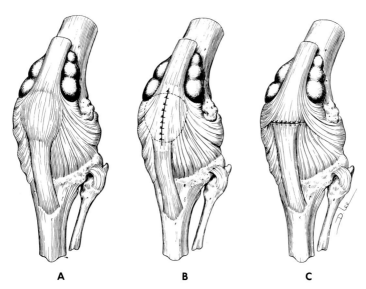

Fig. 12-3. A, Patella links quadriceps tendon directly to patellar ligament. This most anterior portion of quadriceps mechanism is farthest from knee flexion axis and therefore acts on a longer moment arm than any other part of extensor mechanism. B, After total patellectomy and longitudinal closure, quadriceps tendon and patellar ligament separate, allowing resting length of quadriceps muscle fibers to shorten, thereby placing muscle at a physiologic disadvantage. In addition, loss of direct link between quadriceps tendon and patellar ligament diverts pull of quadriceps muscle belly into medial and lateral patellar retinacula. Average course of medial and lateral patellar retinacular fibers is posterior to patellar ligament. Therefore force acting through retinacula acts on shorter moment arm and produces less knee extension torque than identical force acting on patellar ligament. C, Transverse closure of patellectomy defect approximating quadriceps tendon and patellar ligament restores muscle fibers' resting length. It also restores direct link between quadriceps tendon and patellar ligament, which maintains muscle pull in portion of extensor mechanism farthest from flexion axis.

Table 12-1. Patellar contribution to quadriceps moment arm

Knee flexion angle	Patella present*	Patella absent†	Patellar effect‡
0°	5.8	4.0	1.8
30°	5.1	3.9	1.2
60°	4.6	3.8	0.8
90°	4.0	3.5	0.5
120°	3.8	3.25	0.55

*Experimentally determined quadriceps moment arm (in centimeters) for various degrees of knee flexion in intact cadaver knee with patella present.
†Experimentally determined quadriceps moment arm (in centimeters) for the same knees following patellar excision.
‡Difference between figures in "patella absent" and "patella present" columns; represents patella's contribution (in centimeters) to total quadriceps moment arm of knee.

contractile force and its cross sectional area,[2] the observed postpatellectomy atrophy must be associated with decreased muscle belly contractile force.

Contractile force is also influenced by the muscle fiber's prestimulus resting length.[2] Longitudinal closure of the patellectomy defect shortens the muscle fiber's resting length (Fig. 12-3) and therefore decreases the fiber's active tension and total tension. If the patellectomy defect is closed transversely, thus approximating the patellar ligament and quadriceps tendon, the muscle fiber's resting length is increased. Although increased fiber resting length does decrease the force of active contraction, there is relatively less negative effect on the muscle's total tension because of the force contribution of passive stretch produced by increasing the muscle fiber's resting length.[2] In addition to its effect on the quadriceps cross sectional area and its effect on the physiology of muscle contraction, patellectomy also has a negative effect on the mechanics of knee extension because it decreases the extensor moment arm (Fig. 12-2). The quadriceps moment arm has been determined by biomechanical studies on cadaver legs.[7,10] The patella's contribution to the knee extension moment arm is variable. It is quite small when the knee is flexed but increases as the knee is extended. At full extension the patella accounts for nearly one third of the entire extensor moment arm (Table 12-1). The patella increases extensor torque by its linking effect as well as by direct contribution to the moment arm.

The patella links the quadriceps tendon directly to the patellar ligament (Fig. 12-3). Quadriceps force is thus concentrated in the patellar ligament, which is the most effective portion of the extensor mechanism because it is farthest from the knee flexion axis. One can substitute for the patella's linking effect by suturing the patellar ligament directly to the quadriceps tendon (Fig. 12-3). A variety of specialized repairs of the postpatellectomy defect have been described and advocated as methods to enhance the mechanical advantage of the quadriceps.[9,12,16,22] Although transverse repairs are definitely mechanically superior to longitudinal repairs, laboratory studies indicate that all varieties are mechani-

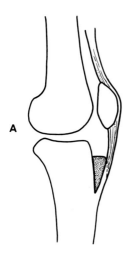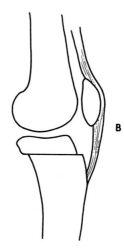

Fig. 12-4. **A,** Elevation of tibial tubercle lengthens extensor moment arm, thus neutralizing mechanical deficit that follows patellectomy. Excised patella is excellent source of bone graft for elevation of tibial tubercle. Elevation of more than 1 cm should be avoided because it is likely to cause difficulty with wound closure. **B,** Anterior displacement proximal tibial osteotomy also lengthens extensor moment arm. This procedure can readily be combined with correction of varus or valgus deformity.

cally equivalent to simple transverse repair, and all varieties of longitudinal repair are mechanically equivalent to simple longitudinal repair.[10] Approximation of the quadriceps tendon and patellar ligament is the common feature of all mechanically superior varieties of postpatellectomy repair. However, these maneuvers do not completely restore extensor torque because the patella also contributes directly to the quadriceps moment arm by displacing the patellar ligament farther from the knee's flexion axis (Fig. 12-2). The amount of displacement is proportional to the thickness of the patella.

Surgical elevation of the tibial tubercle (Fig. 12-4) can displace the patellar ligament anteriorly and thus substitute for the patella's direct contribution to the quadriceps moment arm.[10] It has been shown that approximation of the quadriceps tendon directly to the patellar ligament, combined with elevation of the tibial tubercle 1.5 cm, can completely correct the mechanical defect produced by patellectomy.[10]

Maquet[13] has shown that anterior displacement proximal tibial osteotomy can similarly neutralize the mechanical effect of patellectomy. Either elevation of the tibial tubercle or anterior displacement proximal tibial osteotomy can be performed with or without patellectomy to provide a mechanical boost to knee extension. The Maquet procedure has the advantage that it can be easily combined with varus or valgus correction. Bandi[1] has recommended tibial tubercleplasty without patellectomy for treatment of patellar chondromalacia. Although I have no personal experience with this approach to patellar chondromalacia, the Bandi procedure is based on sound biomechanical principles and certainly decreases patellofemoral contact stress.

Although it is possible to completely compensate for the *mechanical* effect of patellectomy,[10] the previously discussed physiologic effects of patellectomy cannot be neutralized completely. One must therefore expect some loss of knee extensor power after patellectomy regardless of operative technique and postoperative treatment regimen. This opinion is supported by clinical studies that report frequent postpatellectomy extensor lag and 30% to 50% loss of extensor power.[3,6,11,18] One must recognize however, that some of the observed postpatellectomy loss of extensor power may be an effect of the prepatellectomy pathologic condition.

STABILITY

Patellectomy has no direct effect on the passive or ligamentous stability of a knee; however, "giving way" and a subjective feeling of instability are common postpatellectomy complaints.[11,18] Although it is tempting to assume that giving way is simply a reflection of extensor lag caused by decreased extensor power, a recent study showed no correlation between extension lag and giving way.[11] This suggests that postpatellectomy subjective instability may be a complex phenomenon, related more to pain and apprehension than simply to decreased extensor torque. Physical examination does, however, frequently show some degree of objective laxity of the patellectomized knee as compared to the contralateral knee. Although it is likely that the observed laxity is caused, at least in part, by the preoperative pathologic condition, it is possible that late ligamentous laxity may be a secondary effect of patellectomy because decreased extensor power may upset the balance of flexors versus extensors, thus interfering with the stabilizing effect of balanced muscle antagonists as primary joint stabilizers. There would therefore be greater demand placed on the secondary ligamentous joint stabilizers, which would lead to stretching and the observed postpatellectomy ligamentous laxity.

MOTION

Recognized effects of patellectomy on knee motion include extensor lag and loss of flexion range.[3,6,11,21] Electrogoniometry has shown decreased midstance-phase flexion as well as decreased flexion in ascending and descending stairs,[18] and instant center studies show a distortion of the path of instant centers.[17]

Laboratory studies have demonstrated that, depending on the technique of repair, complete extension of a patellectomized knee requires 15% to 30% more quadriceps force than full extension of an intact knee.[10] If the patient is not able to generate the necessary increase in quadriceps pull, he may be unable to fully extend the leg against gravity even though his knee has sufficient passive extension range; this would account for the observed extensor lag. Postpatellectomy extensor lag is therefore likely in patients whose age or local or systemic patho-logic condition compromises the ability to increase quadriceps force. Extensor lag is most likely in patients with preoperative extensor lag. Procedures that im-prove the extensor moment arm (previously described) are most clearly indi-cated for this group of patients.

Although full flexion is possible after patellectomy, many patellectomized knees show a 10° to 20° loss of flexion range.[11,18] This loss of flexion range is the result of operative shortening of the extensor mechanism and postoperative fibro-sis and adhesions as well as preoperative pathologic condition. Excessive post-operative immobilization may also contribute to loss of flexion range. The average postoperative flexion loss is 20°.[11,18] This amount of flexion loss may interfere with certain athletic activities but should have no effect on usual activities of daily living. Longitudinal closure of the patellectomy defect tends to preserve flexion range.

Decreased midstance-phase flexion and decreased flexion in ascending and descending stairs[18] is most likely a consequence of decreased knee extensor torque. The amount of knee extensor torque necessary to maintain upright pos-ture increases rapidly with the knee flexion angle.[5] Patients with impaired ability to generate knee extensor torque will therefore decrease their knee flexion angle while bearing weight.

The recently observed distortion of the path of instant centers[17] in postpatel-lectomy patients is an intriguing phenomenon that could help to explain progres-sive arthrosis of the knee, which is sometimes seen in postpatellectomy patients. It is tempting to attribute the alteration in path of instant centers to postpatel-lectomy change in the direction of quadriceps pull; however, at least some of the observed alteration in path of instant flexion centers may be the result of pre-patellectomy pathology.

• • •

Although patellectomy has multiple undesirable effects, operative techniques are available to decrease the undesirable functional and cosmetic effects of patel-lectomy. Careful attention to extensor mechanism alignment and tendon track-ing should help to minimize postpatellectomy persistence of symptoms in those patients who have a patellectomy for treatment of recurrent patellar dislocation or abnormal patellar tracking.[22] Theoretically the undesirable effects of patel-lectomy can be neutralized best through use of a patellar prosthesis.[14] Although there is considerable enthusiasm for patellar prostheses and/or total patello-femoral joint arthroplasty with or without total knee replacement, the fact is that these devices have an unknown service life and there is ample reason for apprehension about a foreign body in a subcutaneous location subject to trauma. Therefore at the present time patellectomy without prosthetic replacement re-mains the best choice for treatment of knees in which patellectomy is indicated.

References

1. Bandi, W.: Chondromalacia patellae und femoro-patellare Arthrose Atiologie, Klinik und Therapie, Helv. Chir. Acta 39(Suppl. 11):1, 1972.
2. Bechtol, C. O.: Muscle physiology. In American Academy of Orthopaedic Surgeons: Instructional course lectures, vol. 5, Ann Arbor, Mich., 1948, J. W. Edwards.
3. Boucher, H. H.: Patellectomy in the geriatric patient, Clin. Orthop. 11:33, 1958.
4. DePalma, A. F., and Flynn, J. J.: Joint changes following experimental partial and total patellectomy, J. Bone Joint Surg. 40-A:395, 1958.
5. Frankel, V. H., and Burstein, A. H.: Orthopaedic biomechanics, Philadelphia, 1970, Lea & Febiger.
6. Geckeler, E. O., and Quaranta, A. V.: Patellectomy for degenerative arthritis of the knee. Late results, J. Bone Joint Surg. 44-A:1109, 1962.
7. Haxton, H.: The function of the patella and the effects of its excision, Surg. Gynecol. Obstet. 30:389, 1945.
8. Hey-Groves, E. W.: A note on the extension apparatus of the knee joint, Br. J. Surg. 24:747, 1937.
9. Jackson, R.: Personal communication, 1977.
10. Kaufer, H.: Mechanical function of the patella, J. Bone Joint Surg. 53-A:1551, 1971.
11. Lewis, M. M., Fitzgerald, P. F., Jacobs, B., and Insall, J.: Patellectomy, an analysis of one hundred cases, J. Bone Joint Surg. 58-A:736, 1976.
12. Lewis, R. C., and Scholz, K. C.: Cruciate repair of the extensor mechanism following patellectomy, J. Bone Joint Surg. 48-A:1221, 1966.
13. Maquet, P.: Biomechanics and osteoarthritis of the knee, Extrait Onzieme Congres International de Chirurgie Orthopedique et de Traumatologie, Mexico, Oct. 1969, p. 317.
14. McKeever, D. C.: Patellar prosthesis, J. Bone Joint Surg. 37-A:1074, 1955.
15. Scott, J. C.: Fractures of the patella, J. Bone Surg. 31-B:76, 1949.
16. Shorbe, H. B., and Dobson, C. H.: Patellectomy, J. Bone Joint Surg. 40-A:1281, 1958.
17. Steurer, P. A., Gradisar, I. A., Hoyt, W. A., and Chu, M. L.: Patellectomy: a clinical study and biomechanical evaluation, J. Bone Joint Surg. 58-A:736, 1976.
18. Sutton, F. S., Thompson, C. H., Lipke, J., and Kettelkamp, D. B.: The effect of patellectomy on knee function, J. Bone Joint Surg. 58-A:537, 1976.
19. Thompson, J. E. M.: Fracture of the patella treated by removal of the loose fragment and plastic repair of the tendon. A study of 554 cases, Surg. Gynecol. Obstet. 74:860, 1942.
20. Todd, J.: The end results of fractures of the patella, J. Bone Joint Surg. 32-B:281, 1950.
21. West, F. E.: End results of patellectomy, J. Bone Joint Surg. 44-A:1089, 1962.
22. West, F. E., and Soto-Hall, R.: Recurrent dislocation of the patella in the adult, J. Bone Joint Surg. 40-A:386, 1958.
23. Young, H. H., and Regan, J. M.: Total excision of the patella for arthritis of the knee, Minn. Med. 28:909, 1945.

13. High tibial osteotomy for degenerative arthritis of the knee

Robert E. Leach
Stephen Wasilewski
David Segal

Twenty years ago the only operations available to relieve pain secondary to degenerative arthritis of the knee were arthrodesis and joint débridement. Arthrodesis, then as now, has the obvious advantages of providing a stable, strong knee and excellent relief from pain, but at the cost of knee motion. Arguments still rage as to whether the procedure is justified, even with this lack of knee motion, but the popularity of arthrodesis has waned. Joint débridement has enjoyed intermittent rebirths, but the inability to accurately predict which patients would be most helped plus the variability of lasting good results have limited the use of this procedure.

Osteotomy of the upper tibia for degenerative arthritis of the knee was introduced in the late 1950s, with the first published result being by Jackson[7] in 1958 and Jackson and Waugh[8] in 1961. The high tibial osteotomy now most often used was described by Gariepy[5] in 1964, and since that time numerous authors, including Coventry[3,4] and Bauer et al.,[1] have attested to its efficacy in relief of pain.

Soon after tibial osteotomy was introduced, the present wave of enthusiasm for resurfacing procedures of the knee started. Whether it be tibial plateau or femoral condylar prostheses or total knee replacement of some type, resurfacing the degenerative knee appears to be the first thought of many orthopaedic surgeons. However, tibial osteotomy continues to be an important method of alleviating pain from degenerative arthritis and occasionally even rheumatoid arthritis of the knee. We should now reexamine its role in the light of total knee replacement.

INDICATIONS

We consider any operative procedure, including tibial osteotomy, only after a patient with painful degenerative arthritis of the knee has not responded to adequate nonoperative treatment. This includes increasing quadriceps and ham-

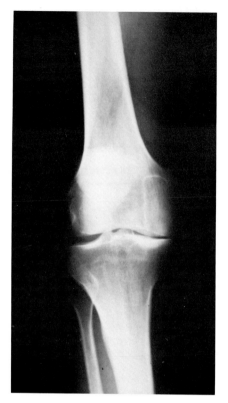 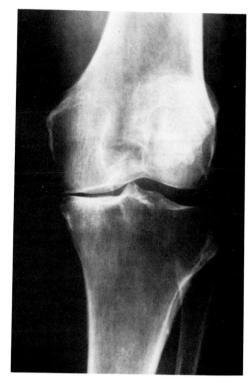

Fig. 13-1   Fig. 13-2

Fig. 13-1. Weight-bearing x-ray film shows mild varus deformity and narrow medial joint space. This patient is a good osteotomy candidate.
Fig. 13-2. Varus deformity plus narrow joint space. However, lateral joint space is "sprung" open, suggesting lateral ligament laxity. This patient is a questionable candidate.

string muscle strength, which may be difficult because of pain and secondary inhibition; the use of anti-inflammatory agents and anodynes such as aspirin, indomethacin (Indocin), and others; decreasing physical activity; and the use of some support such as a cane in the opposite hand. We do not recommend injecting a steroid into a degenerative joint but have at times injected a steroid around the attachments of the medial collateral ligament into the tibia. The rationale for this is as follows. In many patients with a narrow joint space on the medial side, the joint opens and closes in walking, putting stress on the medial collateral ligament. Pain may be pinpointed to this area. Local steroid injections have been helpful in relieving that type of pain but should not be repeated more than several times and must be combined with other conservative measures.

We have found it difficult to make any of the overweight patients lose weight. First, they have established a lifelong pattern and, second, their activity level is low because of pain. They do not adhere well to diets and cannot increase their

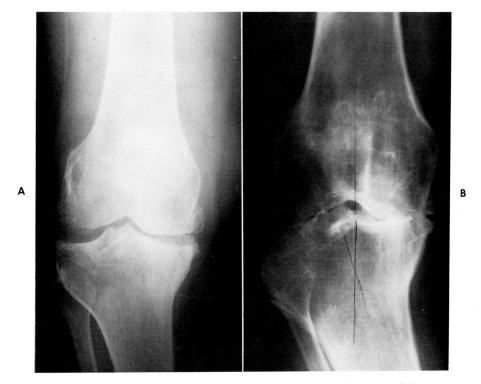

Fig. 13-3. A, Non-weight-bearing film shows mild varus deformity and poor medial joint space. **B,** Weight-bearing film shows severe subluxation producing "teeter" effect. This patient is not an osteotomy candidate.

activities to burn off calories. Refusing to treat them on the basis of their increased weight seems senseless to us, and many patients who have had tibial osteotomy are distinctly overweight.

As a patient begins to have more pain, his ability to walk a long distance and to walk at an increased pace lessens. Both parameters, distance and pace, should be evaluated. If the patient is not responding to conservative treatment and needs surgery, the major question is, In which patient is tibial osteotomy a reasonable operative procedure with a relatively predictable positive outcome? Our best results have been in those patients who have had a varus deformity of the femorotibial articulation. The joint space must be narrowed on the compressed side when viewed on a 14×17-inch weight-bearing film, and the opposite joint space must be relatively normal in appearance (Fig. 13-1). Excessive bone loss on the involved side is a contraindication because, even after osteotomy, some weight must be borne on both tibial plateaus. If osteotomy is done in the face of excessive bone loss, the so-called teeter effect, described by Kettelkamp, will occur. There must be no subluxation of the joint or gross instability of the knee ligaments (Figs. 13-2 and 13-3); knees with ligamentous instability can be subject to lateral thrust in walking, as described by Insall et al.[6] Knee extension must be nearly full, although a flexion deformity of as much as 15° can be compensated for operatively. Knee flexion should be to roughly 90°. Varus deformities appear to be handled more easily than valgus deformities, and we have done osteotomies for patients with varus deformity of as much as 25°.

The major problem is what to do with those patients who start with a valgus deformity. This is roughly 15% to 20% of most published series. Most authorities agree that a patient with a valgus deformity greater than 15° should probably not have a high tibial osteotomy but would be best handled by osteotomy of the lower femur or perhaps even the double osteotomy of Benjamin. Shoji and Insall,[10] in an excellent article in 1973, suggested that osteotomy was far less successful in relief of pain and production of stability in valgus knees than in varus knees. They recommended that, in contrast to a varus deformity, for which over-correction is advised, a valgus deformity requires one to be careful about over-correction. They stated that the postoperative femoral angle should be approximately 175° plus or minus 5°. They called attention to tilting of the tibial plateau

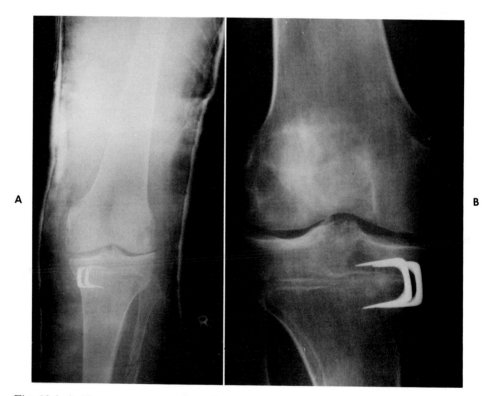

A   B

Fig. 13-4. A, Varus osteotomy performed for valgus deformity and narrow lateral joint space. **B,** Two years later, joint space is increased and joint line obliquity is less than 5°.

and advised that an osteotomy that caused tilting of more than 15° from the horizontal at the tibial plateau would predispose to a poor result (Fig. 13-4).

We have been doing high tibial osteotomy primarily for patients with degenerative arthritis although we have performed some in patients with traumatic arthritis involving one condyle and even in several patients with osteonecrosis involving one condyle. These latter patients are unlikely candidates since they seldom have an angular deformity. Although in the 1960s we did some osteotomies for patients with rheumatoid arthritis, we became disenchanted with this procedure and have found that we can usually realign the leg by one of the resurfacing procedures. Most patients with rheumatoid arthritis have severe valgus deformities and, of course, bicompartmental disease. We have had no personal experience with the double osteotomy involving the lower femur and upper tibia as practiced by Benjamin[2] in England, although his published operative results have been excellent.

Each patient who is being considered for high tibial osteotomy must have the objectives of the operation clearly explained to him. The primary aim is re-

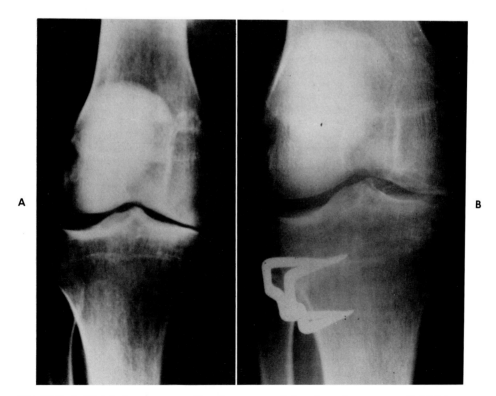

Fig. 13-5. A, Weight-bearing x-ray film shows varus deformity and narrow medial joint space. **B,** Three years after valgus osteotomy, medial joint space is widened.

lief of pain, not increased motion. In fact, most patients can expect a slight decrease in knee motion, although their effective range of motion into extension may be better. The results in most series show that approximately 80% of patients properly selected can expect to have good to excellent relief from pain. This means that 20% of patients probably will not be helped by this surgery.

One worry about tibial osteotomy is that, although the operation might give initial pain relief, there could be a gradual return of this pain. Longer term studies now indicate that the initial relief of pain appears to be long lasting. Kettelkamp and Coventry have shown that even 3 years after surgery approximately 70% of patients have good relief from pain (Fig. 13-5). Some surgeons have the concept that tibial osteotomy buys time by delaying the need for a definitive procedure such as total knee replacement. We do not think that this is a valid concept. Tibial osteotomy is a definitive procedure with a roughly 80% chance of producing good relief from pain, and the vast majority of patients have the opportunity for long-term relief.

OPERATIVE TECHNIQUE

Once we have decided to perform a tibial osteotomy, the 14×17-inch standing films are used to determine the necessary correction. With a varus deformity we want to overcorrect to 6° to 8° of valgus angulation, but with a valgus deformity we plan on ending with a varus angulation of between 0° and 5°. In making this correction we must be sure that the joint line inclination will not be greater than 15°.

In a valgus osteotomy the skin incision is made several fingerbreadths below the joint line, starting at the tibial tubercle and running parallel to the joint line to the posterior aspect of the fibular head and then curving distally 5 to 7 cm down the leg. The incision should extend just beyond the fibular neck distally. The subcutaneous tissues are incised and the muscle dissected by sharp dissection off the proximal aspect of the tibia. A longitudinal incision is made in the ligamentous complex attached to the fibular head, and the fibular head is completely freed by sharp dissection; this forms a sleeve of soft tissues that can be kept intact for simple closure.

Once the fibular head has been dissected free, it is cut at the junction of the head and neck. The ligamentous attachments to the upper tibia must be cut by sharp dissection. This is often the most difficult part of the operative procedure. We remove the fibular head. Occasionally the soft posterior portion of the fibular head may break free, and this has to be removed in piecemeal fashion. The objective of removing the fibular head is to allow easy access to the posterior tibia so that the osteotomy can be done under direct vision. Some authorities prefer to sever the attachments of the fibular head to the tibia, making it possible to lever the fibular head out of the way. After the fibular head is removed, the knee is flexed and a periosteal elevator is used to elevate the soft tissues away from posterior aspects of the tibia. This elevator goes all the way across the posterior portion of the tibia. A small periosteal elevator is then used underneath the patellar ligament, and the medial aspect of the tibia is cleaned anteriorly.

With all tissues cleaned anteriorly and posteriorly and the knee flexed, we are ready to make the first cut. The first cut is parallel to the joint surface of the tibia, but both osteotomy cuts must be planned together. The objective is to have the lower cut skirt the upper edge of the tibial tubercle at the patellar ligament attachment and meet the proximal cut at the medial cortex of the tibia. We agree with Bauer that approximately 1 mm of bone should be removed for each angular degree of correction desired. Generally we may take slightly less than this, since we do not want to remove too much initially. We would like the proximal tibial cut to be as far away from the joint surface as possible to prevent the possibility of an inadvertent fracture into the articular surface of the tibia. Some surgeons drill a Steinman pin across the tibia at the level of the proximal cut and take an x-ray film so that they can see exactly where their cut parallel to the joint surface is going to be. Careful delineation of the joint surface is an absolute necessity for determining where the first cut will go.

Once we have decided where both cuts are going to start, we proceed with the osteotomy, using a large osteotome and cutting one half to two thirds of the way across the tibia. The cuts are continuous anterior to posterior; then the wedge of bone is broken out with the osteotomes or a small curette. Once the wedge of bone is removed, the surgeon can see directly into the osteotomy and finish doing the osteotomy under direct vision. The medial and especially the posteromedial corner of the tibial cortex should be penetrated. If this is not done, the osteotomy may not go through the preferred side but into the tibial plateau instead. We prefer a small osteotome to penetrate the medial cortex several times and are not particularly worried about maintaining a bony hinge at the medial cortex. We think that the soft tissue stability and the use of staples are sufficient to hold the osteotomy well.

Once the osteotomy is completed, the wedge is closed gently and the position of the leg is carefully checked. If correction is perfect, one or two step staples are inserted with pressure applied to keep the cut bone ends in firm apposition. If there is any question about correction, long x-ray films should be taken in the operating room. Careful placement of the staples is necessary since the proximal bony fragment is narrow and it is easy to put a fixation device into the joint surface.

In knees with a flexion contracture prior to surgery, we make a wedge somewhat wider anteriorly to take up for the flexion contracture and bring the knee out into full extension. This may not be a problem at all because the bone is soft enough to allow pressure to compress the bone anteriorly even if no wedge is taken.

Operation from the medial side is more difficult because of the pes anserinus and medial collateral ligament. Thus performing a varus osteotomy means that it is necessary to take up part of the pes anserinus or even dissect away part of the medial collateral ligament and advance it. Sometimes one can work inside the pes tendons, completing the osteotomy by flexing the knee, which allows the pes tendons to drop back a bit.

Vascular damage to the popliteal artery where it passes behind the knee is a potential worry. With the knee flexed and the osteotomy done under direct vision, this should not be a problem. Even in elderly patients, we have used a tourniquet for only 1 hour and have had no difficulty with the postoperative vascularity of the limb.

POSTOPERATIVE CARE

After surgery we place a Penrose drain into the operative wound because of bleeding from the vascular bone. We apply a cylinder or long leg cast with the leg extended in the corrected position; the cast is carefully padded, particularly around the peroneal nerve. We check carefully for both sensation and dorsiflexion of the toes during the first 24 hours. If there is any question of decreased peroneal nerve function or even an anterior tibial compartment syndrome, the cast is promptly bivalved. We window the cast at 24 to 36 hours to remove the drain. The cast is then changed at 6 days for a new long leg cast, and the patient is allowed to bear weight 24 hours later.

Patients are allowed out of bed on the second or third postoperative day but cannot weight bear until the new cast has been applied. Thrombophlebitis is a major worry, and immediate postoperative exercises in the form of quadriceps sets and toe curls are started. Our regular practice has been to give patients aspirin pre- and postoperatively, but patients with a history of severe varicosities or thrombophlebitic problems have been given low-dose heparin postoperatively. We have had some cases of acute thrombophlebitis and one clinically recognizable embolus at this point.

Six weeks following surgery the cast is removed and x-ray films are taken. Almost routinely, union is present at 6 weeks and the patient is brought into the hospital for 5 to 7 days of intensive physiotherapy. We have found hospitalization a more reliable method of getting knee motion and gaining strength than having the patients do outpatient physiotherapy. Many patients are older and some obese, and they find it difficult to move the knee when they do not have hospital personnel to reinforce their physical therapy program. The program includes active range-of-motion knee exercises plus quadriceps sets, and weight bearing on crutches is gradually increased. Gradually the patients move on to progressive weight bearing and then more intensive exercises for the hamstrings and quadriceps. Follow-up examination is performed and weight-bearing films are obtained after 3, 6, and 12 months.

COMPLICATIONS

Complications of tibial osteotomy are varied, common, usually not severe, and mostly preventable. The most common complication is either inadequate correction at the time of surgery or later loss of correction as a result of early weight bearing. We have found that if there is initially overcorrection of varus deformity into valgus angulation, we seldom have a loss of correction later. Again, this must be determined accurately on the operating room table, which may be made difficult by drapes, obese limbs, etc. It is safest to obtain x-ray films on the operating table prior to application of the cast. If correction is inadequate, the surgeon may remove further wedges of bone and obtain correction. If the correction is not adequate postoperatively, the surgeon has a choice of trying to manipulate the leg under anesthesia or reoperating. Inadequate correction must not be accepted. In such instances, pain relief for 1 or 2 years may be adequate, but inevitably loss of correction will lead to further problems.

Our second most common operative problem has been a postoperative peroneal nerve palsy. In the three instances in which this has occurred, it has always been secondary to pressure from the cast, and for that reason we are always ready to bivalve the cast and cut the soft padding postoperatively. During surgery we do not isolate the peroneal nerve, but in no instance have we had an operative problem with the peroneal nerve, as all patients with palsies were able to dorsiflex their foot and toes on awakening from anesthesia. The possibility of an

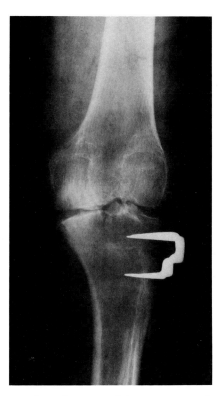

Fig. 13-6. Fracture through intercondylar area; correction is incomplete.

anterior tibial compartment syndrome occurring as a result of bleeding into the compartment must be recognized. This has been reported following a Hauser procedure, which involves even less trauma to the anterior compartment than a tibial osteotomy. Fracture of the proximal tibial fragment has occurred in our hospital in two cases. In each instance the osteotomy was started in the correct place but in one instance it went diagonally up into the joint surface on the medial side (Fig. 13-6). In the other case the osteotomy was completed in the proper position but the medial tibial cortex was not penetrated, and at the time of closure of the two bony surfaces, instead of the medial tibial cortex breaking, the proximal fragment broke at the intracondylar area (Fig. 13-7). In both instances good alignment was obtained and the patients did well. However, internal fixation of the proximal fragment was required in one patient.

Each of these complications is a technical one and should be correctable. Careful attention to operative detail obviates these problems. Infection is not a common occurrence. The blood supply in this area is excellent and even in older patients we have not had problems with infection or soft tissue wound healing.

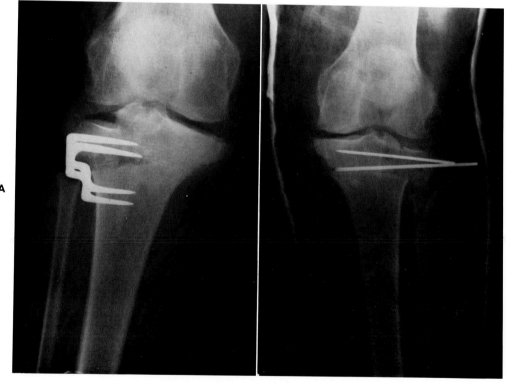

Fig. 13-7. A, Fracture through tibial plateau at surgery was recognized on x-ray film. **B,** Fixation was accomplished by pins. Patient had good results.

Thrombophlebitis is a major postoperative possibility and we think that some type of routine anticoagulation therapy is reasonable.

OTHER CONSIDERATIONS

In several cases that appeared to have had adequate operative correction the correction was lost over a 2-year period. We have no good explanation of why this happened. We have not tightened ligaments at the time of surgery, but in a number of patients who previously had loosening of the ligamentous structures we found that the ligamentous supporting structures tightened once angular bony correction had been achieved.

The question is always raised as to whether or not an operative débridement with removal of degenerative menisci, loose bodies, etc. should be done at the same time as tibial osteotomy. We think that virtually all knees with degenerative arthritis have some degeneration of the menisci and other changes that might legitimately be subjected to joint débridement. However, with proper angular correction after osteotomy, patients do well and do not appear to need intra-articular surgery. We do not enter the joint at the same time we are doing a tibial osteotomy. If the patient's symptoms appear to be primarily those of a torn cartilage, we do a meniscectomy, even in an elderly patient. If symptoms appear to be primarily a result of degenerative arthritis, we do an osteotomy with the possibility of doing another procedure later. We have found that a subsequent intra-articular procedure is seldom needed. Preoperative use of the arthroscope has been recommended by some, and we have used it in several instances. In each instance we found degenerative changes of the meniscus but still elected to go ahead with the osteotomy without doing an intra-articular procedure. Perhaps the arthroscope can be used to get a more definitive idea as to how the joint should look for a tibial osteotomy, and it may be particularly helpful in follow-up of all osteotomy cases, both those that do well and those that fail.

SUMMARY

Proximal tibial osteotomy continues to be a reliable operative procedure giving predictable operative results. It is not a late salvage operation; many knees considered for tibial osteotomy have changes too advanced to allow any benefit from the operation. Knees must be operated on prior to developing lateral subluxation and the teeter effect described by Kettelkamp. Although the majority of our patients have been in their 60s, it may well be that the greater role for tibial osteotomy will be in younger patients in whom joint deterioration and deformity have just started. In these patients we may be able to reverse or arrest the degenerative process by an early tibial osteotomy. It has the advantage of burning no bridges, so that should the case fall into the 20% in which tibial osteotomy fails, another operative procedure may be performed with the leg well aligned.

However, the objective of tibial osteotomy is not simply to align the leg but to relieve pain. It should be considered a definitive procedure.

References

1. Bauer, G., Insall, J., and Koshino, T.: Tibial osteotomy in gonarthrosis (osteoarthritis of the knee), J. Bone Joint Surg. **51-A**:1545, 1969.
2. Benjamin, A.: Double osteotomy for the painful knee in rheumatoid arthritis and osteoarthritis, J. Bone Joint Surg. **51-B**:694, 1969.
3. Coventry, M.: Osteotomy of the upper portion of the tibia for degenerative arthritis of the knee. A preliminary report, J. Bone Joint Surg. **47-A**:984, 1965.
4. Coventry, M.: Osteotomy about the knee for degenerative and rheumatoid arthritis, J. Bone Joint Surg. **55-A**:23, 1973.
5. Gariepy, R.: Genu varum treated by high tibial osteotomy, J. Bone Joint Surg. **46-B**:783, 1964.
6. Insall, J., Shoji, H., and Mayer, V.: High tibial osteotomy, J. Bone Joint Surg. **56-A**:1397, 1974.
7. Jackson, P.: Osteotomy for osteoarthritis of the knee, J. Bone Joint Surg. **40-B**:826, 1958.
8. Jackson, P., and Waugh, W.: Tibial osteotomy for osteoarthritis of the knee, J. Bone Joint Surg. **43-B**:746, 1961.
9. Kettelkamp, D., Leach, R., and Nosea, R.: Pitfalls of proximal tibial osteotomy, Clin. Orthop. **106**:232, 1975.
10. Shoji, H., and Insall, J.: High tibial osteotomy for osteoarthritis of the knee with valgus deformity, J. Bone Joint Surg. **55-A**:903, 1973.
11. Torgerson, W., Kettelkamp, D., Igou, R., and Leach, R.: Tibial osteotomy for the treatment of degenerative arthritis of the knee, Clin. Orthop. **101**:46, 1974.

14. Biomechanics of high tibial osteotomy

Edmund Y. S. Chao

The introduction of the intertrochanteric osteotomy to relieve pain and restore mechanical integrity to the hip joint stimulated the development of various forms of knee osteotomy.* Clinical results were reviewed to establish the basic criteria for patient selection and to determine the efficacy of the procedure according to the specific surgical techniques used. On the basis of an elaborate analysis, Maquet et al.[14] attempted to justify the biomechanical advantages of knee osteotomy. They analyzed force distribution on the plateaus for knees with varus and valgus deformity, as well as for knees with residual flexion contracture. As a result of their study the dome-type osteotomy at the upper tibia with anterior advancement of the patellar tendon was proposed. Steinmann pins and a Charnley compression device were used for fixation.

Kettelkamp and Chao[11] performed a two-dimensional force analysis of the knee joint in the anteroposterior plane for a group of normal persons and a number of selected pre- and postosteotomy patients for the purpose of establishing rational guidelines for determining the proper wedge size to be excised in high tibial osteotomy. In that study the concept of careful preoperative analysis to enhance long-term success of the surgical procedure was emphasized. However, no results based on well-planned prospective study were included to substantiate the theoretical hypothesis. In a recent study the number of normal subjects was expanded and a large group of postoperative patients at various periods of follow-up was included.[12] This study encompassed clinical, functional gait, and plateau force distribution evaluations in the hope of providing a more comprehensive analysis of the procedure. In the light of the current popularity of total joint replacement, the exact role of upper tibial osteotomy can be assessed objectively.

The human knee joint must adapt to high stresses and at the same time maintain a high degree of mobility and stability. This functional demand makes it a common site of traumatic injury and degenerative joint disease. In any reconstructive procedure involving the knee, its complex and demanding functions

---

*References 1, 3-7, 9, 10, 17, 18.

must be taken into account. The following biomechanical factors are important to the long-term success of high tibial osteotomy:

1. Pathomechanics involved in genu varum and genu valgum deformities
2. Tibial plateau contact force redistribution after tibial osteotomy
3. Effects on other anatomic functions of the knee
4. Functional performance of the knee joint in gait and other activities of daily living before and after the surgical reconstruction

This chapter discusses each of these factors on the basis of theoretical concepts. It is hoped that such a discussion can provide helpful information to establish proper guidelines for patient selection, surgical technique, and long-term prognosis in regard to high tibial osteotomy.

Although the ensuing presentation emphasizes the biomechanical aspects of the problem, the clinical advantages of the procedure have been widely appreciated. These advantages can be summarized as follows:

1. The procedure is capable of providing full correction of the deformity.
2. The correction site is near the deformity, thus allowing accurate realignment.
3. The osteotomy is performed at the cancellous bone region, thereby enhancing bony union.
4. Early motion and weight bearing minimize knee functional restriction and muscle atrophy.
5. The surgical procedure is less extensive than other forms of osteotomy at the knee, allowing easy rehabilitation.
6. The procedure provides for convenient exploration of other pathologic conditions of the knee joint.

It is important to recognize these potential advantages so that the following analyses can be put into proper perspective with their clinical significance.

MECHANICS OF TIBIAL OSTEOTOMY

The effects of tibial osteotomy can be discussed in regard to the histologic factors and the biomechanical factors. The histologic factors consist of (1) allowing damaged cartilage to regenerate,[2] (2) retardation of subchondral bone sclerosis and cyst formation, (3) prevention of further capsular-ligamentous laxity, (4) decreasing clinical symptoms and pain, and (5) possible decompression of vascular pressure as a source of pain. The biomechanical factors include (1) correction of knee joint deformity in the anteroposterior plane, (2) realignment of load-bearing axis, (3) increasing joint stability (sometimes involving tightening the contralateral ligament), and (4) altering patellofemoral mechanics, which may be an important factor in causing symptomatic pain. All these factors are intimately related. A clear understanding of the mechanics of the knee joint can be a great help in explaining the deformity associated with joint disease and in analyzing the means of reconstruction.

To study the quantitative mechanics of the knee joint in the frontal plane

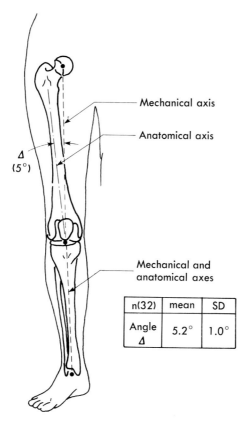

Mechanical axis

Anatomical axis

Δ
(5°)

Mechanical and
anatomical axes

n(32)	mean	SD
Angle Δ	5.2°	1.0°

Fig. 14-1. Definition of anatomic and mechanical axes of femur and tibia. Mean angle difference between the two femoral axes of 32 normal legs is also shown.

during normal standing, it is important to define the mechanical axes of the
femur and tibia in contrast to the clinically determined anatomic axes. As shown
in Fig. 14-1, the mechanical axis of the femur is the line joining the center of the
femoral head to the midpoint of the intercondylar eminence. The anatomic axis
of the femur is the bisector of the distal femoral shaft. The mechanical axis of
the tibia is a line joining the midpoint of the intercondylar eminence and the
centroid of the tibiofibular mortise. The anatomic axis of the tibia is defined in
the same manner as that of the femur. A study of 32 normal anteroposterior x-ray
films showed that the mechanical axis of the femur has a mean varus angle of 5°
(with a standard deviation of 1°), which matches closely with Steindler's finding.[16] In the same control group the mechanical and anatomic axes of the tibia
nearly coincide.

Mechanical axes are more reliable than anatomic axes in defining knee joint
deformity, especially when there are other skeletal deformities away from the
knee joint. These axes provide the precise description of load transmission
through the knee joint. However, in certain clinical circumstances anatomic axes

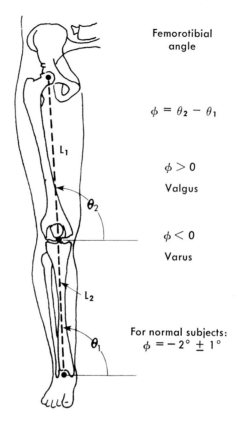

Femorotibial
angle

$$\phi = \theta_2 - \theta_1$$

$$\phi > 0$$

Valgus

$$\phi < 0$$

Varus

For normal subjects:
$$\phi = -2° \pm 1°$$

Fig. 14-2. Definition of femorotibial angle, ϕ, and its mean value and standard deviation for a group of normal subjects. (Minus sign indicates varus angulation.)

would be more convenient to use. In such cases a full appreciation of the inherent difference in orientation between the mechanical and anatomic axes has to be recognized for accurate assessment of load transmission through the knee joint.

The angles of the mechanical axes of the femur and the tibia with respect to the horizontal line of the ground are used to define the knee joint orientation in the frontal plane. As shown in Fig. 14-2, θ_2 is the femoral orientation angle and θ_1 is the tibial orientation angle. The difference between these two angles $(\theta_2 - \theta_1)$, designated as angle ϕ, is used to measure the varus or valgus deformity. In the same group of normal knees studied, a residual varus angle of 2° with a standard deviation of ±1° existed. In essence, a normal knee has a varus angle of about 2°, measured on the mechanical axes of the femur and tibia. If anatomic axes were used, a normal knee would have a 3° valgus angle. These data are limited to normal knees of young men and women. Additional data, including anthropomorphic, age, and sex factors, are required to establish a more reliable reference base.

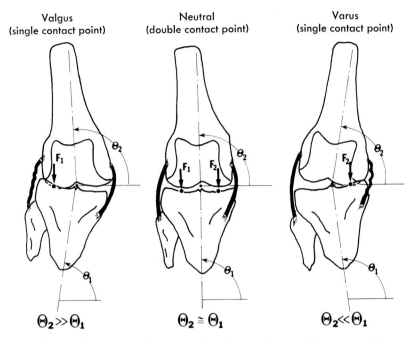

Fig. 14-3. Schematic diagram to show neutral, valgus, and varus deformities of knee joint in anteroposterior plane. Mechanical axes are used for measurement of angles θ_1 and θ_2.

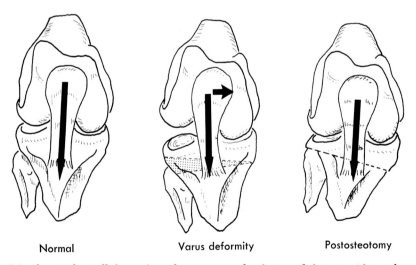

Fig. 14-4. Abnormal patellofemoral mechanics as result of varus deformity. After valgus osteotomy, such abnormal mechanics could be corrected by change of patellar tendon direction.

From such angle definitions, the classic varus and valgus deformities can be quantitated in comparison with neutral orientation of the normal knee joint. Additional features associated with joint deformity can also be defined on the basis of plateau force distribution and the laxity of collateral ligaments. As shown in Fig. 14-3, the normal knee allows contact force on both the medial and lateral plateaus if the collateral ligaments are of a length to allow neutral alignment. In this case, $\theta_1 = \theta_2$. In either deformity there is only one plateau subject to contact force, which causes excessive tension of the contralateral collateral ligament. A correction by upper tibial osteotomy, if done properly, redistributes the forces on the plateaus to resemble those in normal knee orientation. Proper relief of collateral ligament tension can also be achieved.

It is postulated that excessive knee deformity in the anteroposterior plane also alters patellofemoral mechanics, which may cause clinical symptoms. A high tibial osteotomy may correct the pathomechanics of the patella and eliminate one possible source of pain. As illustrated in Fig. 14-4, the varus knee tends to cause a medial pull on the patella, thereby introducing localized patellar cartilage degeneration. Valgus osteotomy alters the dominant medial pull to neutral or even to the lateral direction, which would significantly reduce the pressure sustained by the damaged portion of the patella and allow it to regenerate.

These mechanical factors help to explain the abnormal mechanics associated with knee deformity. Subsequent plateau force distribution would utilize the above definition to predict the quantitative effect of osteotomy in correcting a deformity so that a more accurate correction can be achieved. Other anatomic factors, although not included here, should also be kept in mind since they also contribute to the mechanics of knee joint deformity. These factors consist of joint contact area, tibial plateau geometry, cruciate ligament function, meniscal contribution to stability, and force equilibrium in the saggittal plane. The following analysis did not include these variables merely for reasons of simplicity. However, this simplified analysis should still be able to provide useful information in regard to plateau force distribution.

PLATEAU FORCE DISTRIBUTION

In calculating the tibial plateau forces, the following basic criteria were implied:

1. The knee deformity was defined by the femorotibial angle $(\theta_2 - \theta_1)$, measured on the mechanical axes of the femur and tibia.
2. The force analysis was static and measured in two dimensions[1] in the anteroposterior plane with the patient in a normal standing posture.
3. The geometric data were measured based on a 6-foot long film with load bearing.
4. Both the plateau forces and the collateral ligament forces were considered in the modeling.

The force analysis was based on the free-body diagram shown in Fig. 14-5.

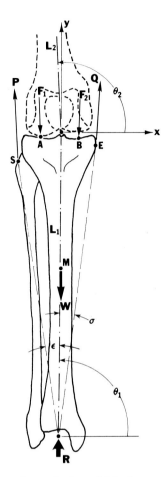

Fig. 14-5. Free-body diagram used to calculate tibial plateau contact forces (F_1 and F_2) and collateral ligament tension (P and Q).

F_1 and F_2 are the lateral and medial plateau contact forces applied at points A and B. P and Q represent the lateral and medial collateral ligamentous forces with the orientation and point of application as illustrated. R is the ground reaction force, which has the value of half the subject's body weight. W is the weight of the leg plus the foot and shoe, which was assumed to be 6.2% of body weight, according to Morrison.[15] L_1 and L_2 are the mechanical axes of the tibia and femur, respectively. All parameters used in this diagram were measured directly from the standing 6-foot long film.

Static equilibrium analysis was based on the input data indicated in Fig. 14-6. The force equations for various cases of knee deformity were derived and presented in a previous publication,[11] and thus are not included here. The solutions of these equations provide the plateau and collateral ligament forces, which can be plotted against the femorotibial angle, ϕ. A typical force plot for a normal sub-

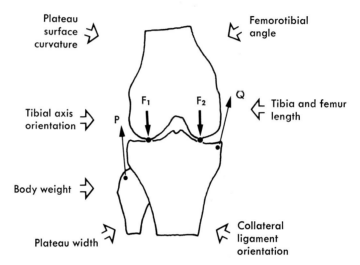

Fig. 14-6. Anatomic and geometric parameters required in determining plateau and collateral ligament forces.

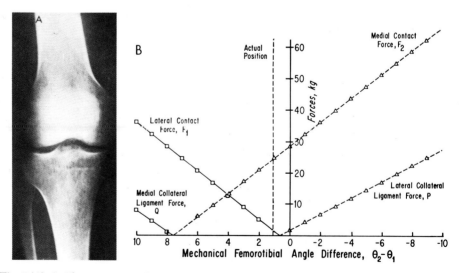

Fig. 14-7. A, Plateau contact force and collateral ligament tension for normal subject. **B,** Variations of these forces are plotted against femorotibial angle, $\theta_2 - \theta_1$.

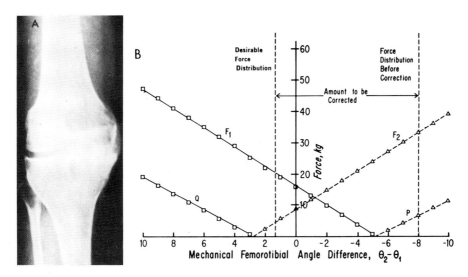

Fig. 14-8. **A,** Plateau contact force and collateral ligament tension for knee with varus deformity. **B,** Variations of these forces are plotted against femorotibial angle, $\theta_2 - \theta_1$.

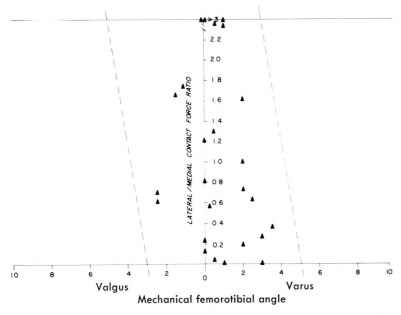

Fig. 14-9. Distribution of normal plateau forces for 26 knees. Region enclosed by dashed lines is defined as normal range.

ject is shown in Fig. 14-7. From this diagram it was found that in standing more force is applied to the medial plateaus and the collateral ligaments carry virtually no load. Fig. 14-8 depicts an abnormal knee with approximately 7° varus deformity in which all plateau force is on the medial compartment (F_1) with significant lateral collateral ligament force (P) present. For proper correction a wedge of 10° is to be excised.

To establish the normal plateau contact forces during standing, 26 apparently normal knees of 13 persons were analyzed. The results are presented in Fig. 14-9, the lateral-medial contact force ratios are plotted against the femorotibial angle, ϕ ($\theta_2 - \theta_1$). The region bounded by two dashed lines, which includes data from all the normal subjects, is defined as the normal range. The slant of the lines was postulated on the idea that the variation of the femorotibial angle has a certain linear relationship with the contact force ratio. The lower limit of this normal range is full medial compartment weight bearing from 5° varus to 3° valgus angulation. The upper boundary of this region is full lateral plateau weight bearing from 3° varus to 5° valgus angulation. This provides a reliable statistical range for most normal subjects. This range serves as a reference in analyzing proper plateau force redistribution in high tibial osteotomy.

In a separate series 10 preoperative and 41 postoperative patients were stud-

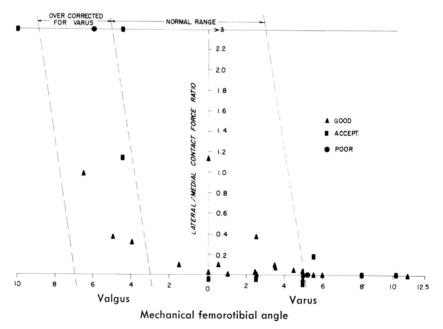

Fig. 14-10. Plateau forces and collateral ligament tension of varus deformity patients after valgus osteotomy. Subjective clinical assessment was used to grade the patients.

ied. The results for the preoperative patients reflect an abnormal plateau force distribution, which obviously requires osteotomy for correction. The postoperative results for the 41 patients were divided into varus and valgus groups based on their preoperative history, as shown in Figs. 14-10 and 14-11. Clinical assessments (to be described in the next section) classified as good, acceptable, and poor were also identified. Of the patients with results classified as good 84% had plateau force distributions either within the normal range or slightly overcorrected. Results for those with undercorrection were reclassified as poor in subsequent clinical evaluations. This reflects the importance of overcorrection in knees with deformity. Similar findings were observed for knees with valgus deformity.

The plateau force distribution among all knees studied can be presented in a simplified diagram, as shown in Fig. 14-12. In this diagram the medial and lateral plateau force difference ($F_2 - F_1$) in units of body weight is plotted against the varus or valgus angle. A neutral zone, similar to the normal region defined previously, can be used to assess the results of the postoperative cases. It can be seen that most of these cases have significant overcorrection. To evaluate the clinical implications of overcorrection, functional evaluation at long-term follow-up is necessary.

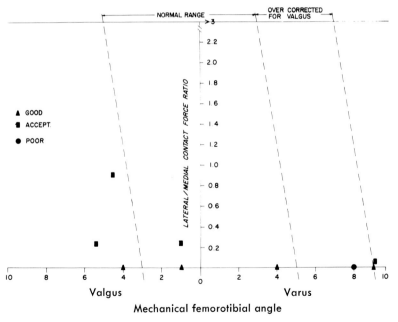

Fig. 14-11. Plateau contact force and collateral ligament tension of valgus deformity patient after varus osteotomy. Subjective clinical assessment was used to grade the patient.

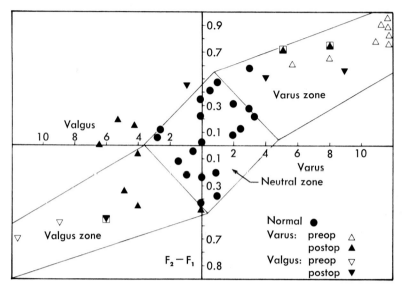

Fig. 14-12. Plateau force distribution of normal, preoperative, and postoperative knees based on femorotibial angle and plateau contact force difference. Neutral zone is defined on basis of the normal population studied.

CLINICAL AND BIOMECHANICAL EVALUATION

The characteristics of the patients included in clinical and biomechanical evaluations (functional gait and activities of daily living) and subjected to plateau force analysis were as follows. The control group consisted of 13 persons with normal knees (26 knees). The patients studied were 25 men and 32 women, of whom 54 had unilateral involvement and 3 had bilateral involvement (a total of 60 knees in 57 patients). Thirty-eight patients had degenerative disorders. Long-term results were available after 39 months and 63 months. The clinical evaluation rating scale is defined as follows:

Good	No support required and no pain present with activity
Acceptable	No support required but some pain present
Poor	Support required and persistent pain present

The evaluation results for the two follow-up series are summarized here:

	1972	1974
Good	32	24
Acceptable	16	16
Poor	12	20

A significant deterioration of results is clearly shown. When the results were studied according to the degree of overcorrection, an interesting finding was observed (Table 14-1). In knees with varus deformity that had overcorrection of 5° or greater the long-term results are more stable, which reflects the importance of overcorrection for valgus osteotomy.

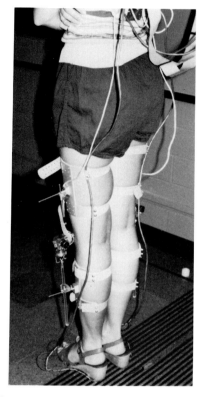

Fig. 14-13. Knee electrogoniometer system used for functional gait evaluation.

Table 14-1. Results of overcorrection of varus deformity

Results	Less than 5° overcorrection		5° overcorrection	
	39 mo	63 mo	39 mo	63 mo
Good or acceptable	15	9	25	23
Poor	5	11	3	5
Poor (%)	25%	55%	11%	18%

Table 14-2. Results of postoperative evaluation of changes in gait

Clinical result	Swing-phase flex.-ext.	Stance-phase flex.-ext.	Abduction-adduction	Rotation	Cadence	Stride
Good	NS	Increased	NS	Decreased	Increased	Increased
Acceptable	NS	NS	NS	Decreased	Increased	Increased
Poor	NS	NS	NS	NS	NS	NS

NS = Not significant.

An electrogoniometer of the type shown in Fig. 14-13 was used in evaluation of level walking and activities of daily living. The evaluation procedure and the definition of gait parameters can be referred to in previous publications.[8,12,13] The most significant gait parameters were found to be (1) swing-phase flexion, (2) stance-phase flexion, (3) range of abduction and adduction, (4) range of axial rotation, and (5) cadence and stride length. The gait evaluation results classified by clinical assessment are presented in Table 14-2. A close correlation between gait evaluation results and the subjective clinical assessments was found.

DISCUSSION

In view of the well-established clinical advantages and the results of bio-mechanical analysis, high tibial osteotomy is certainly a justified reconstructive surgery of the knee for a selected group of patients who have unicompartmental osteoarthritis with acceptable ligamentous stability and minimal bone loss. The results of long-term clinical and biomechanical gait evaluation further sub-stantiate the efficacy of this procedure when it is performed for well-established indications. However, since the longevity of such a procedure in treating varus deformity is very much dependent on overcorrection, careful preoperative analy-sis of joint deformity as shown on 6-foot weight-bearing long film is essential. An ideal correction for various degrees of varus or valgus angulation can be deter-mined according to the diagram shown in Fig. 14-14. In the case of genu varus, overcorrection to 3° to 5° of valgus angulation is recommended. Valgus deformity

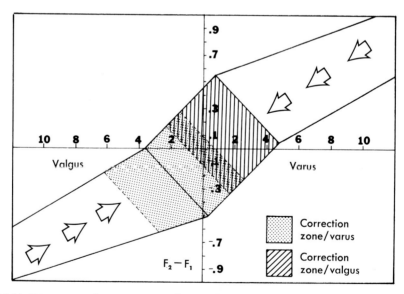

Fig. 14-14. Diagram used to estimate wedge size based on concept of overcorrection for knees with varus deformity and neutral correction for knees with valgus deformity.

should be corrected only to neutral because of the residual varus angle inherent in normal knee geometry. In addition, there is a varus thrust existing in normal walking that tends to shift the plateau force medially during stance-phase motion. Naturally this conclusion is only based on biomechanical analysis. However, the existing patient evaluation results seem to substantiate this theory.

Among other potential advantages of high tibial osteotomy, altering patello-femoral mechanics can contribute to elimination of pain. However, if rotatory de-formity is involved, a three-dimensional wedge may be more beneficial and take into account the change of patellar tendon force direction, as well as the correc-tion of rotation. Additional analysis in this respect is certainly warranted to ex-pand the scope of knee osteotomy. Collateral ligament tightening is also an im-portant factor that is often controversial. From a purely mechanical standpoint, tightening the contralateral ligament is a good practice to enhance joint stability after osteotomy.

For excessive valgus deformity, lower femoral osteotomy may be more de-sirable and effective in shifting the plateau force medially. This can be explained by the simple diagram shown in Fig. 14-15. If the osteotomy site is more proximal, the lower leg is brought closer to the body center line, which would provide the required load transfer medially without significantly altering the tibiofemoral joint line orientation. The common problem of bony nonunion experienced in

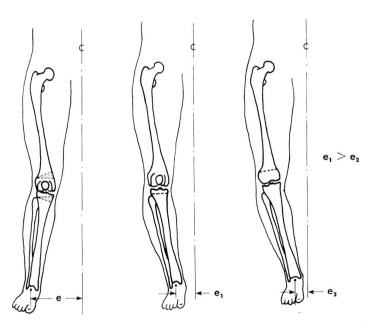

Fig. 14-15. High tibial osteotomy versus lower femoral osteotomy in transmitting plateau load medially. Parameter *e* depicts distance between foot-floor contact point and center line of body gravity.

such cases may be avoided by applying the Hoffman device. However, if the patient has an abnormal hip on the same side, particularly with pronounced adduction, proper correction at the hip is essential in maintaining the effectiveness of tibial or femoral osteotomy.

It may seem misleading and improper to correlate clinical evaluation results with biomechanical force and gait analyses, since there are many other factors that could affect the outcome of osteotomy. These factors are largely anatomic and pathologic. They consist of soft tissue reconstruction, vascular status, nerve impingement and tension, etc., which can only be assessed subjectively by clinical means. However, the present results show a strong correlation between biomechanical evaluation and clinical observation. Valuable information of prognostic significance can then be quantitated by objective analysis of patient function.

For example, if a patient begins to have symptoms of functional deterioration, it can easily be detected by biomechancal evaluation procedures using force analysis and level walking examination as the main criteria. These results should suggest the proper therapeutic course for that patient. Biomechanical evaluation should be incorporated in any clinical study for the purpose of providing guidelines for indications, treatment, and prognosis of high tibial osteotomy. Improvement in surgical technique can also be studied on the basis of retrospective and prospective protocols involving biomechanical analyses.

The question of whether high tibial osteotomy could be used as a prophylactic surgery in younger patients with excessive varus deformity but without clinical symptoms of pain or instability is interesting but controversial. Such a question cannot be answered easily without considering many medical and socioeconomic factors. The age of the individual is also important and should be considered in the light of the current development of joint replacement. Many experienced orthopaedic surgeons believe that if a relatively young patient is asymptomatic, regardless of his knee joint deformity, tibial osteotomy would be contraindicated. For older patients demanding a high level of activity, such a corrective procedure may be indicated to retard cartilage and subchondral bone degeneration. This question should probably be answered on the individual merits of each case. Patients with pronounced knee deformity but no symptoms should be examined frequently. Any slight complaint of pain or discomfort may be an early warning sign of pathologic changes as a result of uneven loading at the plateaus. In such a circumstance, proper therapeutic precautions should be recommended, and performing a high tibial osteotomy at a later time should be considered a strong possibility. It should be remembered, however, that if a joint is allowed to deteriorate, the articular surface and ligamentous structure may experience excessive damage that can make any reconstructive procedure difficult and less effective. These thoughts suggest that prophylactic osteotomy may have its value in orthopaedic surgery. More studies are needed to justify such a radical concept.

CONCLUSIONS

The following conclusions may be drawn from the results of previous studies, as presented in this chapter. Application of these statements should be carefully weighed against other clinical and surgical factors in each individual case.

1. Biomechanical principles justify high tibial osteotomy as a surgical procedure to redistribute knee plateau forces.
2. In determining proper wedge angle the mechanical axes, rather than the anatomic axes, should be used for the femur and tibia. If only anatomic axes are available, careful correction for the residual valgus angle of the femur should be considered.
3. For varus deformity a slight overcorrection of approximately 5° is recommended; the patient's preoperative condition should be taken into account.
4. For moderate valgus deformity the osteotomy should bring the anatomic axes for the tibia and femur in line, which produces a slight varus angle for the load-transmitting mechanical axes because of the residual valgus angle of the anatomic axis of the femur.
5. Distal femoral osteotomy may be indicated for excessive valgus deformity with an inclined plateau line, but a better means of enhancing bony union without loss of mass should be used. If the hip is abnormally adducted, correction at the hip is essential to ensure the desired postoperative result after osteotomy at the knee joint.
6. For rheumatoid arthritis patients with flexion contracture and rotatory deformity in addition to genu varum, a dome-type osteotomy may be more effective in providing three-dimensional correction.
7. Careful patient selection through preoperative analysis can improve the operation results greatly, thereby enhancing long-term success.
8. Objective evaluation methods should be applied when available, to improve patient selection, surgical technique, and postoperative management and follow-up.

Both clinical and biomechanical evaluation results indicate that high tibial osteotomy is acceptable—perhaps the procedure of choice for certain groups of patients with degenerative unicompartmental disease. The many clinical advantages inherent in this reconstructive surgery make it appealing, even in the wake of the present enthusiasm for total knee arthroplasty. Consequently knee osteotomy should be seriously considered before a more radical operation, such as hemiarthroplasty or total knee replacement, is considered. Even if high tibial osteotomy only provides a limited number of years of pain relief and functional recovery, it is still a safe method to trade for time until some major problems in total knee arthroplasty are satisfactorily resolved. With more study and experience, knee osteotomy may even be regarded as a prophylactic procedure to eliminate knee pathologic changes caused by varus or valgus deformity. Until then careful indications based on clinical criteria should probably be followed.

ACKNOWLEDGEMENT

I wish to thank Mark B. Coventry for his many valuable suggestions and encouragement on the preparation of this chapter. Through his help and inspiration I am beginning to understand the various clinical aspects of the operative procedure. I also wish to acknowledge my former colleague and friend, Donald B. Kettelkamp, for his unfailing collaboration, which made this study possible.

References

1. Bauer, G. C., Insall, J., and Tomihisa, K.: Tibial osteotomy in gonarthrosis (osteo-arthritis of the knee), J. Bone Joint Surg. **51-A:**1545, 1969.
2. Coventry, M. B.: Personal communication, May, 1977.
3. Coventry, M. B.: Osteotomy of the upper portion of the tibia for degenerative arthritis of the knee. A preliminary report, J. Bone Joint Surg. **47-A:**984, 1965.
4. Coventry, M. B.: Osteotomy about the knee for degenerative and rheumatoid arthritis. Indications, operative technique, and results, J. Bone Joint Surg. **55-A:**23, 1973.
5. Devas, M. B.: High tibial osteotomy for arthritis of the knee. A method specially suitable for elderly, J. Bone Joint Surg. **51-B:**95, 1969.
6. Gariépy, R.: Correction du genou fléchi dans l'arthrite. In Huitième Congrès International de Chirurgie Orthopédique, New York, September 4-9, 1960. Rapports, discussions et communications particuliéres publiés par M. A. Bailleux, Secrétaire général, Burxelles, 1961, Imprimerie des Sciences.
7. Gariépy, R.: Genu varus treated by high tibial osteotomy. Paper read at the Fourth Combined Meeting of the American, British, and Canadian Orthopaedic Associations with the Orthopaedic Associations of South Africa, New Zealand, Australia, and France. Vancouver, British Columbia, Canada, June 18, 1961.
8. Györy, A. N., Chao, E. Y., and Stauffer, R. N.: Functional evaluation of normal and pathologic knees during gait, Arch. Phys. Med. Rehabil. **57:**571, 1976.
9. Harris, W. R., and Kostuik, J. P.: High tibial osteotomy for osteoarthritis of the knee, J. Bone Joint Surg. **52-A:**330, 1970.
10. Jackson, J. P., and Waugh, W.: Tibial osteotomy for osteoarthritis of the knee, J. Bone Joint Surg. **43-B:**746, 1961.
11. Kettelkamp, D. B., and Chao, E. Y.: A method for quantitative analysis of medial and lateral compression forces at the knee during standing, Clin. Orthop. **83:**202, 1972.
12. Kettelkamp, D. B., Wenger, D. R., Chao, E. Y., and Thompson, C.: Results of proximal tibial osteotomy. The effects of tibiofemoral angle, stance-phase flexion-extension, and medial-plateau force, J. Bone Joint Surg. **58-A:**962, 1976.
13. Kettelkamp, D. B., Johnson, R. J., Smidt, G. L., Chao, E. Y., and Walker, M.: An electro-goniometric study of knee motion in normal gait, J. Bone Joint Surg. **52-A:**775, 1970.
14. Maquet, P., Simonet, J., and de Marchin, P.: Biomécanique du genou et gonarthrose. In Symposium, les gonarthroses d'origine statique, Rev. Chir. Orthop. **53:**111, 1967.
15. Morrison, J. B.: The forces transmitted by the human knee joint. Thesis, University of Strathclyde, Glasgow, Scotland, 1967.
16. Steindler, A.: Kinesiology of the human body, Springfield, Ill., Charles C Thomas, Publisher, 1955, p. 331.
17. Wardle, E. N.: Osteotomy of the tibia and fibula, Surg. Gynecol. Obstet. **115:**61, 1962.
18. Wardle, E. N.: Osteotomy of the tibia and fibula in the treatment of chronic osteoarthritis of the knee, Postgrad. Med. J. **40:**536, 1964.

15. Arthrodesis of the knee

Theodore N. Siller
A. Hadjipavlou

Arthrodesis of the knee has almost always been undertaken as a last resort. At present it is even less considered, and is performed primarily for implant failure. This reliance is now beginning to be strongly questioned.

INDICATIONS

Previous reasons for arthrodesis, such as pain relief, sepsis, and instability, have been replaced by salvage, which includes failure of total knee arthroplasty and postoperative sepsis. Lack of facilities or facilities inadequate for other surgery are still factors in some parts of the world.

METHODS

Many methods have been described. They all have a basic technique of denuding articular surfaces and immobilizing the joint until fusion occurs. With time and sophistication these methods have stressed increasingly rigid immobilization. Conversely others have suggested intermittent pressure as being more conducive to fusion. The former have included the use of plating or compression such as described by Charnley.[2] The intermittent pressure can be achieved with the use of an intermedullary rod as advocated by Chapchal.[1] More recent modifications have tended to increase both size and complexity of apparatus. Others have added simpler refinements.[4]

The advantages of the compression method include technical ease, accuracy, rigidity, comfort, early ambulation, and rapid fusion. However, Key[6] abandoned his method of compression because of difficulties in obtaining fusion with poor tuberculous bone. The modern surgeon has added more apparatus, possibly as a challenge to the more complicated changes of the tissue involved. Generally fusion is more easily obtained as bone approaches normal. At best, fusion takes longer to occur than most authors have indicated.[11]

COMPLICATIONS

Complications of arthrodesis include the following:

Early complications
Local: Osteomyelitis, pressure sores, neuroma, foot drop

161

Table 15-1. Recommended positions for knee fusion

Author	Position (degrees of flexion)
Charnley[2]	0-5
Chapchal[1]	20-25
Green et al.[5]	0-30
Moore and Smillie[8]	0-30
Nelson and Evarts[9]	
Male	5-10
Female	10
Siller and Hadjipavlou[11]	15-20
Stewart and Bland[12]	10-20

General: Thrombophlebitis, pulmonary embolus, pain at donor graft site, crutch walking neuritis

Late complications
Local: Persistent knee pain, fractures
General: Back pain, hip arthritis, psychiatric problems

Complications are more common than expected. Persistent knee pain can occur in up to 36% and back pain in 44% of cases.[11] The back pain may be related to the position of the fused knee and the resultant gait. Fractures can occur more easily. The aging process with its decreased activity, resultant osteoporosis, and stiffness contributes to the increasing number of fractures with time. Neuroma rarely causes the knee pain, and it is impossible to differentiate between a learned behavior pattern from primary disease and malingering.[3]

GAIT AND POSITION OF FUSED KNEE

Fusion of· the knee in extension, even with some shortening, causes a gait with excessive pelvic rise. This results in the patient bouncing up and down more than is normal, probably increasing energy consumption and predisposing the patient to a lumbosacral strain. Fusing the knee in flexion improves the gait. This is mediated by a "gait-en-fauchant" in which the patient abducts the limb at the hip joint and swings the affected leg out sideways, forming a scythelike curve. This results in less pelvic rise and bounce. The recommended positions for knee fusions have ranged from 0° to 30° of flexion; there is no consensus as to the best position (Table 15-1).

After energy consumption studies Mazzetti[7] suggested 15° to 20° of flexion as optimal for fusion, and we agree. Flexion places the leg in a more favorable position to increase propulsive thrust at the expense of vertical thrust (Fig. 15-1). Besides improving the gait, this makes sitting easier and is cosmetically more acceptable.

GENERAL PROBLEMS

After arthrodesis activities of daily living can present difficulties that increase with time. Heavy work cannot be done, and transportation problems may restrict

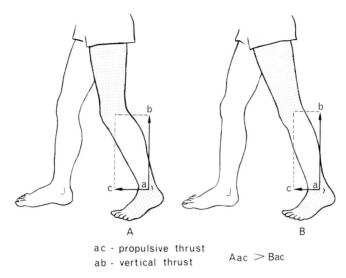

ac - propulsive thrust

ab - vertical thrust

Aac > Bac

Fig. 15-1. Forces in gait. Horizontal or propulsive thrust increases with flexion, at the expense of vertical thrust.

other types of work. Specially equipped automobiles become impractical because of expense or lack of interest. Social activities are greatly curtailed because of the preparation required for transportation and seating at public events. Even at home, simple things require increased awareness, such as rugs, ladders, and stairs. Simple dressing may be hindered, such as when trouser legs cannot be reached without some form of instrument for assistance.

FAILED ARTHRODESIS

In the implant era there is some promise that, in a young person, arthrodesis can be osteotomized and an implant inserted to allow motion. Even with weak or little quadriceps muscle activity, function can be quite adequate with passive extension.[10] In the event of further failure of such an implant, repeated arthrodesis may not be feasible.

SALVAGE OF IMPLANT SURGERY

The premise that a failed total arthroplasty is easily treated by arthrodesis is wrong. The marked changes in the tissues minimize osteoblastic potential. Sepsis may provide an adequate fibrous ankylosis if drainage subsides, but this cannot be counted on. If large amounts of bone are removed, as for a stem-type implant, the problem is greatly magnified. A not untypical case illustration follows.

On October 19, 1971, a Shiers type of prosthesis was inserted in a 60-year-old woman who had had a total hip procedure on the same side and a lipectomy in the same year. After immobilization for 10 days in a posterior slab, she was al-

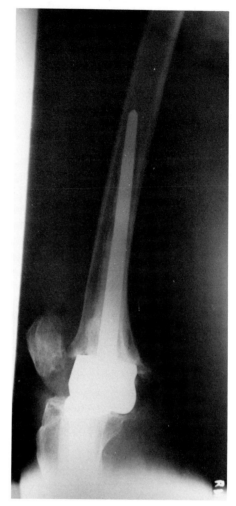

Fig. 15-2. Radiograph taken 4 years after Shiers-type total knee replacement in 64-year-old woman.

lowed movement; she was discharged to a convalescent hospital several weeks later. The patient was without complaint until the onset of pain in the right knee on September 8, 1975, after a twisting injury (Fig. 15-2). Because of the persistence and severity of the pain, an arthrotomy was done, and a grossly infected prosthesis was removed on October 6, 1975. Closed suction irrigation was instituted at the same time; 2½ weeks later débridement and packing were done. The patient attempted walking on crutches with little activity, but drainage continued. In April, 1976, a weight-bearing caliper was tried, but the patient was unable to tolerate it. On April 23, 1976, a compression type of fusion was attempted with a contemporary external compression apparatus (Figs. 15-3 to 15-5). A skin

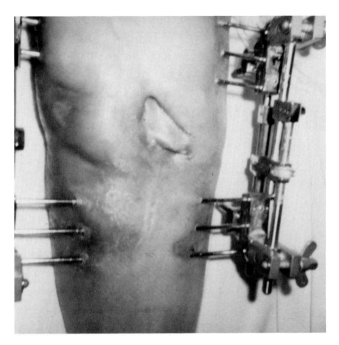

Fig. 15-3. Appearance of knee in Fig. 15-2, 6 months later. After compression type of fusion, drainage is present.

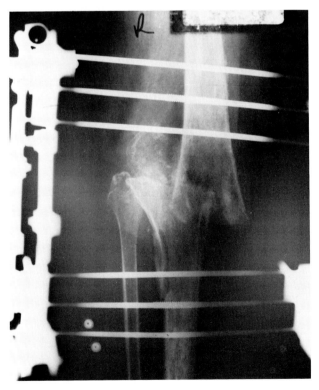

Fig. 15-4. Radiograph of knee shown in Fig. 15-3.

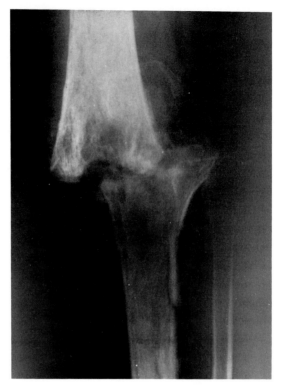

Fig. 15-5. Radiograph of same knee after attempted fusion. Drainage persists.

graft was applied at the same time by a plastic surgeon. On July 8, 1976, after no signs of healing and deterioration of position, the decision was made to amputate. A drug-induced hemolytic anemia postponed this until September 3, 1976, when an above-knee amputation was performed. The second stage was completed several weeks later. Even with adequate healing, it is doubtful that this patient will be active enough after such a long period of illness to efficiently use a prosthesis.

PRESENT STATUS OF FUSION

What is the status of fusion today? It has been unpopular throughout history, but it may increase in popularity, even if not in efficiency. The problem now is that a new type of fusion is required, not new apparatus. Early attempts at fusion using suction drainage for infection have been done with some success. Because of lack of normal tissue, some simple extra-articular type of fusion would be helpful for future use. Improved implants requiring even less removal of bone will be required. More important, rigid indications for implant surgery have to be followed in the present state of our knowledge. Fusion as a treatment for the knee may again have a place in orthopaedic surgery.

SUMMARY

1. Arthrodesis of the knee is still rarely required.
2. The compression method is the best, the most widely used, and the most widely modified.
3. Problems are many—physical, social, and economic.
4. In selected cases of failed fusion, a total knee arthroplasty can be considered.
5. Arthrodesis cannot always be relied on to salvage failed implant surgery. The "last resort" may have been passed.

References

1. Chapchal, G.: Intramedullary pinning for arthrodesis of knee joint, J. Bone Joint Surg. **30-A**:728, 1948.
2. Charnley, J. C.: Positive pressure in arthrodesis of knee joint, J. Bone Joint Surg. **30-B:** 478, 1948.
3. Clawson, D. K., Bonica, J. J., and Fordyce, W. B.: Management of chronic orthopaedic pain problems. In American Academy of Orthopaedic Surgeons: Instructional course lectures, vol. 21, St. Louis, 1972, The C. V. Mosby Co.
4. Cloutier, J. M., and Fortin, R.: Arthrodèse du genou avec un long clou de Kuntscher, Union Med. Can. **101**:1842, 1972.
5. Green, D. P., Parkes, J. C., and Stinchfield, F. E.: Arthrodesis of knee, follow-up study, J. Bone Joint Surg. **49-A**:1065, 1967.
6. Key, J. A.: Positive pressure in arthrodesis for tuberculosis of knee joint, South Med. J. **25**:909, 1932.
7. Mazzetti, R. F.: Effect of immobilization of knee on energy expenditure during walking. In Proceedings of Western Orthopaedic Association, J. Bone Joint Surg. **42-A**:533, 1960.
8. Moore, F. H., and Smillie, I. S.: Arthrodesis of knee joint, Clin. Orthop. **13**:215, 1959.
9. Nelson, C. L., and Evarts, C. M.: Arthroplasty and arthrodesis of knee joint, Orthop. Clin. North Am. **2**:245, 1971.
10. Siller, T. N.: Arthrodesis in the treatment of degenerative arthritis of the knee. In Surgical management of degenerative arthritis of the lower limb, Philadelphia, 1975, Lea & Febiger.
11. Siller, T. N., and Hadjipavlou, A.: Knee arthrodesis: long term results, Can. J. Surg. **19**:217, 1976.
12. Stewart, M. J., and Bland, W. G.: Compression in arthrodesis: comparative study of methods of fusion of knee in ninety-three cases, J. Bone Joint Surg. **40-A**:585, 1958.

PART FIVE

Ligamentous reconstruction of the knee

16. Classification and diagnosis of knee instabilities

Kenneth E. DeHaven

Chronic ligamentous instability of the knee continues to present a formidable challenge to the orthopaedist. The first step to successful management of these problems is the accurate assessment of the type or types of instability. Although considerable confusion and controversy continue to exist in regard to some aspects of ligamentous instability, certain features of classification and diagnosis are emerging as general principles that form the basis for agreement in understanding the nature, if not the underlying causes, of instability. The various instabilities are named according to the movement of the tibia in relation to the femur. Simple instability refers to abnormal motion in one plane, either on the horizontal or vertical axis, and complex instability involves abnormal motion in two or more axes.

Knee instability can be classified into four basic categories—straight instabilities, rotatory instabilities, patellar instabilities, and combined instabilities:

Straight
   1. Medial
   2. Lateral
   3. Anterior
   4. Posterior

Rotatory
   1. Anteromedial
   2. Posteromedial
   3. Anterolateral
   4. Posterolateral

Patellar

Combined

STRAIGHT INSTABILITIES
Medial

Straight medial instability is defined as widening of the medial joint space with the application of valgus stress (Fig. 16-1). This is diagnosed clinically by

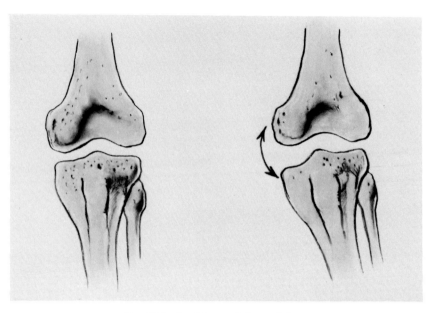

Fig. 16-1. Straight medial instability.

applying valgus stress to the knee first in full extension and then with the knee in 20° to 30° flexion. The degree of medial joint space widening can be quantitated and documented on stress x-ray films.[2]

Lateral

Straight lateral instability is defined as widening of the lateral joint space with the application of varus stress (Fig. 16-2). The clinical diagnosis is made by applying varus stress with the knee in full extension and then repeating the test with the knee flexed 20° to 30°. Stress x-ray films can also be useful in quantitating and documenting the amount of straight lateral laxity.

Anterior

Straight anterior instability is defined as the tibia moving anteriorly in relation to the femur with no differential excursion between the medial and lateral tibial condyles (Fig. 16-3). The clinical diagnosis is made by performing the classic anterior drawer test with the tibia in neutral rotation and observing anterior displacement of the tibia. The degree of anterior displacement can be documented by stress x-ray films obtained in the lateral projection.[2]

Posterior

Straight posterior instability is defined as the tibia moving posteriorly in relation to the femur with no differential excursion between the medial and lateral

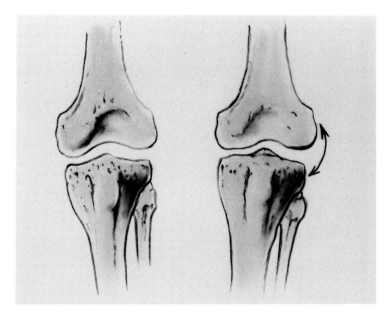

Fig. 16-2. Straight lateral instability.

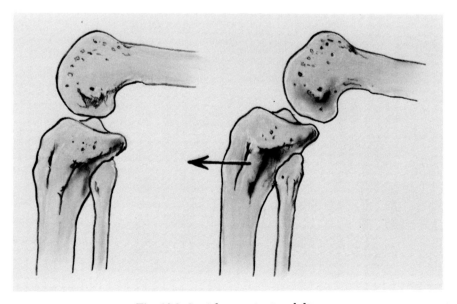

Fig. 16-3. Straight anterior instability.

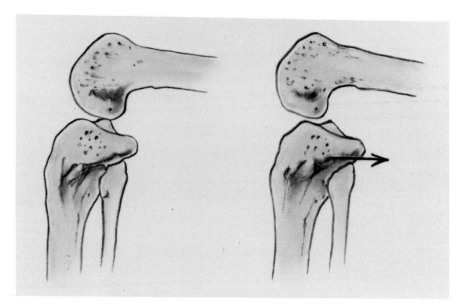

Fig. 16-4. Straight posterior instability.

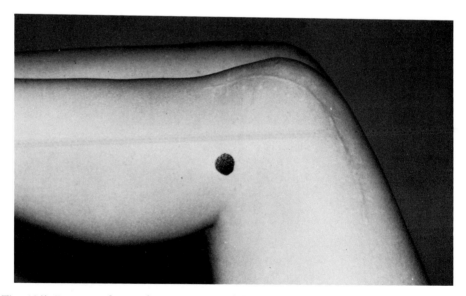

Fig. 16-5. Patient with straight posterior instability demonstrating posterior sag of proximal tibia on affected side when relaxed legs are supported with hips and knees flexed 90°.

tibial condyles (Fig. 16-4). Straight posterior instability is diagnosed clinically by performing the classic posterior drawer test and observing posterior displacement of the tibia. Straight posterior instability is frequently misinterpreted as being straight anterior instability, as the tibia sags posteriorly before the drawer test is performed, and displacement back to its normal neutral position gives the impression of anterior instability. The situation can usually be clarified by supporting the relaxed legs by the heels with the hips and knees flexed 90°. In the presence of straight posterior instability, a posterior sag of the proximal tibia can be observed in the involved leg (Fig. 16-5).

ROTATORY INSTABILITIES
Anteromedial

Anteromedial rotatory instability is defined as abnormal tibial rotation that causes the medial tibial plateau to displace anteriorly in relation to the femur. This is associated with a shift of the vertical axis of rotation anteriorly and laterally (Fig. 16-6). Anteromedial rotatory instability is diagnosed clinically by observing that the medial tibial plateau has a greater anterior excursion than the lateral when the anterior drawer test is performed in neutral rotation and noting enhancement of the anterior drawer sign when it is performed with the tibia externally rotated as described by Slocum and Larson.[7]

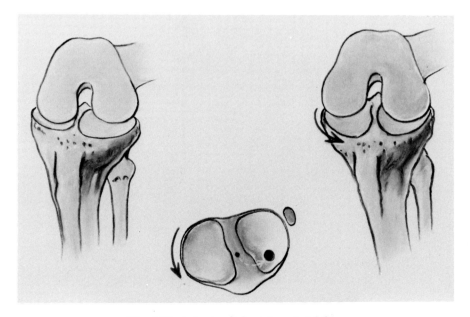

Fig. 16-6. Anteromedial rotatory instability.

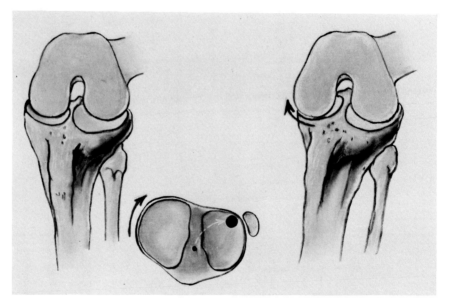

Fig. 16-7. Posteromedial rotatory instability.

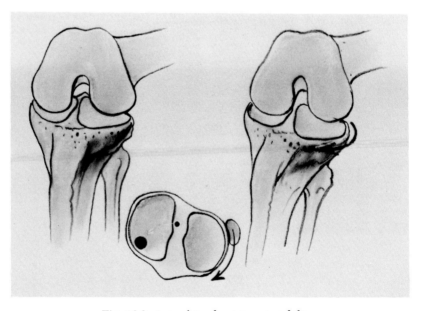

Fig. 16-8. Anterolateral rotatory instability.

Posteromedial

Posteromedial rotatory instability is defined as abnormal rotation of the tibia permitting posterior displacement of the medial tibial plateau in relation to the femur; it is associated with a posterior and lateral shift of the vertical axis of rotation (Fig. 16-7). This uncommon instability can be diagnosed by observing posterior displacement of the medial tibial condyle when the knee is placed in a position of relaxed hyperextension and by noting the medial tibial condyle to be displaced posteriorly to a greater degree than the lateral tibial condyle in the posterior drawer test.

Anterolateral

Anterolateral rotatory instability is defined as abnormal tibial rotation with the lateral tibial plateau moving anteriorly in relation to the femur with a concomitant shift in the vertical axis of rotation anteriorly and medially (Fig. 16-8). There are two types of anterolateral rotatory instability; one is diagnosed by performing the anterior drawer test with the tibia internally rotated and assessing the anterior excursion of the tibia as described by Slocum and Larson.[7]

The other, more common type of anterolateral rotatory instability is diagnosed clinically with the knee nearer to full extension; it is described as the "lateral pivot shift" by MacIntosh[3] and as the "jerk sign" by Hughston et al.[1] Slocum and Larson have also described a method of demonstrating this type of anterolateral rotatory instability.[7]

The common features of all of these tests are the application of internal rotation and valgus stress to the totally relaxed knee as it nears full extension and the production of an anterior subluxation of the lateral tibia plateau, which then reduces as the knee is flexed.

Posterolateral

Posterolateral rotatory instability is defined as abnormal tibial rotation that results in posterior displacement of the lateral tibial plateau in relation to the femur, and it is associated with a concomitant shift of the vertical axis of rotation medially and posteriorly (Fig. 16-9). Posterolateral rotatory instability is diagnosed clinically by the presence of an abnormal hyperextension external rotation sign and positive posterolateral drawer sign as described by Hughston et al.[1] The involved knee sags into a position of increased hyperextension and slight varus, and the lateral tibial plateau is noted to rotate posteriorly in relation to the femur.

The posterolateral drawer sign refers to the seemingly positive posterior drawer sign in these patients, which in reality is posterior rotation of the lateral tibial plateau when the posterior drawer sign is performed with the tibia in neutral rotation. The posterior displacement is increased when the posterior drawer sign is repeated with the tibia externally rotated.

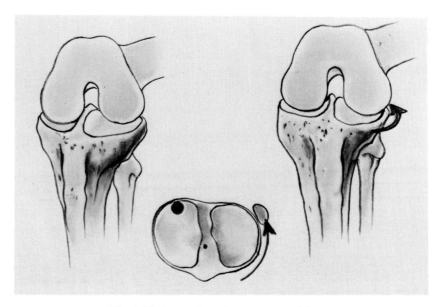

Fig. 16-9. Posterolateral rotatory instability.

PATELLAR INSTABILITY

Patellar instability is almost always lateral, but on occasion it may be medial or both medial and lateral. The diagnosis of lateral instability of the patella is based on the observation of valgus alignment of the extensor mechanism (increased quadriceps angle), excessive lateral mobility of the patella, pain or apprehension with lateral displacement of the patella, facet tenderness, and pain with dynamic patellofemoral compression. In addition there are x-ray abnormalities suggesting lateral patellar instability; these include patella alta and laterally placed patella seen on standard lateral and anteroposterior projections and several abnormalities that can be seen on the Hughston patella view, including hypoplastic patella, shallow patellar groove of the femur (increased sulcus angle), low-lying lateral femoral condyle, and lateral tilting of the patella.

COMBINED INSTABILITIES

Two or more of these instabilities can and commonly do exist in the same knee, forming various types of combined instability. Virtually any combination could occur, but certain combinations are more frequently encountered. These are medial-anteromedial rotatory, medial-anteromedial-anterolateral rotatory, anterior-anteromedial-anterolateral rotatory, anterolateral-posterolateral rotatory, and lateral-anterolateral rotatory instabilities.

SUMMARY

A general scheme of classification and diagnosis of ligamentous instability of the knee has been presented. Certain basic principles are applicable in approaching the evaluation of an unstable knee. Each knee should be examined for all types of instability. Each component of the instability should be assessed separately before sequential integration of the various component parts and analysis of the knee as a whole. Accurate analysis of ligamentous instability is the essential first step toward effective ligamentous reconstruction of the knee. One must first determine the type or types of instability present, correct coexisting internal derangements, and then select the appropriate reconstructive procedure or procedures, many of which will be discussed in the following chapters.

References

1. Hughston, J. C., Andrews, J. R., Cross, M. J., and Moschi, A.: Classification of knee ligament instabilities. Part I, the medial compartment and cruciate ligaments. Part II, the lateral compartment, J. Bone Joint Surg. **58-A:**159, 1976.
2. Kennedy, J. C., and Fowler, P. J.: Medial and anterior instability of the knee. An anatomic and clinical study using stress machines, J. Bone Joint Surg. **53-A:**1257, 1971.
3. MacIntosh, D. L.: The lateral pivot-shift, Paper presented at American Academy of Orthopaedic Surgeons postgraduate course on reconstructive surgery of the knee, Cleveland, Ohio, 1974.
4. Nicholas, J. A.: The five-one reconstruction for anteromedial instability of the knee, J. Bone Joint Surg. **55-A:**941, 1973.
5. O'Donoghue, D. H.: Reconstruction for medial instability of the knee, J. Bone Joint Surg. **55-A:**941, 1973.
6. Slocum, D. B.: A test for anterolateral rotatory instability, Paper presented at American Academy of Orthopaedic Surgeons postgraduate course on reconstructive surgery of the knee, Cleveland, Ohio, 1974.
7. Slocum, D. B., and Larson, R. L.: Rotatory instability of the knee. Its pathogenesis and a clinical test to demonstrate its presence, J. Bone Joint Surg. **50-A:**211, 1968.

17. Medial instability of the knee

H. Royer Collins

Chronic knee instability is a difficult problem for both the patient and the orthopaedic surgeon who must correct the disability. This is particularly true when the patient is an athlete who must be able to change directions suddenly and whose performance depends on an almost perfect result from surgery. To achieve the best possible result, the surgeon must first make the correct diagnosis and be aware of the type or types of instability that exist. Many classifications have been proposed, and Hughston et al.[5] have attempted to correlate the pathologic lesions and deficiencies with the subsequent type of instability. This chapter deals only with instabilities involving the medial side of the knee.

If the surgeon were present each time an injury occurred, could see the mechanism of injury and the direction and severity of forces, and could examine the patient immediately, repair would probably be undertaken immediately and subsequent chronic instability would not exist. Most commonly, however, the patient is seen some time after the injury has occurred. The cause of injury may vary from a simple cutting maneuver, at which time the athlete felt or heard a pop with subsequent giving way, to severe trauma with a force from the lateral side with or without rotation. Often the patient is unable to tell just what happened. He is aware, however, of giving way and instability of the knee. Physical examination may reveal opening with valgus stress of varying degrees. If the knee opens when it is in full extension, the surgeon must assume that fairly extensive damage has been done to the capsular structures and that either or both of the cruciate ligaments may be involved. If the knee does not open in full extension but does so when the knee is flexed 20° to 30°, the damage may not be as extensive, but there is still laxity of the medial structures and there may be associated anterior cruciate ligament damage. There may be associated instability in a rotatory plane as described by Slocum and Larson,[9] and the surgeon must examine carefully for this. Other associated instabilities must be examined for.

Once the disability has been classified, the surgeon must decide how best to treat the problem. Such factors as the age of the patient, the amount of disability, pain, effusion, degenerative change, and the general condition of the

180

patient are all important in determining if surgical intervention is indicated. The strength of the involved extremity must also be assessed; if it is found to be inadequate, an extensive rehabilitation program should be initiated first. If this does not improve the stability of the knee and if the disability is sufficient, then surgery is indicated.

ANATOMY

Stability on the medial side of the joint depends on the medial ligaments, the medial meniscus, the anterior and posterior cruciate ligaments, as well as the musculature that crosses the joint. Slocum and Larson[9] described three portions of the medial capsule, which they called the medial capsular ligament. The anterior portion consists of the anterior capsule and the vastus medialis retinaculum. The middle portion is the deep layer of the medial collateral ligament, and the posterior portion is the posterior capsule. The capsular ligament is reinforced by the tibial collateral ligament, which is often referred to as the superficial portion of the medial collateral ligament. The anterior fibers of this structure move posteriorly with flexion, causing the anteromedial aspect of the joint to be weakest at that time. The oblique fibers of the tibial collateral ligament give support to the posteromedial aspect of the femoral condyle and the tibia, and this is reinforced by the semimembranosus. Hughston and Eilers[2-4] have stressed the importance of this posteromedial corner of the joint in achieving stability.

SURGICAL PROCEDURES

Various surgical techniques have been used in the past to stabilize the knee with varying degrees of success. Mauck advised distal displacement of the tibial

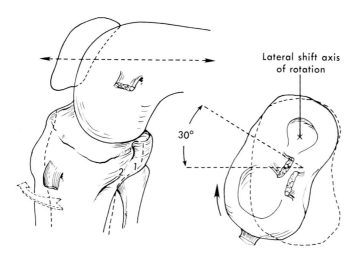

Fig. 17-1. Excursion of medial tibia in anteromedial rotatory instability. (From Slocum, D. B., and Larson, R. L.: J. Bone Joint Surg. **50-A:**211, 1968.)

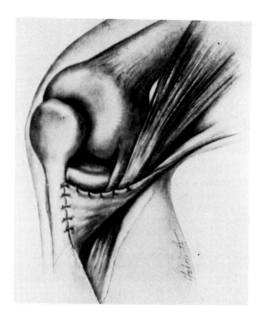

Fig. 17-2. Completed pes anserinus transfer. (From Slocum, D. B., and Larson, R. L.: J. Bone Joint Surg. **50-A**:226, 1968.)

Fig. 17-3. O'Donoghue advancement of medial capsular ligament, illustrating sutures in medial capsular ligament, which is being advanced. (From O'Donoghue, D. H.: J. Bone Joint Surg. **55-A**:941, 1973.)

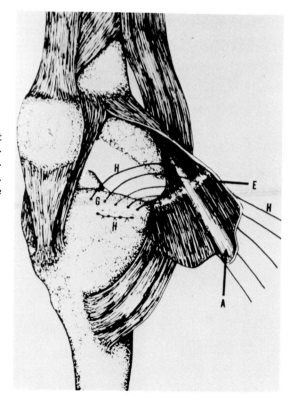

attachment of the medial collateral ligament, and some have reversed this procedure.[1] Sage overlapped the transversely cut medial collateral ligament.[1] Blair used strips of fascia lata crossed extra-articularly to support the posteromedial side of the joint.[1] Hey-Groves in 1917 advised the use of fascia lata to reconstruct the medial collateral ligament and the anterior cruciate ligament.[1] McMurray used the semitendinosus to replace the medial collateral ligament, and Helfet modified his procedure to allow this tendon to run in a groove in the medial side of the femur and support this side of the joint.[1] Along with these techniques, synthetic materials have also been used. The large number of procedures attests to the fact that none of these procedures was universally successful and most were just attempts to replace or reinforce the medial collateral ligament while ignoring the remaining structures of the joint.

Since the introduction of the dynamic concept of rotatory instability by Slo-

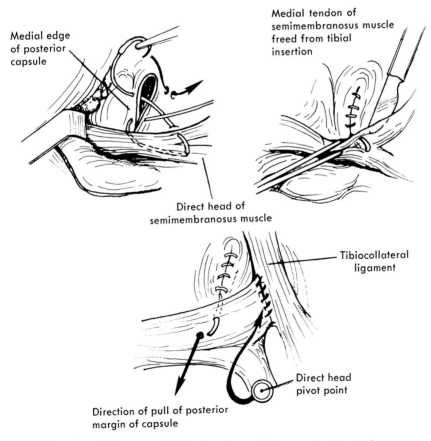

Fig. 17-4. Slocum and Larson method of posteromedial reconstruction tightening posterior capsule and backing up with semimembranosus. (From Slocum, D. B., Larson, R. L., and James, S. L.: Clin. Orthop. No. 100, p. 23, May 1974.)

cum and Larson[9,10] (Fig. 17-1) and the need for muscular reinforcement of static repairs, most orthopaedists have attempted to back up their repairs with some type of dynamic stabilization such as the pes transfer.

New procedures

Pes anserinus transfer as described by Slocum and Larson[10] for anteromedial instability with little or no medial laxity has proved a satisfactory solution to this problem (Fig. 17-2). It is important, however, to adhere to the techniques and indications advocated by these authors. Although this procedure may improve mild medial collateral ligament laxity, because of the cowl effect, it must be combined with other procedures in cases in which there is a marked amount of medial laxity.

At the present time there are several procedures that are popular for repair of medial instabilities. O'Donoghue[8] has advocated distal advancement of the entire medial capsular ligament (Fig. 17-3), starting from the anterior tibia and extending all the way around the joint to the midportion of the tibia posteriorly. This capsular sleeve is then fixed into bone with sutures passed through drill holes, and the repair is dynamically supported by a pes transfer.

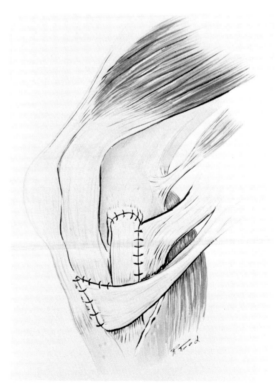

Fig. 17-5. Nicholas five-one procedure showing advancement of medial collateral ligament, semimembranosus and pes transfer.

Slocum et al.[11] have advocated a procedure in which the posteromedial corner of the joint is imbricated using fascia lata, the capsule is advanced, and the repair is reinforced by the semimembranosus and pes anserine transfer to give further dynamic stabilization (Fig. 17-4).

Nicholas[7] has described his five-in-one operation, which includes removal of the medial meniscus, advancement of the medial collateral ligament, distal advancement of the vastus medialis obliquus, and pes transfer. I have attempted to leave the meniscus intact if it is not damaged and to advance the medial collateral ligament either proximally or distally depending on where the laxity exists (Fig. 17-5). The medial meniscus helps to give stability, and the posterior capsule can usually be mobilized well by freeing all areolar tissue around the posteromedial corner of the joint without removing the meniscus. It is obvious that if the meniscus is damaged or stability cannot be achieved with the meniscus in place, it should be removed.

POSTOPERATIVE CARE

Postoperatively the patient is treated in a plaster cast with the knee in 45° flexion. A silesian belt around the waist helps take some of the weight of the cast off the repair and has been found useful. The cast is worn for 8 weeks, during which time straight leg raising exercises and isometrics may be carried out. Once the cast is removed, an intensive progressive resistance exercise program is undertaken to regain strength in the quadriceps, hamstrings, hip flexors, adductors,

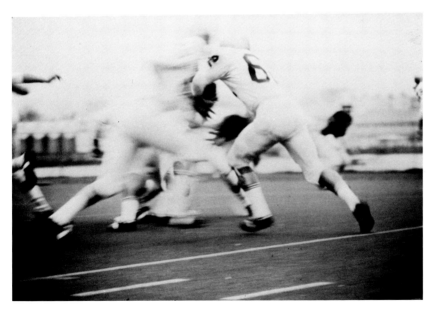

Fig. 17-6. Lenox Hill brace in use.

and abductors, as well as the gastrocnemius. To prevent stretching of the repair, a Lenox Hill brace is worn at all times until muscular strength is equal to that of the opposite leg. It is thought that the collagen tissue in areas of repair does not attain its previous strength for at least 6 months, so I usually do not allow the athlete back to competition for 1 year after surgery and then strongly advise that additional support with the Lenox Hill brace be used for contact sports (Fig. 17-6).

SUMMARY

The surgeon dealing with problems of medial side instability should be familiar with all of the repairs used, as he may find it necessary to use any one of them or combinations of these procedures in a given case. The basic principles in all of these procedures must be followed. Attention must be paid to the posteromedial corner of the joint. There must be good tissue that is tightened and fixed firmly to bone. Repairs should be backed up by dynamic transfers to prevent stretching out of the repair. There should be an adequate length of immobilization. Postoperative rehabilitation should be extensive, and the repairs should be protected for an adequate period of time by an external appliance such as a Lenox Hill brace until there has been complete maturation of the scar tissue and repair.

References

1. Collins, H. R.: Reconstruction of the athlete's injured knee: anatomy, diagnosis, treatment, Orthop. Clin. North Am. 2:207-230, March 1971.
2. Hughston, J. C.: A surgical approach to medial and posterior ligaments of the knee, Clin. Orthop. 91:29, 1973.
3. Hughston, J. C., and Eilers, A. F.: The role of the posterior oblique ligament in repairs of acute knee ligament tears, J. Bone Joint Surg. 53-A:1018, 1971.
4. Hughston, J. C. and Eilers, A. F.: The role of the posterior oblique ligament in repairs of acute medial collateral ligament tears of the knee, J. Bone Joint Surg. 55-A:923, 1973.
5. Hughston, J. C., Andrews, J., Cross, M., and Moschi, A.: Classification of knee ligament instabilities. Part 1. The medial compartment and cruciate ligaments, J. Bone Joint Surg. 58-A:159, 1976.
6. Larson, R. L.: Dislocations and ligamentous injuries of the knee. In Rockwood, C. A., Jr., and Green, D. P., editors: Fractures, vol. 2, Philadelphia, 1975, J. B. Lippincott Co.
7. Nicholas, J. A.: The five-one reconstruction for anteromedial instability of the knee: indications, technique and the results in fifty-two patients, J. Bone Joint Surg. 55-A:899, 1973.
8. O'Donoghue, D. H.: Reconstruction for medial instability of the knee: techniques and results in sixty cases, J. Bone Joint Surg. 55-A:941, 1973.
9. Slocum, D. B., and Larson, R. L.: Rotatory instability of the knee, J. Bone Joint Surg. 50-A:211, 1968.
10. Slocum, D. B., and Larson, R. L.: Pes transfer, J. Bone Joint Surg. 50-A:226, 1968.
11. Slocum, D. B., Larson, R. L., and James, S. L.: Reconstruction of ligamentous injuries of the medial compartment of the knee, Clin. Orthop. No. 100, p. 23, May 1974.

18. Acute and chronic lateral instabilities of the knee: diagnosis, characteristics, and treatment

James A. Nicholas

Although anteromedial and medial instability have been known, studied, and discussed now for three decades, lateral instability has been popularly diagnosed only in the past 5 to 10 years.[3,4,6,10] The role of the meniscus-cruciate complex in instability was described five decades ago[3] (Fig. 18-1), but its frequency has not been appreciated until recently. As anteromedial reconstruction became popular, it became evident that a number of knees were not made stable by this type of repair. Some of these cases were examples of undiagnosed lateral instability. A large number of observers including MacIntosh,[10] Kennedy,[8] Ellison,[2] and others[7,11,12,14,15] have identified the multiple components of lateral instability.

The failure to recognize the importance of lateral rotatory instability for more than three decades has been most intriguing. What happened in all those years to patients who had it unbeknownst to their doctors? How were they treated? How did they manage? These patients were diagnosed as having "trick knees" and were forced to give up active sports participation. Now with our ever-increasing leisure time and the successful return to active top-level performance of certain athletes, this method of treatment has become unacceptable to the knowledgeable public.

TYPES OF INSTABILITY

In acute lateral instability there is varus instability. It can be associated with peroneal nerve neuropraxia, biceps tendon rupture, lateral collateral ligament laxity, and fractures of the tip of the fibular styloid. There is usually lateral meniscus pathology.

Lateral instability that develops from a chronic bowleg is usually caused by gradual relaxation of the lateral capsular structures, particularly the lateral ligament, which permits subluxation of the tibia to develop. Medial compartment arthritis is present early, and lateral arthritis occurs later. Instability in the lateral

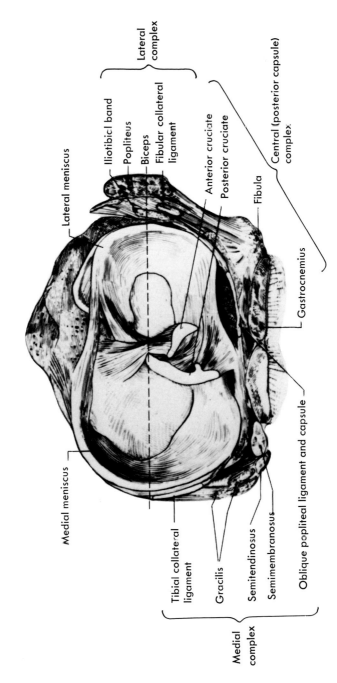

Fig. 18-1. Horizontal and vertical axes of tibia in relation to femur are used to denote rotatory instability of tibia. Note three anatomic complexes (lateral, central, and medial), which control interior and medial-lateral corners of knee, by which muscles, tendons, and ligaments harmoniously act to control rotational stability.

Table 18-1. Comparison of lateral instabilities

	Anterolateral	Posterolateral	Combined (anteromedial-anterolateral)
Mechanism	Internal rotation, flexion, and extension	External rotation and hyperextension	All
Tibiofemoral subluxation	Anterolateral	Posterolateral	Both sides of tibia forward
Internal rotation	↑	0	↑
External rotation	0	↑	↑
Characteristic signs			
Pivot shift	+	0	+
Recurvatum	0	+	0
External rotation	0	+	+
Valgus stress	Trace	0	+
Dropback	0	+	0
Anterior draw sign	+	0	+
Posterior draw sign	0	Trace	0
Sites of pathology			
Capsule supportive area	Mid third	Posterior third	Posterior third (medial and lateral)
Iliotibial band	+	+	+
Popliteus	0	+	0
Lateral ligament	0	+	0
Arcuate-gastrocnemius system	0	+	0
Patella	+	0	+
Torn meniscus	+	±	± (medial and lateral)
Surgical repair			
Site aim	Iliotibial band to posterior capsule (mid third)	Posterior capsule to iliotibial band	Bilateral (mid and posterior third of capsule)
Pes anserinus	0	+	+
Medial complex	0	±	+
Fascial repair	0	+ (Occ.)	± ?
Biceps plasty	+ ?	0	± ?
Iliotibial band	+	0	+
Posterior capsule	±	+	±
Anterior cruciate	?	0 (Posterior cruciate?)	?

±, Rarely; Occ., occasionally.

side can be classified into three types: (1) anterolateral, (2) posterolateral, and (3) combined (Table 18-1).

Lateral instability may be associated with developmental laxity, such as is seen in congenital recurvatum or epiphyseal dysplasia, or with malaligned hip, knee, or ankle rotational axes, or it may be acquired from trauma. Whenever the instability is in only one plane, and this is unusual, it is called *simple* instability.[12] It is not bothersome and the patient may not even notice it, but it can be seen in the stance phase of gait, particularly in midsupport, when the patient begins to push off and there occurs a small lateral thrust in the posterolateral corner of the knee. Many ballet dancers acquire this thrust.[9] However, the most common types of instability are the acquired types, caused by accidents such as automobile or motor bike accidents or athletic injuries such as in skiing or basketball.

There are two common traumatic causes for lateral rotatory instability. One is a varus thrust of the leg when there is force driving the tibia backward and in external rotation, in which case there is posterolateral disruption. If the knee is flexed and a force drives the tibia forward while internally rotating it, an anterior cruciate tear is produced and results in anterolateral instability.

ANTEROLATERAL INSTABILITY
Characteristics

Anterolateral instability is produced in three ways: (1) with the tibia internally rotated, (2) with the femur externally rotated, and (3) with the femur externally rotated and the tibia flexed or extended (Fig. 18-2). The internal rotation is such that the vertical axis of rotation passes toward the medial side. At the same time the anterior cruciate ligament is disrupted, or it may be inadequate from previous trauma. At arthrotomy or arthroscopy the anterior cruciate ligament may appear to be intact and have substance. In this instance the integrity of its function has been impaired, which produces anterior instability. Loss of function in this vital structure results in altered contact areas and altered load transmission on maneuvers such as running and jumping. As a result of this, both static and dynamic stabilizers of the lateral compartment are stretched in early cases by repeated injury. The result may be a tear of the lateral meniscus or loosening of the posterolateral capsule. The gastrocnemius, which influences the posterior capsule, and the popliteus and biceps muscles are impaired by such gradual stretching and weakening. At the same time the normally tight (especially in flexion with internal rotation) lateral collateral ligament may stretch. The result is that the capsule between the posterolateral complex and the iliotibial band is impaired. A true laxity has developed. We have sought to document a mid-third lateral capsule injury but have not found any true isolated lateral capsular tears.

Patients operated on for acute anterolateral instability are characterized by rather significant ruptures that are diagnosable. But most patients are seen later, when the anterolateral compartment of the tibia subluxes forward and internally

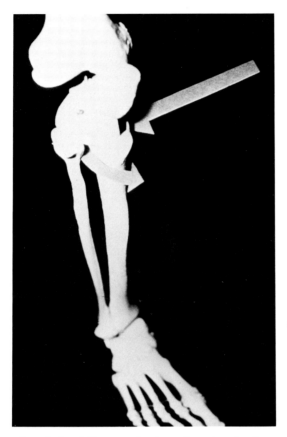

Fig. 18-2. In anterolateral instability, mechanism of action is characterized by internal rotation of tibia with medial or posteromedial force directed to tear anterior cruciate ligament and stress lateral capsular ligaments. Posterior half of lateral meniscus tears, but posterolateral corner (lateral complex) remains intact.

rotates, with the tibial tubercle moving medially, and with little varus deformity. In anterolateral instability, internal tibia rotation is increased and external rotation is not (Fig. 18-2). The clinical diagnosis is often aided by a history of a buckling of the knee, particularly on jumping with the leg internally rotated in slight varus alignment. Snowplowing in skiing is a common way in which this is produced. Note, however, that it is easy for the patient to confuse this with the external rotation (valgus) type of mechanism, which has been associated with anteromedial laxity.

Pivot shift. In time a characteristic phenomenon develops and has been noted by a number of investigators.[2,3] A "pivot shift," as described by Gallway,[4] is pathognomonic of anterolateral rotatory instability. By the time this develops, the lateral meniscus has probably been torn or the lateral femoral condyle has become eroded as a result of anterior cruciate insufficiency. In addition, there is increased tibial internal rotation that is not checked by the dynamic structures of the posterolateral capsular component and the damaged posterolateral meniscal region. Slocum describes anterolateral rotary instability as the ALRI sign and describes a different method of eliciting the shift than the way described by MacIntosh. Essentially the pivot shift is a jerklike (Fig. 18-3, A) phenomenon characterized by a sudden clicking subluxation of the tibia forward on the femur while the tibia is abducted, internally rotated, and moved from flexion to extension.

The reader should be cautioned to recognize that (a) relaxation on the part of the patient is required; (b) it is best done with the patient on his side; (c) it does not require much force; (d) in early cases it often is absent on repeated maneuvers, only to reappear again at other times; and (f) it disappears in late cases after severe arthritis develops. I think that there has to be some degree of medial vastus weakness, or slight medial laxity, for this sign to be best demonstrated. As the anterolateral laxity increases, it is easy to thrust the fibula forward, secure the tibia, hold the leg in slight abduction and internal rotation, and notice the movement back and forth of the tibia on the femur by pushing behind the fibula.

The presence of a pivot shift indicates that the anterior half of the iliotibial band has become an extensor rather than a flexor and that it can no longer hold the tibia backward. The reason for this is that the iliotibial band no longer is controlled by the dynamic posterior capsular muscles (biceps, gastrocnemius, and popliteus). The popliteus, which acts on the femur in this instance as an insertion point rather than as its origin, also depresses the femur, because of laxity that develops in the posterolateral compartment and because of the cartilage tear. Some patients with significant problems can produce their own ALRI sign. They draw the tibia forward with the quadriceps and tense the gastrocnemius, popliteus, and biceps to produce this maneuver.

A discoid meniscus can simulate the click of pivot shift, but in flexion, and a shift can occur in cases of developmental laxity without any pathology in individuals born with lateral thrust. I have seen this repeatedly.[5] The presence of a shift therefore may not require surgery. A shift is also seen in individuals who have an abnormal femorotibial axis with internal rotation of the tibia and external rotation of the femur that stretches the lateral capsule.

Other diagnostic signs. There are other findings often present with anterolateral instability (Table 18-1). When the patient seeks medical advice because of the buckle, in many instances a simple meniscectomy has already been done. Usually this operation was performed on the basis of a positive arthrogram and physical examination. The anterior drawer sign may then increase and the pivot shift reduce. Such operations done without recognition of anterolateral instability produce some improvement, but in time increased laxity and more buckling occur. Some patients never develop these findings. These patients are tightly structured or muscular and have developed mechanisms to prevent the buckle. Specifically, there is practically no recurvatum. External rotation has not increased. Physical examination reveals that there is no dropback of the tibia, since the posterior cruciate is normal and the posterior drawer test is negative. There is a positive anterior drawer test. There is usually a trace of valgus deformity, presumably caused by mild stretching of the medial collateral ligament and posteromedial complex.

Converted instability

Instability that is thought to be anteromedial instability but is actually complex can be converted to anterolateral instability by anteromedial repair with pes plasty and posterior capsule advancement. Unrecognized posterolateral compartment pathology may have occurred at the time of the original injury, caused by a cutting action. This occurs with the abducted leg externally rotated and the foot fixed; the lateral posterior meniscus is compressed and the lateral capsules are damaged. However, the symptoms on the medial side are so predominant as to lead one to do an anteromedial repair, since there is valgus deformity and an anterior drawer sign. This operation does not work if there is combined anterolateral and anteromedial instability. This has been all too common in my experience with medial reconstruction when the anterolateral instability has not been diagnosed.

Pathology

Treatment of this condition is based on an understanding of the pathology and the mechanism of injury. First, the mid-third capsular structures are loosened, and laxity there may be ascribed to an old tear that has healed. The iliotibial band is a prime stabilizer of the lateral side of the knee, but it is not usually affected until late chronic instability develops. However, it has lost its ability to flex and smoothly aid in extending the knee. Instead it shifts forward as the leg internally rotates to become a rather marked extensor. It can be seen to bow out as described by both Ellison and MacIntosh (Fig. 18-3). Second, there is lateral-facet patellar disease. Third, the lateral meniscus is almost always torn in the posterolateral compartment and, depending on the length of time and frequency of injury until the operation is done, there is a variable amount of articular damage that develops into rather large lateral condyle defect. Again the most important factor is that there is no functioning anterior cruciate ligament shown in a buckling phenomenon with the tibia *internally rotated* (an outside cut or crossover step).

Ultimately an untreated knee with anterolateral instability tends to stabilize by developing arthritic changes. These changes occur along the lateral femoral condyle and in the medial and lateral patellar facets. The end result is a reduction of tibiofemoral rotation. Some persons get along for a time by not stressing the knee. Some patients do not quit decelerating and accelerating movement in sports, such as in tennis and running up and down hills, and they experience pain and swelling.

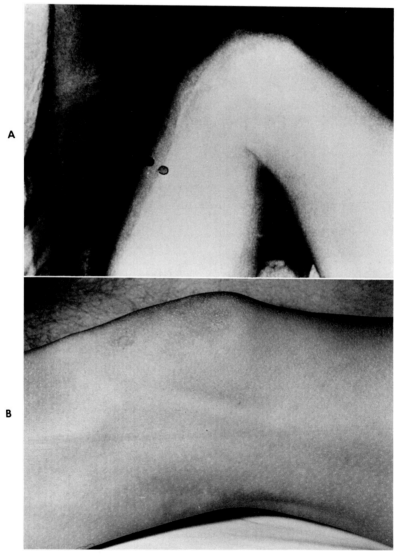

Fig. 18-3. A and **B,** Iliotibial band has altered its function and become an extensor. Pivot shift develops as result of loss of restraint by posterolateral capsule and as result of anterior instability and increased internal rotation. **C,** Incision preparing Gerdy's tubercle for turn up and attachment through lateral ligament (Ellison).

This chronic instability is a significant problem. Surgery in middle-aged athletes may lead to further surgery. These patients have an anterolateral instability that has been constrained by an almost "benevolent" arthritis.

Treatment

Treatment first requires a correct diagnosis. The initial treatment should be a power program to strengthen the abductors of the hip and the iliotibial band. The details of this rehabilitation are not the subject of this chapter, but essentially the aim is to build up the abductor mechanism and the linkage in the foot to the hip.[5] Assuming that power has been restored, as much as possible, under no circumstances should five-one reconstruction, pes anserinus transfer, or other type of medial reconstruction be done on the medial side as a treatment for anterolateral laxity. Instead, the objective of surgical intervention is to hold the tibia back as the knee extends.

When there is marked anterior displacement with the internal rotation, one has to restore the pull of the posterolateral capsular back to the iliotibial band. This can be accomplished by transfer of the iliotibial band through the lateral collateral ligament and then back on itself, as described by MacIntosh. It should be pointed out that if there is gross anterior laxity, this is not likely to improve function for an extended period. As motion is restored, the knee may loosen. The meniscus should be taken out.

A second method, the Ellison method, probably is the most common. The iliotibial tubercle is taken out. A wide flap of the iliotibial band is dissected,

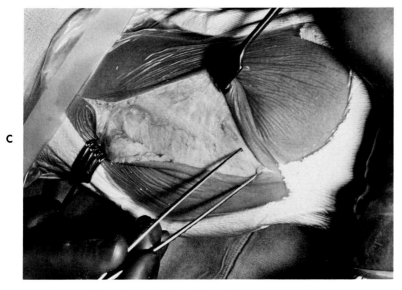

Fig. 18-3, cont'd. For legend see opposite page.

passed through the lateral collateral ligament, brought forward, and refixed to the tibia, which is displaced backwards. The flap then holds the tibia back. However, if the patient is an individual with loose joints, deterioration occurs in time. My experience is that lateral compartment pain or discomfort develops at the site where the tendons pass deep to the lateral ligament.

Patients who have a loose capsular structure may also have a flimsy lateral collateral ligament that cannot act as a pulley required in the dynamic action of the well-designed Ellison operation. In such instances, we remove the iliotibial band from Guerdy's tubercle. We look at the joint, explore it, and determine the integrity of the anterior cruciate ligament. At the same time, we advance anteriorly that portion of the posterolateral capsule anterior to the arcuate ligament, which is intact. To accomplish this, the leg is externally rotated and the iliotibial band is attached with a barbed staple just behind its previous origin on the tibia. At the same time the iliotibial band is sutured to the advanced capsule and lateral ligament, or it can be passed under and through the intercondylar notch and the bone block fixed anteriorly on the floor of the tibia with a screw.

This repair requires bracing (with a reversed Lenox Hill brace) postoperatively. The reversed derotation strap prevents internal rotation and forward displacement of the tibia and lateral laxity. Unfortunately one of the problems with these types of anterolateral instabilities is that there is usually already considerable arthritis in the lateral femoral and tibial condyles. Nevertheless, with the pivot shift removed and the leg rehabilitated over 9 to 12 months, especially if the reverse type of derotation brace (or some other appliance to limit anterior displacement of the tibia) is used with the leg in external rotation, a number of these individuals do quite well. This operation was first performed in 1967.[13] The patient remains satisfied 10 years after the operation.

As in all other types of instability, a diagnosis is extremely important, and the intent of operation is to restore the half-bucket hold of the posterior capsule on the lateral side and the medial side to the middle *horizontal capsular axis*. If the anterior cruciate ligament is still extremely lax in spite of the transfer, one has to decide whether there should be some attempt to stabilize anterior cruciate laxity.

Some patients have required further reconstruction for this problem. In these patients we lukewarmly prefer a modification of MacIntosh's patellar tendon "over the top" repair. A ¾- to 1-inch strip of medial quadriceps tendon is used. A ½-inch hole is drilled in the tibia. The tendon strip is passed through the hole, through the notch, and over the top of the posterior lateral femoral condyle. The strip is then attached to the posterolateral capsule. The patient should be warned that the functional effect of this procedure is to produce some loss of motion if it is to be satisfactory. This occurs frequently because the transarticular graft within the joint, as it is attached to the lateral intermuscular septum and lateral capsule, restrains motion.

We have not encouraged this operation except in gross anterolateral instability; we prefer to hold it as an alternative method of passing the iliotibial band, detached at Gerdy's tubercle, behind the lateral femoral condyle and through the intercondylar notch and fixing it with a screw to the anterior tibial plateau. Operative results from long-term follow-up of patients with lateral instability are few. We estimate that between 75% and 80% of our first 60 patients are satisfied with this operation and can play sports other than basketball. If they are to play tennis on a hard surface, they must have a brace.

Conservative treatment. It must also be pointed out that derotation bracing for anterolateral instability, combined with a thorough rehabilitation program, can sometimes be quite effective. Indeed, one patient is a professional football player who for 3 years has declined surgery in spite of obvious anterolateral instability diagnosed by arthroscopy, with minimal lateral meniscus pathology but with femoral articular cartilage defect and a definite pivot shift. He is remarkedly able to control this and has been able to play well without missing a game and without complaints. We do not advocate this as a method of treatment. I simply want to point out the fact that pivot shifts have been present before our recent increased sophistication, probably for generations. Patients got along with it in many instances without our knowledge of what the condition was, although Whitman unknowingly described it in his book in 1909.

Every case must be analyzed carefully before surgery is recommended. We have found the success rate for knee reconstruction to be no better than 80%, even though we are analytical and careful in selection. For this reason the indications for reconstruction are removal of the dynamic causes of painful developing pathology and provision of dynamic support for rebuilding the leg. We are pessimistic with some patients. We do not expect such patients to achieve superior athletic performance. We encourage them to divert themselves from those sports capable of causing further injury. In professional athletes, careers are in jeopardy, but we do perform the operation. There are no promises, and it is explained that stopping the knee in internal rotation with sudden deceleration, such as in running into a wall or a fence, or a sudden acceleration gain (or jump) may end a career. Nevertheless, most athletes can expect to function quite well although they may need a brace. They are also informed that arthritis will develop in time. Proper exercise programs are a must, and the patient must continue to exercise.

POSTEROLATERAL INSTABILITY
Characteristics

Posterolateral instability is less common than anterolateral instability. It too can be difficult to treat. There is little experience in the literature to draw from. Professional hockey players and football linemen have had it without sufficient impairment of function to warrant any except conservative treatment. Their careers were limited in time, however, by arthritis. Posterolateral instability usually occurs when the leg is externally rotated and a blow from the front causes it to

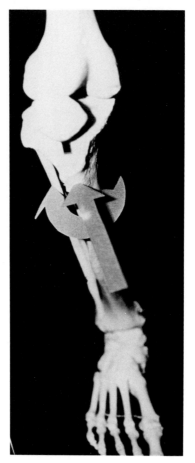

Fig. 18-4. Mechanism of posterolateral instability produces tear of posterolateral corner at arcuate-quadruple complex and allows tibia to drop back with fibula into recurvatum and external rotation.

hyperextend. Maintenance of the integrity of the medial compartment and the posterior cruciate ligament occurs at the expense of posterolateral corner disruption (Fig. 18-4). Ultimately a moderate posterior laxity develops. This is especially true when there is recurvatum. This recurvatum develops because of the injury to the posterolateral arcuate complex.

Acute posterolateral instability caused by hyperextension and external rotation is sometimes obscured by the swelling and cruciate integrity, but it can be diagnosed easily in an anesthesized or relaxed patient. Obvious tenderness, swelling, and rotational laxity of the tibia posteriorly in flexion as well as hyperextension, without tibiofibular diastasis in the posterolateral compartment, indicate its presence. Surgery performed soon after injury shows substantial hemorrhage and tearing of the lateral quadruple complex as far back as the arcuate-gastroc-

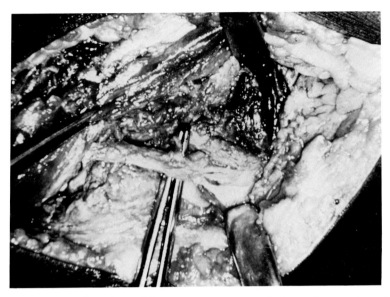

Fig. 18-5. Acute posterolateral instability. Note extensive pathology of posterolateral capsule under lateral collateral ligament. All components of posterolateral quadruple complex, arcuate ligament and lateral meniscus, and peroneal nerve have been injured.

nemius capsular attachment (Fig. 18-5). A popliteal, lateral collateral ligament, or lateral meniscal tear or a combination thereof is present and should be repaired. Early repair can produce successful results. In this sense acute posterolateral instability may be easier to diagnose than acute anterolateral laxity, which does not have such obvious pathology initially.

Chronic posterolateral instability. Chronic posterolateral instability is characterized by a tibiofemoral hyperextension and subluxation backward (Fig. 18-6). In flexion the fibular head moves back toward the popliteal space, rotating with the lateral tibial condyle posteriorly on the flexed knee at 90°, with the fulcrum of the transverse knee axis at the anteromedial corner. Since the medial compartment is stable and the anterior cruciate ligament may not be positive in the drawer test or is functionally intact, the rotation is limited to a dropback of only the lateral femoral condyle. The tibial tubercle moves laterally and backward. Recurvatum is quite obvious, especially at the posterolateral corner. Internal rotation and external rotation are increased. This has been called the hyperextension–external rotation sign. In such cases, when the relaxed extremity is held on the examiner's palm, tibial rotation backward on the femur occurs in external rotation and in hyperextension.[7]

As time progresses not only do patients have external rotation–hyperextension dropback of the tibia but also with 90° flexion they develop a 1+ posterior drawer sign and further external rotation dropback. There is no pivot shift, there is no increase in valgus stress, and there is no anterior drawer sign of any consequence,

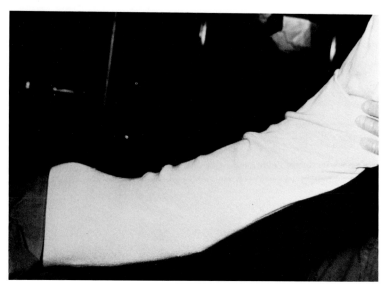

Fig. 18-6. Posterolateral instability. Note recurvatum and sag at posterolateral corner with external rotation as tibia and fibula have dropped back on femur because of loss of sling supporting function of posterior and lateral capsule.

even if an anterior cruciate tear exists (Table 18-1). Varus stress in extension can develop.

The pathology in this region runs from the posterior third of the capsular supportive area and the posterolateral complex to the lateral femoral attachments of the posterior capsule. What happens is that the iliotibial band is no longer able to keep the arcuate complex drawn forward with the attached lateral head, the gastrocnemius. This sling (or lateral half-bucket) capsular hold normally prevents tibial dropback laterally, together with the intimate bands of attachment of the popliteus and lateral collateral ligament. With posterolateral instability, dissociation of the functional attachments of these structures at the popliteal notch occurs. The capsule of the arcuate-gastrocnemius system at the posterolateral corner loosens. The result is that the sling effect is lost, producing recurvatum and increased dropback. The patella is usually not involved, and the lateral meniscus may or may not be torn. In our experience it is usually intact. Chondral fractures are rare early, but loose bodies form in time because of the dropback, and they often lodge in the pouch just in front of the popliteus muscle behind the tibia.

Left on its own to recover with a cast or no treatment, this instability in time produces lack of pushoff, and a posterior drawer sign develops. Additional injury occurs to the entire posterior capsule and menisci anteriorly. Yet several football linebackers have played without braces and functioned remarkably well over 5 or 6 years without having progressive dropback. (These individuals played at their own risk, against medical advice.) Heavy calf and quadriceps musculature and the ability to learn not to push off this leg excessively probably accounted for this survival. But it is not possible to play a charging type of position in any sport (for example, running back or shortstop) with any efficiency for very long. It is dangerous to jump and decelerate, as in rebounding in basketball; if the leg is in valgus alignment at the same time, the associated posterolateral instability can cause a dislocated knee.

Treatment

The aim of surgery is to bring the posterior capsule forward so that it can reassert its hold on the iliotibial band, which is usually intact, producing the posterolateral cowl-sling effect again. The tibia has to be rotated forward after the arcuate-gastrocnemius complex is brought forward. This may require fascial repair occasionally, if there is little arcuate ligament scar to work with, and this can be taken from the fascia lata above the leg. In these patients a large cavity noted behind the knee joint is caused by the posterolateral laxity (Fig. 18-7, A) and by the capsule and the arcuate ligament being torn off the femur (Fig. 18-7, B). The popliteus is usually scarred, as well as the lateral collateral ligament.

For this reason we take the iliotibial band together with Gerdy's tubercle off at the start of the operation to get a good view of the anterior and posterior aspects of the knee. This permits a complete assessment of the lateral and posterior capsule, all the structures of the quadruple complex, and the degree of scarring and defects. After the back of the femoral condyle and its large mass are exposed, one can see the posterior cruciate ligament. It may be stretched and can sometimes have a fragment of bone at its tibial attachment, which can be advanced down and back and refixed.

Then one has to restore the posterolateral complex by anterior advancement. The key to repair of posterolateral instability is to reestablish the connections of the pull of the iliotibial band and quadriceps muscles by reattachment of the torn posterolateral capsule behind the intact iliotibial band, to the mid transverse axis (Fig. 18-8). We usually take the popliteus off and advance it at the same time, using it as a bed for the advancement of the posterolateral corner. Just as in the five-one procedure, we use the medial ligament as a bed for advancement of the posteromedial capsule.

During the entire operation and postoperatively for 6 to 8 weeks, the tibia must be held forward and in internal rotation while the knee is held in flexion and attached to a cast with a pelvic band or some other support to control movement of the proximal femur by the pelvis. After cast removal, a flexion contracture of a few degrees is a favorable indication. Sometimes, we have done pes anserinus transfer at the same time, especially if there is some tendency of the leg to externally rotate excessively even when it is held forward.

After the cast is removed, we use a Lenox Hill brace for 6 weeks with the knee held in flexion, internal rotation, and abduction, with a lock to control these motions at first. Extralarge calf cuffs are used; flexion is held to 90° and not permitted beyond that. No weight bearing is permitted until extension is accomplished. The brace is used with a posterior support to keep the femur and tibia from dropping back. The derotation brace is used with double straps on either side and a stop at 90° for 3 months more. It takes up to a year to get a satisfactory result, and motion in flexion beyond 120° is usually not possible.

Our results have not been studied long enough to endorse this operation as

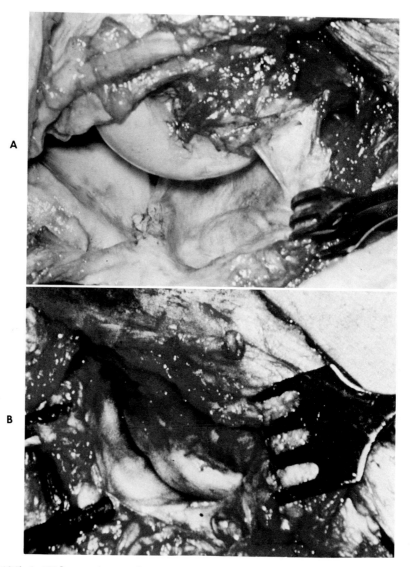

Fig. 18-7. **A,** Wide gap that can be seen in posterolateral instability due to avulsion of posterolateral corner. **B,** This has to be closed, as noted in Fig. 18-8 and in text, but it allows thorough scan for loose bodies, posterior cruciate stability, and popliteus muscle integrity and to plan closure.

a routine procedure. We have some good results in some tightly muscled athletes who have been able to go back to playing tennis and softball, and we have had several football players who have gone back to play. Indeed, the first patient on whom we performed this operation played on special teams on three professional football teams for 8 years after the surgery and is still doing well. However, this is rare and requires an especially motivated patient.

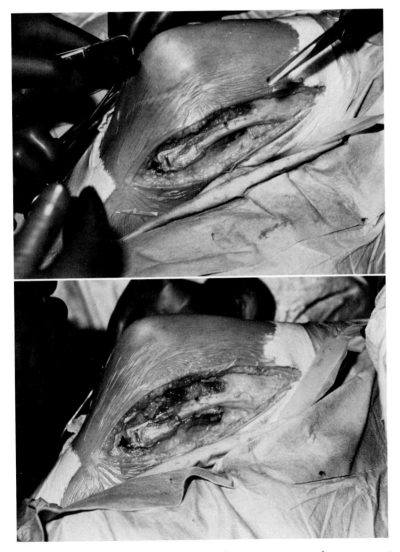

Fig. 18-8. Reconstruction in posterolateral instability. Here arcuate ligament, posterolateral capsule, and gastrocnemius have been pulled forward, while tibia is held forward. It has been stapled to advanced popliteus and iliotibial band, which is reinserted to its tibial attachment with a barbed stable. Note that opposite side has been done by advancement of posterior capsule also. (Top of knee shows open wound.)

COMBINED INSTABILITY

It is not the purpose of this chapter to discuss combined anterolateral and anteromedial instability, which is discussed in Chapter 19. However, it should be reiterated that a combination of anteromedial and anterolateral instability is extremely common. The tibia comes forward and there is increased internal and external rotation with the pivot shift, as well as anteromedial laxity with valgus stress. The pathology is in both sides of the knee. There is laxity in the lateral posterolateral capsule structures as well as the medial collateral ligament and posteromedial corner.

Surgical treatment by simultaneous advancement of both sides is involved in repair, with or without anterior cruciate reconstruction. In some instances these reconstructions have been most satisfactory, but only in patients with an intact posterior cruciate ligament and posterior capsule complex, so that most of the pathology is in the mid third of the transverse axis and forward.

In more severe cases, especially those that also involve posterolateral laxity, we have used O'Donoghue's or Hey Grove's procedure to control severe anterior laxity (Fig. 18-9); we have also used an iliotibial band passed through the intercondylar notched and fixed with a bone block by a screw, as developed by my associate Dr. Jeffrey Minkoff and myself. We are encouraged by the early results.

We have also used the popliteus tendon as a substitute in a few cases of posterior laxity. Early results are encouraging, but these remain too early to report.

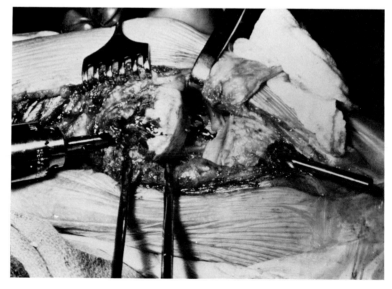

Fig. 18-9. In combined instability, we prefer modified Hey-Groves or O'Donoghue procedure with posterior capsular advancements as well or, better still, iliotibial band passed behind lateral femoral condyle into anterior surface of tibia and fixed with screw.

No repairs in reconstruction should be taken lightly. Even when surgery is done under the best of circumstances, with good technique, a sound preoperative analysis of what surgery can do, and a long postoperative period of rehabilitation, a certain number of knees loosen up readily regardless of what is done.

The aims of reconstruction should be realistic. The articular surfaces should be in relatively good condition, the patient should be muscular and tightly structured, and immobilization should be dynamic, permitting active exercises. Ligaments take a long time to remodel, and there is much to be learned about how reconstruction affects these knees in later years. We know that some have done extremely well and have developed few arthritic changes over a decade. But others are worse than when we started; multiple incisions increase the ever-present possibility of loss of strength, infection, peroneal nerve irritation, and phlebitis.

Each case must be assessed on its own merits and discussed candidly with the patient; limited goals should be outlined: (1) relief of buckling and (2) preservation of the ability to walk up and down stairs. Sports involving stop-and-go variations in throwing, running, and jumping movements are better off abandoned, and the operations are not designed for patients with this in mind. The fact that they are done on professional and highly skilled amateur athletes does not mean that everyone should have them. Conservative measures, adequate total rehabilitation, bracing, and redirected activity must be tried in most patients first. Special evaluations do exist, however, for such repairs.

References

1. Abbott, L. C., Saunders, J. B., Bost, F. C., and Anderson, C. E.: Injuries to the ligaments of the knee joint, J. Bone Joint Surg. **32-A**:721, 1950.
2. Ellison, A. E., Wieneke, K., Benton, L. J., and White, E. S.: Preliminary report, results of extra articular cruciate reconstruction, paper presented at annual meeting, American Academy of Orthopaedic Surgeons, New Orleans, February 3, 1976.
3. Galeazzi, R.: Clinical and experimental study of lesions of the semi-lunar cartilages of the knee joint, J. Bone Joint Surg. **9**:515, 1927.
4. Galway, R. D.: Pivot shift syndrome, J. Bone Joint Surg. **54-B**:558, 1972.
5. Grossman, R., and Nicholas, J. A.: The common disorders of the knee in sports, Orthop. Clin. North Am. **8**:619, 1977.
6. Helfet, A. J.: Disorders of the knee. In Nicholas, J. A.: Rehabilitation of the knee, Philadelphia, 1974, J. B. Lippincott Co.
7. Hughston, J. C., Andrews, J. R., Cross, M. J., and Moschi, A.: Classification of knee ligament instabilities, J. Bone Joint Surg. **58-A**:159, 1976.
8. Kennedy, J. C., and Swan, W. J.: Lateral Instability of the knee following lateral compartment injury, J. Bone Joint Surg. **54-B**:762, 1972.
9. Liebler, W.: Personal communication, Institute of Sports Medicine and Athletic Trauma, Lenox Hill Hospital, 1976.
10. MacIntosh, D. L.: Acute tears of the anterior cruciate ligament, Paper presented at annual meeting, American Academy or Orthopaedic Surgeons, Dallas, 1974.
11. Marshall, J. L., and Rubin, R. M.: Knee ligament injuries, Orthop. Clin. North Am. **8**:641, 1977.
12. Nicholas, J. A.: The five-one reconstruction for anteromedial instability of the knee, J. Bone Joint Surg. **55-A**:899, 1973.
13. Nicholas, J. A., and Liebler, W.: A surgical operation for the treatment of anterior

lateral instability, Movie presented at annual meeting, American Academy of Ortho-paedic Surgeons, Chicago, January 30, 1970.

14. O'Donoghue, D. H.: Surgical treatment of fresh injuries to the major ligaments of the knee, J. Bone Joint Surg. **32-A**:721, 1950.
15. Slocum, D. B., Larson, R. L., and James, L. S.: Late reconstruction procedures used to stabilize the knee, Orthop. Clin. North Am. **4**:679, 1973.

19. Combined instabilities: combinations of surgical procedures

Robert L. Larson

Failure to recognize the presence of more than one type of instability is one of the factors that produces a less favorable result after reconstruction of the knee. It is often difficult to make this determination, particularly when the laxity does not allow a stable neutral point. As with testing for anteroposterior laxity, when there is sometimes a question as to whether the laxity is all anterior, all posterior, or degrees of each, recognition of combinations of rotary excesses with or without anteroposterior laxity may be difficult. Unless the examiner recognizes the true neutral point, he may be misled.

CLASSIFICATION AND ASSESSMENT

The classification of knee instabilities[7,8,10,13] includes straight instability, in which the excess motion is in one plane only. This category includes medial or lateral and straight posterior or anterior instability. The second classification is rotary instability, which includes anteromedial, anterolateral, posterolateral, and posteromedial instability. Hughston[6] questions whether there is actually posteromedial rotary instability; he thinks that for this type of instability to be present, the posterior cruciate ligament must be deficient and therefore no rotary component is possible because no axis of rotation exists. Combined instabilities, the third category, may be combinations of any of the above-mentioned instabilities.

It is important when evaluating a patient with an instability problem to assess the functional deficiency that exists. There are many persons who have relaxed knees. Some knees tolerate instability, whereas some do not. It is the functional loss that produces a disability in desired activities that demands attention to determine if a surgical correction will be beneficial. For an active individual, for instance, it may be inability to participate in desired recreational activities such as tennis or golf; for a sedentary individual it may be problems with the knee buckling or an inability to go up or down inclines for fear of the knee giving way.

We therefore are attempting to restore a function and to rid the patient of a disability. Stability in all degrees of passive motion is often impossible. It is the dynamic function of the knee and the ability of the individual to participate in activities that we are attempting to improve.

"Priorities" therefore becomes a meaningless term because it suggests doing one thing at the expense of not doing another. The knee is a complicated joint that requires flexion, extension, and rotation, as well as a gliding, rocking action, in its normal function. When attempting to correct combined instabilities, we cannot direct our attention to restoring only one plane of instability while not improving or correcting the other plane or planes of instability. The surgical correction of the combined instabilities is to reconstruct the dynamic function of the knee. This requires as much stability as possible in all planes of knee motion.

The problem is not one of priority, but one of assessment and recognition that a combined instability exists and of definition of all components of instability so that correction can be attempted. This is sometimes difficult. In a normal knee the axis of rotation is near the attachment of the posterior cruciate ligament to the inner aspect of the medial femoral condyle. If the medial structures have been stretched or torn, the axis of rotation is allowed to shift laterally, increasing the external rotation of the tibia on the femur. If in addition to deficiency of the medial structures there is also deficiency of the anterior cruciate that allows increased anterior translation of the tibia on the femur, a second plane of instability is present. With involvement of these two structures, there is likely to be an excess medial opening of the knee with valgus stress, giving another plane of instability. Recognition of all the planes of instability is therefore necessary before the surgical procedures to correct them can be undertaken.

One of the common combined instabilities is an anteromedial laxity associated with an anterolateral laxity. The medial laxity may actually be the first to develop after injury. The secondary lateral laxity develops with the continuing stresses to the anterior cruciate ligament, which no longer has the restraints of the medial structures to protect it. If the initial injury is severe enough, stabilizing ligaments on both the medial and lateral aspects of the knee may be torn as well as the anterior cruciate. This is often seen with posterolateral and anteromedial laxity in combination with anterior instability. There may be components of anteromedial, anterolateral, and posterolateral instability, producing an even more difficult task in evaluation and treatment.

SURGICAL PROCEDURES

When the combinations of instabilities have been recognized, the disability ascertained, and the functional demands evaluated, the surgical correction can be determined. Correction of all planes of instability at the time of reconstruction should be attempted. Should the surgical reconstruction be too extensive, it may be necessary to consider a two-stage procedure.

Reconstructive procedures for chronic instability should include dynamic muscular backup to decrease the stretching stresses on retightened ligamentous and capsular tissue.[12,16,17] Palmer,[14] in his original treatise of 1938, described the functional overlap of muscles and ligaments about the knee. The ligaments surrounding the knee have two functions. They act first as a guiding rein for knee motion. Their second function is as a stabilizer through a dual action. Stabilization is first accomplished by the ligamentomuscular reflex. This reflex, as explained by Palmer, allows the myelin-free nerve endings in the ligament to react to tension, causing increasing tonicity of the muscles about the knee. Muscle strength is therefore the first line of defense in protecting the knee. Should these muscles fail or become overstretched, the ligaments then act as mechanical stabilizers through their firm, inelastic tissue.

In chronic instability there has been disruption of the ligamentomuscular reflex. It is necessary therefore to restore a muscular backup to provide the dynamic tightening necessary to protect these ligaments. To omit this step leaves the ligaments more prone to continued stretching with stresses, with ultimate return of the instability over a period of time. Free and fascial substitutes for ligament stability lead to stretching and recurrence of the disability. DuToit[3] points out that such new ligaments suffer a loss of proprioceptive nerve endings with loss of the feedback mechanism and reflex postural tone of muscles. Even when muscle transfer has been done, the surgeon cannot always be certain that the transferred muscles will provide the dynamic support necessary. Certainly unless there is a rigorous and religious rehabilitation program, they will not take over the desired function.

Medial, anterior, and external rotary instability

The combination of a valgus opening of the knee with stress, anterior play of the tibia on the femur, and an increased external rotation of the tibia on the femur involves the deep capsular ligaments on the medial aspect of the knee, the superficial tibial collateral ligament, the anterior cruciate ligament, the medial meniscus, and the anterior medial retinaculum. There also may be patellar instability and possibly involvement of the medial half of the posterior capsule.

Surgical exposure to allow reconstruction for this combination instability is through a medial curved incision (Fig. 19-1). The incision begins at the medial femoral epicondyle and extends anteriorly to the midpatellar area medially, extends thence distally along the patellar tendon to the tibial tubercle, and curves slightly posteriorly at this point to below the pes anserinus insertion. This produces a large medial flap that can be reflected, allowing inspection of the entire medial aspect of the knee from the posteromedial corner to the patellar tendon.

One of the more important areas to tighten in this type of instability is the posteromedial corner, which has been called by Trillat "the keystone of the knee." Hughston and Eilers[6] have recently coined the term "posterior oblique ligament" to differentiate this important stabilizing structure in the posteromedial aspect of the knee. Posterior capsular laxity is first corrected. A slightly oblique incision is made in the posteromedial capsule at its soft spot (Fig. 19-2). This is

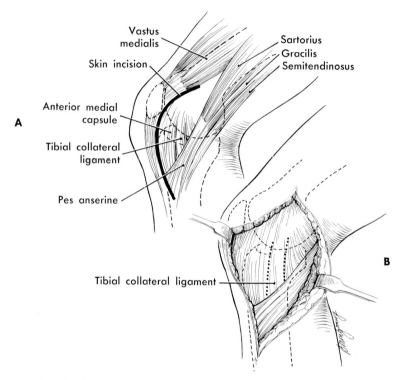

Vastus medialis

Sartorius
Gracilis
Semitendinosus

Skin incision

Anterior medial capsule

A

Tibial collateral ligament

Pes anserine

B

Tibial collateral ligament

Fig. 19-1. A, Medial skin incision and underlying medial structures. (See text.) **B,** Posterior skin flap allows visualization of medial side of knee from patellar tendon to posteromedial corner. (From Larson, R. L.: In Rockwood, C. A., Jr., and Green, D. P., editors: Fractures, Vol. 2, Philadelphia, 1975, J. B. Lippincott Co.)

defined by palpation posterior to the trailing edge of the tibial collateral ligament. When the knee is opened in this area the posterior aspect of the joint can be inspected.

An incision should be made into the anteromedial aspect near the medial edge of the patellar tendon so that the joint can be inspected anteriorly for a full evaluation of the medial meniscus as well as the internal structures of the knee such as the cruciate ligaments. If the meniscus is damaged, it should be removed. The importance of the meniscus as a stabilizing structure has, however been stressed in more recent studies.[9,11,18,19] When there is no definite tear in the body of the meniscus or if there is only separation on its periphery that can be resutured, then I think that the meniscus should be left in place. One exception to this rule, however, is when there is considerable laxity of the posteromedial capsule that requires an anteromedial advancement of the posterior capsule. The medial meniscus may have to be removed since the posterior aspect of the meniscus attaches to the posterior capsule through the semimembranosus muscle. The meniscus must be removed to allow the mobility of this capsule for its anterior advancement.

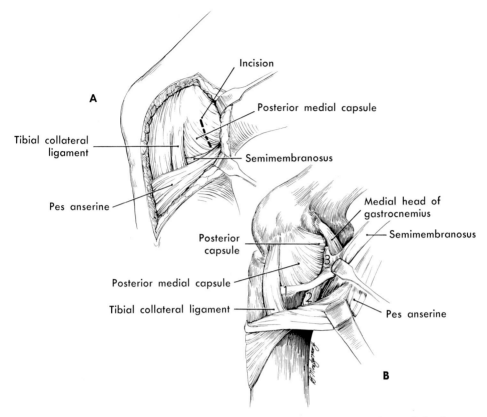

Fig. 19-2. A, Elective incision to inspect posteromedial joint is through soft area behind strong oblique band that forms trailing edge of posteromedial capsular ligament (posterior oblique ligament). **B,** Posteromedial structures: posteromedial capsule, posterior capsule, and three of tendons of semimembranosus. *1,* Anteromedial tendon; *2,* direct head inserting into posterior tubercle of tibia; *3,* lateral expansion, which becomes oblique popliteal ligament. (From Larson, R. L.: In Rockwood, C. A., Jr., and Green, D. P., editors: Fractures, Vol. 2, Philadelphia, 1975, J. B. Lippincott Co.)

Excess laxity may require distal advancement of the posterior capsule on the tibia. Fixation can be accomplished by drilling holes through the proximal tibial area and passing sutures through the posterior capsule and through the drill hole, bringing them out either anteriorly or medially and pulling the capsule downward (Fig. 19-3). Care must be taken to ensure that the knee can be nearly extended after this tightening has taken place. I think that a lack of 5° or 10° of complete extension is allowable since this can be stretched out with use.

After the laxity of the posterior capsule has been corrected, the posteromedial corner is tightened by advancing the anterior edge of the posteromedial capsule, bringing it forward, and imbricating it into the trailing edge of the tibial collateral ligament. To provide the necessary dynamic backup of this repair, the semimembranosus conjoined tendon is used. The conjoined tendon is advanced

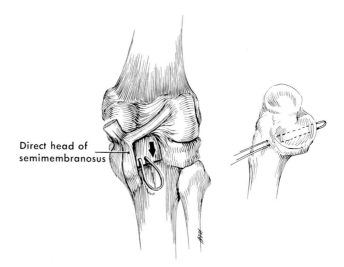

Direct head of
semimembranosus

Fig. 19-3. Posterior capsule should be repaired if it is torn. When detached from posterior tibia, it can be reattached through drill holes in proximal tibia placed lateral to direct head of semimembranosus. (From Larson, R. L.: In Rockwood, C. A., Jr., and Green, D. P., editors: Fractures, Vol. 2, Philadelphia, 1975, J. B. Lippincott Co.)

anteriorly and proximally and sutured into this repair. When this is done slack develops in the anteromedial limb of the semimembranosus, which travels beneath the attachment of superficial collateral ligament (Fig. 19-2). This insertion is detached by elevating the trailing edge of the superficial tibial collateral ligament. The free tendon is then brought superficially to the tibial collateral ligament and sutured to the ligament in the direction of the proximal muscle fibers. This allows a more direct pull when the semimembranosus contracts, a broader area of fixation, and increased efficiency in stabilization of the posteromedial corner.

It is wise to close the anteromedial incision prior to closure of the posteromedial aspect, since if the latter is closed too tightly, it may be difficult to completely close the anteromedial capsule. The effect of the closure of these two portions of the capsule is to tighten the half sleeve of the medial capsule to decrease the tendency of the tibia to externally rotate.

Should the medial opening on valgus stress still persist, the tibial collateral ligament can be advanced either proximally or distally. Bartel et al.[2] have suggested that mechanically the best procedure is to advance the tibial attachment of the tibial collateral ligament distally and anteriorly with the knee at 30° flexion. A transfer of the sartorius muscle can also be added. This is done by isolating the sartorius muscle, leaving it attached at its anterior attachment to the tibia, and swinging the sartorius tendon and muscle anteriorly along the direction of the tibial collateral ligament (Fig. 19-4). It is sutured in this line using the tendinous portion of the muscle for the anchoring sutures; anchoring points are pro-

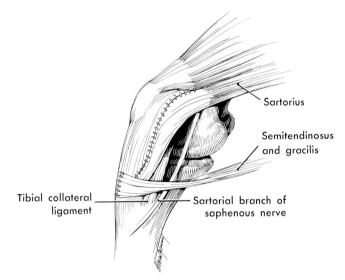

Fig. 19-4. Sartorius advancement. Tibial collateral ligament can be reinforced by mobilizing sartorius and suturing it along anterior border of tibial collateral ligament and into distal edge of vastus medialis fascia. Distal insertion of sartorius is left attached. Care is taken in mobilizing muscle to protect sartorial branch of saphenous nerve. Remaining two components of pes anserinus, semitendinosus and gracilis, are reflected proximally and attached to medial border of patellar tendon, as in usual pes anserinus transfer. (From Larson, R. L.: In Rockwood, C. A., Jr., and Green, D. P., editors: Fractures, Vol. 2, Philadelphia, 1975, J. B. Lippincott Co.)

vided near the tendinous portion of the vastus medialis and distalward along the line of the tibial collateral ligament. When this is done, care must be taken to protect the sartorial branch of the saphenous nerve and avoid causing any entrapment of this nerve in sutured tissue. The sartorial muscle transferred in this manner will then help to provide dynamic tightening of the medial side of the knee with contraction. The two remaining muscles of the pes anserinus, the gracilis and semitendinosus, are then freed in their lower two thirds from their attachment to the tibia anteriorly. They are turned on themselves, reflected proximally, and sutured to the medial border of the patellar tendon. This provides a dynamic constraint to excess external rotation of the tibia on the femur.[15]

Should the anterior cruciate be absent or deficient so that an anterior play of the tibia as in a straight instability is present, a substitution of this ligament should be considered. A method described in the Scandinavian literature[1] is to use the medial third of the patellar tendon (Fig. 19-5). This is detached with a small block of bone from the anterior surface of the patella and redirected through a drill hole in the proximal tibia, exiting near the normal attachment of the anterior cruciate, and thence into the notch area. A bed is created in the posterior aspect of the lateral femoral condylar area and two drill holes, spaced approximately 1 to 2 cm apart, are drilled from the inner aspect of the notch

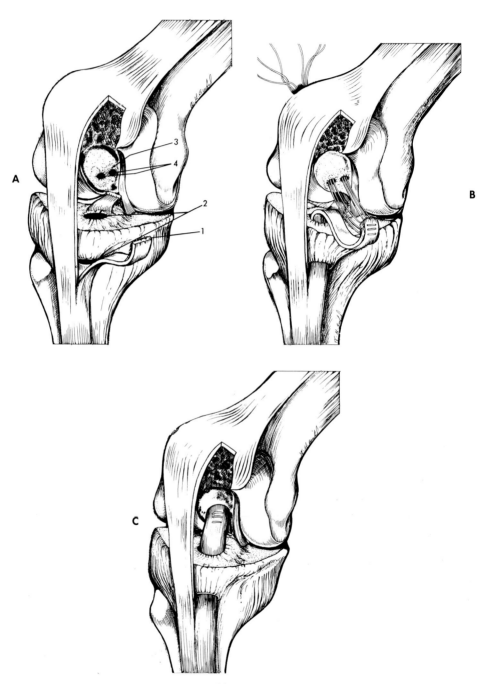

Fig. 19-5. For legend see opposite page.

area to the lateral aspect just above the lateral femoral condyle in the region of the intermuscular septum.* The tendinous tissue is then brought into this bed by multiple sutures to fix it in a tightened position to constrain the tibia from being displaced anteriorly.

Whether this tendinous tissue will eventually stretch out, as has been noted with previous types of repairs done in this manner, has not been determined. However, it is thought that having the constraint of this ligament while the other transferred dynamic tissues are healing may allow a better chance for these tissues to heal without undue stress for a longer period of time.

Another method using the gracilis tendon has been described by Lindemann[3] (Fig. 19-6). The gracilis tendon is detached from its tibial insertion, with care to preserve the other attachments of the pes anserinus group. The tendon is freed proximally to the back of the knee medially. The free end of the tendon is then brought through the posterior capsule and medial attachment of the gastrocnemius muscle into the notch area. It is then passed through a drill hole in the anterior tibia. This hole is directed from the area just medial to the tibial tubercle into the notch area at the tibial attachment of the anterior cruciate ligament. The gracilis tendon, after being passed through this hole, is sutured to the surrounding tissue or stapled in place on the tibia.

If patellar instability accompanies the other instabilities on the medial side of the knee, steps must be taken to correct this deficiency. A tightening of the medial retinaculum by direct distal advancement of the vastus medialis helps to provide dynamic stability to the medial aspect of the patella and retinaculum. It is important not to advance the vastus medialis distal to the midportion of the patella. Muscular action on the distal portion of the patella may cause it to rotate in the sulcus and give problems with the normal tracking of the patella in its femoral groove.

If there is considerable laxity of the medial retinacular structures from tear or previous stretching injuries, a split patellar tendon advancement can be done

---

*I now drill only one hole for one bundle of sutures and pass the second bundle of sutures posteriorly, to exit through the capsule near the intermuscular septum.

Fig. 19-5. **A,** *1,* Medial one third of patellar tendon is detached proximally with thin block of bone from anterior surface of patella. *2,* Drill hole is made from tibial tubercle region into notch near tibial attachment of anterior cruciate ligament. *3,* Bed of raw bone is curreted in posterior aspect of inner aspect of lateral femoral condyle. *4,* Two small drill holes, spaced 1 to 2 cm apart, are drilled to exit on the outer aspect of lateral femoral condyle near intermuscular septum. **B,** Free edge of detached medial one third of patellar tendon is passed through tibial hole into notch. Sutures are placed transversely across free end of patellar tendon. Sutures from each side of tendon are passed through appropriate drill hole as a group. It helps to identify each end of a suture by a different number of small knots or using different colored sutures. **C,** Sutures are pulled up and tied independently. Most proximal suture is tied first, then the next, then the next, to tighten tendon into its bed with each successive suture.

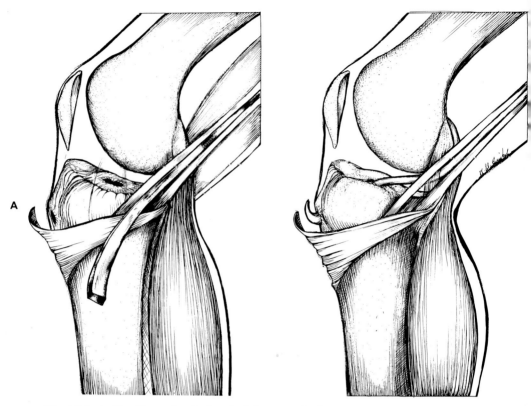

Fig. 19-6. A, Gracilis tendon is detached from its tibial insertion and freed proximally to behind posteromedial aspect of knee. **B,** Free end of tendon is then delivered through back of knee into notch area. This requires penetration of medial portion of gastrocnemius and posterior capsule. Care is taken not to go too far laterally in the notch and risk injury to neurovascular structures. Free end is then directed through drill hole in proximal tibia. This hole is made from just medial to tibial tubercle to tibial attachment of anterior cruciate ligament. After this tendon is passed through the hole its free end is secured to surrounding tissue.

(Fig. 19-7). In this situation the medial one third of the patellar tendon is dissected free and detached from its attachment to the tibial tubercle. The medial retinaculum and capsule are then brought anteriorly and laterally and sutured to the remaining edge of the patellar tendon to tighten up the medial retinaculum and capsular half sleeve of the medial side of the knee. The detached third of the patellar tendon is then reattached more medially by elevating a small subperiosteal tunnel of tissue on the proximal tibia in the area medially where it will fit firmly. The patellar tendon end is passed beneath this subperiosteal bridge and either stapled or sutured into this position. This should be done before the pes anserinus transplant since the pes anserinus transplant may then overlap this transferred patellar tendon. The resultant vector force is then in a more medial direction to lessen the likelihood of the patella displacing laterally.

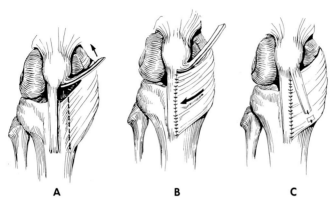

Fig. 19-7. Method to reinforce anteromedial corner of knee by splitting patellar tendon. **A,** Patellar tendon is split and medial half is reflected proximally. **B,** Anteromedial capsule is advanced laterally to edge of attached portion of patellar tendon. **C,** Split end of patellar tendon is reattached medially to tibia to reinforce anteromedial corner and stabilize patella from lateral displacement. (From Larson, R. L.: In Rockwood, C. A., Jr., and Green, D. P., editors: Fractures, Vol. 2, Philadelphia, 1975, J. B. Lippincott Co.)

Summary. The reconstructive procedures that are available for the medial aspect of the knee include the following: (1) tightening of the posteromedial aspect (posterior oblique ligament with advancement of the semimembranosus tendon into the repair), (2) sartorial advancement along the line of the tibial collateral ligament to provide dynamic support to the medial side of the knee, (3) pes anserinus transfer to decrease excess external rotation of the tibia and to provide a sling beneath the tibial condyle for increased medial instability, (4) advancement of the medial gastrocnemius head and posterior capsule to a more anterior and medial position to further reinforce the posteromedial corner of the knee, (5) patellar tendon split with advancement of the medial retinaculum and capsule and medial transfer of the medial third of the patellar tendon, and (6) vastus medialis advancement to correct medial retinacular laxity and provide dynamic tightening of the anterior aspect of the medial retinaculum. If additional stability is required in an anterior plane, use of the medial third of the patellar tendon or the gracialis tendon is added.

Lateral instability

Lateral instability with increased internal rotation of the tibia on the femur is sometimes associated with medial instabilities. The deficency of the anterior cruciate ligament, along with incompetence of the lateral capsule, allows the tibia to rotate anteriorly. As the knee is extended the quadriceps mechanism pulling on the tibial tubercle, along with the iliotibial band pulling on Gerdy's tubercle and migrating anteriorly as the knee is extended, enhances the forward translocation of the lateral tibial condyle, allowing the femur to slip posteriorly in a subluxated position. This subluxation as the knee is extended has been described by MacIntosh[5] as the pivot shift. It has various names: MacIntosh sign, jerk test, anterolateral instability, and anterior-internal rotary instability. The goal in correcting this is to prevent the anterior migration of the lateral tibial condyle as the knee is extended.

MacIntosh originally described the procedure in which he fashioned a band of tissue involving approximately 1 to 2 cm of the midportion of the iliotibial tract. This band is detached 15 to 20 cm proximally. This tissue is then rerouted beneath the fibular collateral ligament, up through the intermuscular septum on the lateral aspect of the femur, and thence back on itself; it is then sutured into the band of transferred tissue. Tightening of the band is done with the knee flexed. This provides a static restraint to the forward displacement of the tibia.

Several modifications were then introduced. Slocum modified the procedure by directing the iliotibial tissue through a vertical drill hole in the lateral femoral condyle for fixation. Ellison's[4] modification is to detach the iliotibial tract distally with a small button of bone, still fashioning the band approximately 1 to 2 cm wide. This tissue is then redirected beneath the fibular collateral ligament and reattached to its previous bed or slightly anteriorly and distally to again provide a restraint to anterior displacement of lateral tibial condyle.

When these procedures are done, the lateral capsule is incised, the lateral meniscus is inspected, and appropriate measures are taken if any pathology of the meniscus exists. Some knees with a chronic anterolateral instability have meniscal changes in the posterior horn because this structure is pinched beneath the femur and tibia with the subluxation that occurs. If such changes are noted, with tearing of the meniscal body, its removal is indicated. On the other hand, if the meniscal tissue appears to be intact and no definte pathology is noted, I think that it is better to preserve the meniscus since it does provide a stabilizing action to the knee.

After the interior aspect of the joint has been inspected, the lateral capsule is closed; care should be taken to imbricate and tighten the capsule as much as possible.

It is often necessary to direct one's attention to the posterior lateral aspect of the joint and to tighten this area also. The lateral gastrocnemius and arcuate structures are brought forward and sutured to the popliteus. The lateral head of the gastrocnemius may be detached with a small flake of bone. The lateral aspect of the femoral condyle is roughened just posterior to the popliteal tendon. The lateral gastrocnemius tendon and underlying posterolateral capsule are pulled anteriorly and laterally and attached to this surface. Their anterior edges, which include the arcuate structures, are sutured to the popliteus tendon proximally and then to the lateral capsule beneath the fibular collateral ligament.

When the transferred iliotibial tract is directed beneath the fibular ligament, it is kept outside the capsule since the fibular collateral ligament is exterior to the synovium. The bony block taken from Gerdy's tubercle is attached to the tibia by a staple. The knee is extended after fixation to see that adequate extension and flexion are possible.

Following the transfer of the band of iliotibial tract, the defect created in the iliotibial tract is closed by bringing the freely movable posterior edge anteriorly to the posterior edge of the remaining anterior fibers of the iliotibial tract. This also advances the biceps anteriorly. Care should be taken to avoid too tight a closure, which may produce patellar problems if the patella is pulled too tightly into the sulcus. If it appears that this closure would produce too tight a closure, the biceps is mobilized more proximally to allow closure. The lower edge of the biceps tendon is then dissected and the peroneal nerve identified. The biceps tendon is removed from its attachment to the fibular head, with care to prevent any injury to the fibular attachment of the lateral collateral ligament. The short head of the biceps is also protected and its attachment to the posterior lateral complex left intact. The biceps is then transferred either by flipping it proximally or by moving it proximally and reattaching it to the transferred portion of the iliotibial tract to provide a dynamic muscular action on this transferred tissue.

Anteromedial and anterolateral instability

In a situation in which there is both anteromedial and anterolateral instability, both the pes anserinus transplant and the iliotibial band transfer with the biceps transplant are done at the same time. This provides a checkrein from both sides of the tibia that keeps the tibia from advancing anteriorly either from the lateral or the medial side. When there is marked deficiency of the anterior cruciate with a straight anterior drawer sign, the medial third of the patellar tendon or the gracilis is also transferred through the proximal tibia and into the joint area as described previously.

Posterolateral instability

Posterolateral laxity allows an excess external rotation of the lateral tibia posteriorly on the femur. This may occur in combination with the other instabilities mentioned. Combinations of anteromedial and posterolateral; anterolateral and posterolateral; or anteromedial, anterolateral, and posterolateral instabilities may occur. Laxity of the posterolateral corner involves some stretching of the posterior capsule and sometimes the posterior cruciate. I think that instability of this type is the most difficult to adequately correct. The attempt is made to tighten the posterolateral structures, at the same time taking away any posterior pull on the tibia. The entire posterolateral complex is tightened by detaching the gastrocnemius insertion of the lateral head from the femur, taking a small plate of bone. This is then pulled anteriorly and proximally to tighten the posterolateral corner of the knee. It is reattached by roughening an area just behind the femoral attachment of the popliteus tendon and either stapling or suturing it in this area to tighten up the posterior lateral capsule. The arcuate complex and lateral head of the gastrocnemius are then sutured to the posterior edge of the top of the popliteus tendon and the posterior edge of the fibular collateral ligament and lateral capsule to reinforce the posterolateral corner. The biceps tendon is detached from its fibular attachment to lessen the posterior pull from the lateral side of the tibia. It is advanced anteriorly, slightly above or at the joint line area, and reattached to the iliotibial tract tissue near Gerdy's tubercle.

If the posterior cruciate ligament is involved with straight posterior displacement of the tibia on the femur, this should also be corrected. A medial incision is necessary to advance the posterior capsule on the tibia distally and to provide some substitute for the deficient posterior cruciate ligament. Several methods have been advocated. A method that I have used is to take the medial third of the medial head of the gastrocnemius tendon, detaching it from its femoral attachment and directing it through the posterior capsule and into the posterior aspect of the notch. The tendinous free end is directed into a bony bed on the inner aspect of the medial femoral condyle at the normal attachment of the posterior cruciate ligament. This is tightened by the use of multiple sutures through two drill holes spaced to provide a wide insertion into its new bed.

Summary. Procedures used on the lateral aspect of the knee include the following: (1) transfer of a band of the iliotibial tract by the manner of Mac-Intosh or Ellison; (2) anterior advancement of the biceps tendon to provide a change in pull on the lateral side of the knee, either reinforcing its posterior pull on the tibia or decreasing its posterior pull on the tibia by advancing it more proximally; (3) transfer of the lateral gastrocnemius tendon insertion more laterally and proximally along with its posterior capsular attachment; and (4) tightening of the arcuate ligament complex to the posterior edge of the fibular collateral ligament. In addition, when marked varus laxity is present the fibular collateral ligament can be advanced either proximally or distally to tighten this structure. Posterior cruciate substitution using the medial third of the gastrocnemius tendon is added when straight posterior instability is also present.

SUMMARY

The various components of instability in the knee and their combinations must be appreciated to take appropriate steps to correct each component. As the reconstruction of the unstable knee proceeds, a check for residual instability in the various planes is necessary. Additional procedures may be added to reinforce areas where deficiency still exists. It must be emphasized that a normal, completely stable knee is usually impossible to produce by reconstruction of a chronically unstable knee with various combinations of instability. The goal is to provide as much stability as possible in an attempt to improve the functional capabilities of the knee.

References

1. Alm, A., and Gillquist, J.: Reconstruction of the anterior cruciate ligament by using the medial third of the patellar ligament, Acta Chir. Scand. **140:**289, 1974.
2. Bartel, D. L., Marshall, J. L., Schieck, R. A., and Wang, J. B.: Surgical repositioning of

the medial collateral ligament. An anatomical and mechanical analysis, J. Bone Joint Surg. **59-A:**107, 1977.

3. DuToit, G. T.: Knee joint cruciate ligament substitution. The Lindemann (Heidelberg) operation, S. Afr. J. Surg. **5:**25, 1967.

4. Ellison, A. E.: A modified procedure for the extra-articular replacement of the anterior cruciate ligament, Paper presented at annual meeting, American Orthopedic Society for Sports Medicine, New Orleans, July 28-30, 1975.

5. Galway, R. D., Beaupre, A., and MacIntosh, D. L.: Pivot shift: a clinical sign of anterior cruciate instability, J. Bone Joint Surg. **54-B:**763, 1972.

6. Hughston, J. C., and Eilers, A. F.: The role of the posterior oblique ligament in repairs of acute medial (collateral) ligament tears of the knee, J. Bone Joint Surg. **55-A:**923, 1973.

7. Hughston, J. C., Andrews, J. R., Cross, M. J., and Moschi, A.: Classification of knee ligament instabilities. Part I. The medial compartment and cruciate ligaments, J. Bone Joint Surg. **58-A:**159, 1976.

8. Hughston, J. C., Andrews, J. R., Cross, M. J., and Moschi, A.: Classification of knee instabilities. Part II. The lateral compartment, J. Bone Joint Surg. **58-A:**173, 1976.

9. Johnson, R. J., Kettelkamp, D. B., Clark, W., and Leaverton, P.: Factors affecting late results after meniscectomy, J. Bone Joint Surg. **56-A:**719, 1974.

10. Kennedy, J. C.: A preliminary working classification of knee joint instability, Unpublished manuscript.

11. Krause, W. R., Pope, M. H., Johnson, R. J., and Wilder, D. G.: Mechanical changes in the knee after meniscectomy, J. Bone Joint Surg. **58-A:**599, 1976.

12. Larson, R. L.: Fractures and dislocations of the knee. Part 2. Dislocations and ligamentous injuries of the knee. In Rockwood C. A., Jr., and Green, D. P., editors: Fractures, Vol. 2, Philadelphia, 1975, J. B. Lippincott Co.

13. Nicholas, J. A.: The five-one reconstruction for anteromedial instability of the knee, J. Bone Joint Surg. **55-A:**899, 1973.

14. Palmer, I.: On the injuries to the ligaments of the knee joint, Acta Chir. Scand. **81**(Suppl.):3, 1938.

15. Slocum, D. B., and Larson, R. L.: Pes anserinus transplant. A simple surgical procedure for control of rotary instability of the knee, J. Bone Joint Surg. **50-A:**226, 1968.

16. Slocum, D. B., Larson, R. L., and James, S. L.: Late reconstruction procedures used to stabilize the knee, Orthop. Clin. North Am. **4:**679, 1973.

17. Slocum, D. B., Larson, R. L., and James, S. L.: Late reconstruction of the medial compartment of the knee, Clin. Orthop. **100:**23, 1974.

18. Walker, P. S., and Erkman, M. J.: The function of the menisci of the knee, J. Bone Joint Surg. **57-A:**1028, 1975.

19. Wang, C., and Walker, P. S.: Rotary laxity of the human knee joint, J. Bone Joint Surg. **56-A:**161, 1974.

PART SIX

Current status of total knee joint reconstruction

20. UCI and other knee joint replacements: present problems and future development

Theodore R. Waugh

With the almost daily addition of still another knee replacement prosthesis to orthopaedics, one cannot help but be confused by the claimed advantages of the many types. In spite of Riley's attempts to bring order to this chaos by subdividing the prostheses according to their degree of constraint, it remains axiomatic of orthopaedic surgery that when multiple surgical procedures exist for a given pathologic state, no procedure is clearly superior to others.[14] This may also be true of total knee replacement arthroplasty.

Our experience at the University of California, Irvine, has been, for the most part, with the UCI prosthesis replacement, but the number of other devices we have seen because of failure, suggests that our own problems are not unique.[5,18] It would appear that most of these share common features, which can be subdivided into those of surgical technique, biology, and biomechanics. In addition, based on these problems and some possible solutions to them, we believe that the present hundreds of designs will be replaced by second-generation prostheses embodying significant improvements. By the same token, however, it is important to recognize that the great majority of patients in our series, about 80%, are much improved by knee replacement, and we should not lose sight of the great benefit that most patients enjoy as a result of this new surgery.

PROBLEMS OF SURGICAL TECHNIQUE

Most authors have published their recommended technique for insertion of their own prosthetic design, but experience and the passage of time have led to less publicized improvements.[2,6,9,10] Accordingly the average surgeon is somewhat handicapped by the available instructions for a procedure that may require significant technical skill. By and large, it appears that most devices are more easily inserted through a medial parapatellar incision. The transverse approach has caused difficulty because removal and reattachment of either the origin or the insertion of the patellar tendon has necessitated a significant period of immobilization, which seems to interfere with the achievement of excellent motion. Where the joint has not been protected, patella alta usually results. When the

225

surgeon elects a lateral parapatellar approach to protect sensation and possibly improve wound healing, considerable difficulty has resulted in preparing the medial compartment of the knee. The meniscus is attached to the medial side of the tibia by the deep portion of the medial collateral ligament. This is frequently sacrificed in the performance of total knee replacement, but from the lateral aspect it is an easy matter to cut the superficial portion of the ligament as well when preparing the tibial plateau.

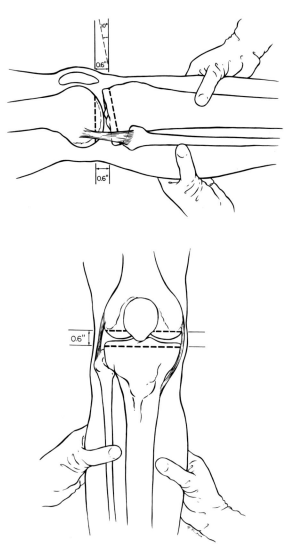

Fig. 20-1. During arthroplasty procedure joint must be passively corrected and ligament slack removed.

Surgeons performing knee arthroplasty not only seek to correct the gross varus or valgus deformity secondary to loss of joint space, but also strive to finish the procedure with tight ligaments and a stable replacement. To accomplish this objective it is essential that the surgeon ascertain the amount of laxity present in the ligaments that can be corrected passively at the time of surgery (Fig. 20-1). If this is not done, inordinate amounts of bone are resected, resulting in a loose joint or the necessity of correcting the error by utilizing an extrathick tibial prosthetic component. Both templates and exact measurements are of value in this regard, as removal of the correct amount of bone initially not only shortens the duration of the surgical procedure but also avoids complications. In those knee replacement procedures, such as UCI, in which the posterior condyles of the femur are removed in a precise manner, exact spacing is in turn used for the location of slots for the prosthetic fins.[18] The necessity for subsequent trimming of the distal femur should be avoided, as this can cause significant difficulty with the placement of the prosthesis. Replacement of the femoral prosthesis in most knee replacements is fairly critical if the load is to be borne correctly and evenly on both sides of the joint. Where the prosthesis is too far posterior, a tendency develops for hyperextension and increased pressure on the tibial component during the initial part of the stance phase of gait. Attempts to rectify placement of a femoral component too far posteriorly have resulted in the need for additional trimming of the posterior condyles of the femur and the cutting of additional slots in the femur, all of which can on occasion result in complete excision of the origin of the cruciate ligaments.

Additionally, attempts to rectify inadequate bone removal of prosthetic insertion have led to further trimming of the proximal tibia to accept this component. Unfortunately such a solution not only provides a poorer foundation for the prosthesis, as will be dealt with subsequently, but also results in the prosthetic component being placed too far distal to the intercondylar eminence, with resulting impingement of this bone on the femoral component. This causes a fairly painless range of active non-weight-bearing motion but significant pain on weight bearing on the extended knee.

Although the problem of insufficiently anterior placement of the femoral components has been discussed, more frequently problems occur when the femoral component is placed too far anteriorly. This results in impingement of the patella on the anterior surface of the prosthesis, a circumstance that is made more likely by the failure of some manufacturers to provide a radius of curvature on the femoral component to blend into the normal radius of curvature of the femoral articular surface. Patellar impingement generally does not interfere with normal level walking, which is often pain free, but does cause significant problems in the greater degrees of flexion necessitated by stair climbing. Often the easiest solution to this problem is patellectomy rather than the large amount of surgery necessary to accomplish a repositioning of the prosthetic components or to insert another design.

BIOLOGICAL PROBLEMS

One of the most fascinating aspects of knee arthroplasty has been the recognition in the past few years that technically well-performed prosthetic replacements may fail. The reasons for this are poorly understood, but it is becoming apparent that the strength of the upper tibia is dependent largely on the outer cortical shell and very little on the cancellous bone that underlies it. In the past it was customary, while performing prosthetic replacement, to remove the subcondylar bone plate to secure a cancellous bed for maximal interlocking of the methacrylate, thereby providing a satisfactory methacrylate-bone interface. Sectional radiographs of the proximal tibia demonstrate that the strength of the proximal tibia varies in an inverse relationship with its distance from the cortical plate (Fig. 20-2). As a result, apparently satisfactory replacements of the tibial components have been noted, with the passage of time, to migrate distally until the prosthesis comes to lie on a level with the upper tibial surface. In this position the ligaments are unstable; the intercondylar eminence butts on the femoral prosthesis, and significant pain may be associated with contact of the residual tibial cortical shell (Fig. 20-3).

Alternatively, in some patients, cancellous bone is noted to hypertrophy, becoming identifiably sclerotic under the medial plateau. Evaluation of long-term results suggests that the cancellous bone is faced with two possibilities, atrophy and hypertrophy; the result appears to be dictated by many factors, but the weight of the patient seems important. Obviously some prosthetic components,

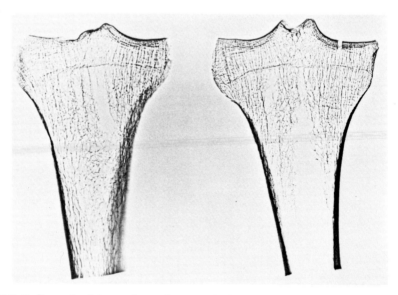

Fig. 20-2. Radiograph of 6 mm slices of a normal tibia indicating poor support providable by cancellous bone.

by their design, have a much smaller area of contact than others. This area of contact and the patient's weight dictate the pressure on the polyethylene component, which in turn results in high pressure on the cancellous structure supporting the knee. Recognition that the excessively heavy patient is more likely to have underlying bone failure has resulted in a general tendency to restrict knee arthroplasty to those weighing less than 200 pounds. Additionally, most orthopaedic surgeons remove less cancellous bone and in some circumstances even retain some of the cortical plate for support purposes. Attempts to bone graft the proximal tibia are still too recent to provide information as to whether this will be of value. Suffice it to say, however, that protection of the knee by use of walking aids in the several months immediately following knee arthroplasty certainly appears to be of theoretical value in biomechanically reducing the stress on the tibial plateau. Support for the concept of bone response by atrophy or hypertrophy has been described by Charnley in regard to total hip replacement arthroplasty.[1] He believes that these changes represent a physiologic response of bone to increased mechanical stress. In the case of the hip a majority of the response is seen in the cortex, although some condensation of can-

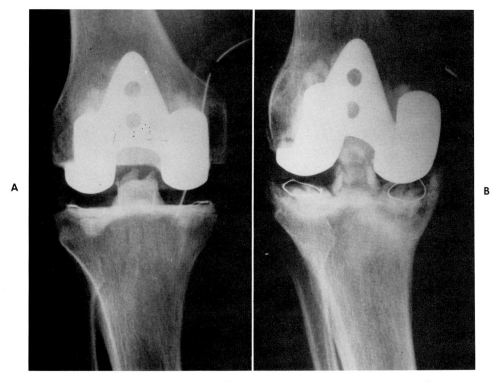

A   B

Fig. 20-3. A, Initial postoperative x-ray films of obese 63-year-old woman with degenerative arthritis. **B,** Radiograph taken 40 months later shows failure of tibial support on medial side.

cellous bone is also seen demarcating the external surface of the cement. According to Charnley, this appearance first became manifest between 1 and 2 years after replacement, which would be temporally similar to those changes seen in the knee.

BIOMECHANICAL PROBLEMS

The implant materials customarily utilized for knee replacement consist of one of two metals, either a stainless steel or a cobalt-chromium-molybdenum alloy, which is generally fabricated by casting. Polymers have been used for the opposite side of the bearing surface because of the galling and fretting motion of metal on metal.[3] Ultrahigh molecular weight polyethylene, with an average weight of 3×10^6, has improved mechanical properties with reduced creep and increased abrasion resistance. However, polyethylene is a weak material; it has poor fatigue life and rapidly develops cracks and pits under cyclic impact loading. Friction and wear experiments made under laboratory conditions indicate that resistance to wear is proportional to the molecular weight of the polyethylene. Wear of total joints occurs predominantly through a surface fatigue mechanism attributable to breaks in the polymer chain beneath the surface, and longer polymer chains are more resistant than shorter ones.[11] Unfortunately the interface between polyethylene and polymethylmethacrylate, the bone cement conventionally utilized, is poor and for the most part is dependent on mechanical interlocking.

In most designs currently available for orthopaedic implantation, the tibial component is of polyethylene and frequently is of relatively thin design. With the weakness of the polyethylene-methacrylate interface, it is not surprising that problems occur. Morrison[12] has analyzed the forces transmitted by the knee joint and has found that maximal values of approximately four times body weight were noted coincidentally with the activity of the hamstrings subsequent to heel strike and the gastrocnemius prior to toe off. Our own wear studies suggest that these forces are concentrated at the anteromedial corner of the tibial component (Fig. 20-4).

Several authors have studied the weight-bearing area of human knees.[4,7,8,16] Their figures vary between 1.8 and 5 cm^2 for the medial condyle and 1.4 and 3 cm^2 for the lateral. Evanski and Krug[4] loaded cadaver knee joints, following ideal replacement, and established total contact areas of 2.5 to 3 cm^2 equally distributed between the two sides. With increasing amounts of anterior subluxation of the femoral component relative to the tibial component there was a progressive decrease in contact area to well below 1 cm^2 (Table 20-1). The yield strength of polyethylene is approximately 250 kg per cm^2, and this figure would be exceeded by those weighing 63 kg or more. However, it is recognized that a prosthetic component may tolerate high levels of force in areas away from the edges because of plastic constraint.

It is evident that success following knee repacement arthroplasty is dependent

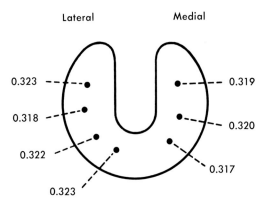

Fig. 20-4. Wear pattern in 1-year-old tibial component subjected to heavy use by small patient weighing 50 kg. Original thickness was 0.325 inch.

Table 20-1. UCI total knee contact area

Displacement (mm)	Contact area (cm²)	
	Average	Range
0	2.77	2.58-3.03
2	2.56	2.45-2.64
4	1.74	1.68-1.80
6	1.10	0.97-1.35
8	0.44	0.44-0.44
10	0.21	0.15-0.26

on proper centralization of the prosthetic components, with correction of varus and valgus deformity, particularly in nonconstrained knee replacement arthroplasty. Failure to correct all aspects of the deformity may well be disastrous in all but the lightest of patients.

Walker et al.[17] have demonstrated that forces applied to the central portion of polyethylene tibial components on cancellous bone result in slight U-shaped bending of the polymer. This bending of the tibial component under load could lead to permanent deformation of the polyethylene.[13] Clinical evidence, however, suggests that loosening alone is not always associated with failure of a joint replacement.

FUTURE DEVELOPMENTS

Under existing federal guidelines, it is assumed that acceptance of new materials for use as implants will require more stringent investigation than has been carried out in the past. However, it is doubtful that these controls will prevent the development of new materials. Several new metals are being tried because of the need to find a material that combines the good ductility of stainless steel with the improved corrosion resistance of cobalt-chromium alloys. MP35N (Protasul-10*) is an alloy of cobalt, nickel, chromium, and molybdenum that does combine excellent corrosion resistance with superior mechanical properties.[3] Steels with transformation-induced plasticity exhibit strength, ductility, and toughness superior to the currently popular 316L stainless steel; however, corrosion resistance is being investigated at the present time. Additionally a multitude of new polymeric materials are under investigation in the hope of finding a substance with good lubricity without toxicity or the poor fatigue life of polyethylene.

Biological fixation is currently being investigated in our own laboratory, as well as others, in an attempt to circumvent the problems engendered with methacrylate.

Sintered powders of 316L stainless steel and cobalt-chromium alloy have been applied to substrates of the same material. We have been able to show good ingrowth of bone with minimal immobilization and the development of excellent resistance to interface shear. Although there has been concern that high rates of corrosion might result from such processes, this has not been found in our laboratory.[3] Similar studies by Spector et al.[15] have indicated excellent bone ingrowth into porous high-density polyethylene.

In view of the obvious disadvantages of many of the present ultrahigh-density polyethylene tibial components, an obvious solution might be the encasement of the polyethylene in a metal shell. Such a device would have significantly im-

---

*De Puy Corp., Warsaw, Ind.

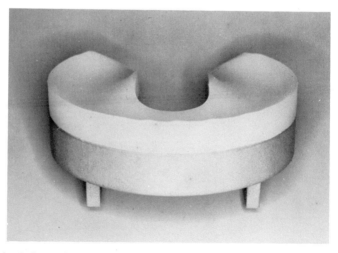

Fig. 20-5. Polyethylene tibial component placed in metal shell to provide better force distribution.

proved fixation potential and greater resistance to deformation of the polyethylene. Similarly, better load distribution by the more rigid metallic material would result in better force distribution on the tibia. Small amounts of motion between the ultrahigh-density polyethylene and the metal would not be detrimental (Fig. 20-5). The majority of present designs for knee replacement arthroplasty employ a concave tibial surface of polyethylene, which is in some measure a reduplication of anatomy. Whether such an arrangement is necessary is unclear, but it is suggested that it is undesirable. Particles of debris from the knee joint tend to congregate in the concave surface of the tibial component, resulting in abrasion of the polyethylene. It should be possible to reverse the materials and design such that the tibial component might be convex and of metal. Our preliminary experimental work with such an alternative may be fruitful.

In summary, it has been the purpose of this presentation to discuss some of the problems being generated by first-stage total knee replacement devices. It is believed that a majority of these problems have solutions and that in the foreseeable future a new generation of knee devices will be developed, permitting further improvement over the present 80% rate of good to excellent results being achieved by those performing knee replacement arthroplasty.

References

1. Charnley, J.: Acrylic cement in orthopaedic surgery, Edinburgh, 1970, E & S Livingstone.
2. Coventry, M. B., Upshaw, J. E., Riley, L. H., Finerman, G. A. M., and Turner, R. H.: The geometric total knee arthroplasty. I. Conception, design, indications, and surgical technic, Clin. Orthop. 94:171, 1973.
3. Dumbleton, J. H., and Black, J.: An introduction to orthopaedic materials, Springfield, Ill., 1975, Charles C Thomas, Publisher.
4. Evanski, P. M., and Krug, A. K.: Contact area with the UCI knee replacement prosthesis. (In press.)
5. Evanski, P. M., Waugh, T. R., Orofino, C. F., and Anzel, S. H.: UCI knee replacement statistics, Clin. Orthop. 120:33, 1976.
6. Gunston, F. H.: Polycentric knee arthroplasty—prosthetic simulation of normal knee movement, Clin. Orthop. 94:128, 1973.
7. Kettlecamp, D. B., and Chao, E. Y.: A method for quantitative analysis of medial and lateral compression forces at the knee during standing, Clin. Orthop. 83:202, 1972.
8. Kettlecamp, D. B., and Jacobs, A. W.: Tibial femoral contact area—determination and implications, J. Bone Joint Surg. 54-A:349, 1972.
9. Marmor, L.: The modular knee, Clin. Orthop. 94:242, 1973.
10. Matthews, L. S., Sonstegard, D. A., and Kaufer, H.: The spherocentric knee, Clin. Orthop. 94:234, 1973.
11. Miller, D. A.: A technical report on ultra-high molecular weight polyethylene and update (B4561), February 20, 1975, Zimmer Corp., Warsaw, Ind.
12. Morrison, B.: Bio-engineering analysis of force actions transmitted by the knee joint, Biomed. Eng. 3:164, April, 1968.
13. Reckling, F. W.: Detailed studies of an ex-vivo geometric total knee prosthesis, J. Bone Joint Surg. 56-A:1302, 1974.
14. Riley, L. H.: Paper presented at Symposium on total knee replacement, American Academy of Orthopaedic Surgeons, San Francisco, March 5, 1975.

15. Spector, M., Fleming, W. R., and Kreutner, A.: An evaluation of bone growth into porous high-density polyethylene, J. Biomed. Mater. Res. 7:595, 1976.
16. Walker, T. S., and Hajek, J.: The loadbearing area in the knee joint, J. Biomech. 5:581, 1972.
17. Walker, P. S., Ranawat, C., and Insall, J.: Fixation of the tibial components of condylar replacement knee prosthesis, J. Biomech. 9:269, 1976.
18. Waugh, T. R., Smith, R. C., Orofino, C. F., and Anzel, S. H.: Total knee replacement operative technic and preliminary results, Clin. Orthop. 94:196, 1973.

21. Unicondylar knee replacement

A. A. Savastano
V. A. Zecchino

Beginning with John Rhea Barton[3] in 1826 and Verneuil[3] in 1860, many surgeons have made attempts to interpose various substances between roughened bone ends of joints in an attempt to relieve pain and render joints functional. These procedures have been successful just often enough to maintain surgical interest in joint replacement.

Degenerative arthritis of the knee joint is essentially a compartmental disease that may involve the lateral tibiofemoral, the medial tibiofemoral, or the patellofemoral articulations in any combination.[5] Involvement of the lateral or medial compartment often results in varus or valgus deformities. Over the years many forms of treatment have been used, with reasonable success in some patients and failure in others. Among the procedures that have been utilized in an attempt to correct the deformity, relieve the pain, and restore joint function are the following:

1. Proximal tibial osteotomy
2. Supracondylar osteotomy
3. Joint débridement
4. Synovectomy
5. Patellectomy
6. Loose body removal
7. Arthroplasties using interposing substances such as the following[3]:
    a. Metallic foil
    b. Pig bladder
    c. Plastic sheets of various types
    d. Fascia lata
    e. Skin

The normal knee joint is a ginglymoid diarthrodial joint that has a range of motion of approximately 145°. The range may extend from approximately 5° of hyperextension to approximately 140° of flexion. In addition the knee also has 10° to 15° of axial rotation. The knee, unlike the hip, depends on its ligaments for stability. It is common knowledge that lesions of the quadriceps mechanism hinder knee joint motion. Thus in knee joint replacement surgery, if a functioning arthroplasty is to result, the quadriceps mechanism must be capable of unrestricted function.

From 1958 through 1970 many reports appeared in the orthopaedic literature regarding the use of the high tibial osteotomy to correct the arthritic process.[4] Many of these reports indicate that when the procedure is properly selected good results can be anticipated in a large percentage of cases. The Mayo Clinic in particular reported extensive use of tibial osteotomy with reasonably good results.[1]

With further reference to high tibial osteotomy, it is generally conceded that a closing wedge osteotomy for a valgus deformity has rather limited use, as osteotomies on knees that have more than 10° to 15° of valgus deformity have not generally produced acceptable functioning knees.[4]

The osteotomies, however, that have been done for varus deformities of knees have generally given better results than the osteotomies done for valgus deformities. Insall states that a valgus osteotomy can be expected to give reasonably good results if the femorotibial angle is less than 190°.[5] On the other hand, this same osteotomy is contraindicated when the femorotibial angle is more than 195°.[5] He describes the femorotibial angle as the angle formed by the longitudinal axes of the femur and tibia at the lateral side of the knee.[5]

It has been stated that unicompartmental replacement of the knee joint is rarely indicated, as the criteria for unicompartmental replacement are often difficult to meet. Therefore bicompartmental replacement should be done in the average case. If one analyzes what high tibial osteotomies and the insertion of McKeever or MacIntosh prostheses accomplish, one will probably come to the conclusion that these procedures in essence are an attempt at a unicompartmental correction. As a matter of fact, the McKeever and MacIntosh procedures replace only one fourth of the knee joint, while the tibial osteotomies shift the weight to the opposite side of the arthritic half of the joint.

Among the procedures that have been used in compartmental replacement in a large series of cases are the sled system of Buchholz and that of Marmor. Each of these systems has produced many good, functioning, painless knees; however, each also has its own peculiar limitations. In the Marmor system sagging of the tibial component is definitely a possible complication; in the Buchholz not only is sagging possible but also fractures of the tibial plateaus may result at the time of the insertion of the system.

Most types of arthroplasties of the knee involve the use of metal-to-plastic nonhinged components. One of my first exposures to knee joint replacement took place at the Hospital for Special Surgery a few years ago when Frank Gunston presented his paper on this subject at one of the alumni meetings. His talk served to further stimulate our interest in joint replacement surgery of the knee. We thereafter visited Professor Hans Buchholz at the St. Georg Hospital in Hamburg, Germany, watching him do a few of his so-called St. Georg sled type of knee replacements. Many types of systems have since appeared in the literature, including the geometric, polycentric, UCI, HSS, and Marmor systems. These are all of the nonhinged variety. For the knee with gross instability many hinge-type systems have been devised, including the Lagrange, Young,[8] Waldius,[6] Letournel, Shiers, Buchholz, Herbert, Guepar, and spherocentric knees.

Since a large percentage of arthritic knees are affected on one side of the joint only, we decided to try to develop a system that could be used either for unicompartmental or bicompartmental purposes. We thought that if MacIntosh and McKeever prostheses and osteotomies relieved the pain and corrected the deformity to some degree, then unicondylar replacement of the knee joint should produce an even better result.

In view of the fact that many of our cases involved one compartment only, we could not bring ourselves to destroy the other nonarthritic or minimally arthritic compartment. Accordingly most of our patients received unicompartmental replacement only.

In developing such a system we concentrated on developing one in which the possibility of sagging of the tibial component or fracturing of one of the tibial condyles would be practically eliminated. This system has been in use at Rhode Island Hospital since January 16, 1972; since that time the operation has been done 178 times. These include both unicompartmental and bicompartmental procedures.

This chapter deals only with the unicompartmental cases.

The requisites for our nonhinged total knee replacement operation in every one of our cases have included most of the following:
1. Pain (with or without swelling)
2. Fairly good bone structure
3. Ligamentous stability
4. Medial or lateral knee compartment changes
5. Competent extensor mechanism

Uncorrectable instability usually requires use of hinged prostheses or even arthrodesis.[8]

The system that we have used has the following features:
1. Ease of insertion
2. Minimal removal of bone stock
3. Tibial component resting on peripheral cortical bone
4. Decreased chances of sagging of the tibial component
5. Some correction of valgus, varus, or flexion deformity
6. Correction of recurvatum when both compartments are involved
7. Versatility
8. Preservation of knee rotation
9. Reduction of the chances of improper insertion
10. Possibility of substitution of other systems in case of failure

The tibial components that we use come in three sizes: small, medium, and large. Each of these sizes comes in four different thicknesses, 6, 9, 12, and 15 mm. Custom-made sizes can be provided. By selection of the proper thickness of the tibial component, a certain amount of correction of varus or valgus is made possible.

The femoral runners come in two different sizes, 18 by 50 mm, and 18 by 60 mm. Correction of moderate or even severe varus or valgus deformity is definitely possible at times.

SURGICAL TECHNIQUE OF IMPLANTING SAVASTANO KNEE PROSTHESIS
Preoperative measures

Whenever possible, photographs should be taken of the entire leg in front and side views. In addition, anteroposterior and lateral x-ray films of the knee should also be taken with the patient supine and with the patient bearing weight. The x-ray films help the surgeon to determine the extent of the disease process and to formulate a plan for the surgery. The x-ray films and the photographs help in correcting valgus or varus deformity as well as extension or flexion deformity. The patient is begun on extensive quadriceps exercises for approximately 1 month prior to the operation.

The irrigating antibiotic solution that has been used at Rhode Island Hospital consists of bacitracin, 50,000 units in 500 ml sterile water. Suction and coagulating units should also be available at the time of surgery. A small bottle of sterile methylene blue should be included in every surgical setup and is used to mark the approximate area of placement of the femoral metallic runner.

The operation may be done with or without the aid of a pneumatic tourniquet. When calcification of the vessels of the extremity is present we do not recommend the use of a tourniquet; however, if no calcification of the vessels is present and pulsation in the popliteal and dorsalis pedis arteries is adequate, we do use a pneumatic tourniquet.

Skin incisions

One incision generally suffices for knee replacement. When only one component is to be replaced, either a straight or a parapatellar incision is used, depending on the component to be replaced. When both components of the joint are to be replaced, two incisions may be required; in certain circumstances only a long medial parapatellar incision is enough.

When two incisions are used the middle portion of the medial parapatellar incision is placed 1¼ inches from the medial border of the patella and the lateral parapatellar incision at least 2 inches from the lateral border of the patella. It is important not to place these two incisions too close together to avoid compromising the blood supply to the skin between the two incisions.

When a knee replacement operation is done in rheumatoid knees, it is usually advisable to do as clean a synovectomy of the knee joint as possible prior to the insertion of the implants. The patient is given 1 or 2 gm of cephalothin (Keflin) intravenously immediately prior to the operation, before the tourniquet is inflated.

Surgical procedure

Once the joint has been opened with a medial or lateral parapatellar incision or both, the knee joint is flexed and inspected and then appropriately prepared for the procedure. A tibial template is inserted into the flexed joint to determine the approximate working space on each side of the knee joint. The tibial plateau is prepared first. If the medial half of the joint is to be replaced, a reciprocating power saw is used to level off the medial tibial plateau. Once this has been done, a trial tibial component is inserted for size and the knee is flexed and extended to determine the working space available. At this point it may become necessary to remove a portion of the non-weight-bearing posterior aspect of the femoral condyle. This can easily be done with a curved osteotome with the knee in as much flexion as possible. It may become necessary to remove ¼ to ½ inch of the posterior femoral condyle.

If the four components of the knee joint are to be replaced, the lateral side of the joint is treated in a similar manner. At times, to get better exposure of the articular surfaces, a laminar spreader is placed between the intercondylar notch and the middle of the tibial plateau.

The tibial template is now placed flat on the tibial plateau and the slot in the tibial template is traced with methylene blue. The opening in the tibial template is 1 inch long and ⅜ inch in width. The area that has been marked on the medial side of the tibial plateau with the methylene blue is now removed with a burr or with a narrow osteotome to a depth of ½ inch and the edges are undermined. This opening is made to receive the keel on the bottom surface of the plastic tibial component.

Femoral preparation

The femoral template is now placed over the middle of the femoral condyle, and the femoral template is traced on the condyle with methylene blue. Drill holes ⅜ inch in diameter are made into the femoral condyle through the holes in the femoral template. These holes accommodate the studs that protrude from the undersurface of the femoral component.

A trial femoral component is tried for size and for proper location on the femoral condyle. If the holes to house the studs are not large enough or are not properly placed, they may be enlarged or their position may be altered with a power dental burr. Once the trial femoral prosthesis has been properly placed, a trial tibial prosthesis is inserted on the plateau of the tibia. The knee is now flexed and extended to check for proper positioning of the femoral runner on the tibial plateau and proper height of the tibial plateau as it pertains to the correction of preexisting varus or valgus deformities.

Final seating

The two openings made into the femoral condyle are undermined and connected, leaving the cortical cartilaginous division between the two holes intact. Once this has been done, methyl methacrylate is prepared; when it is of the proper consistency it is placed into the openings in the femoral condyle and the previously selected femoral component is inserted, tapped firmly into place with a special driver, and held in place until the cement hardens. The joint is carefully irrigated with an antibiotic solution and every particle of cement or debris is removed.

In the placement of the tibial component, methyl methacrylate is prepared; when it becomes of proper consistency it is placed into the cavity on the top of the tibial plateau, and the previously selected tibial component is inserted. The knee is now fully extended and an attempt is made to correct any valgus or varus deformity. The joint is thoroughly irrigated.

The knee joint is flexed and extended several times prior to beginning of closure to be sure that the joint is mechanically stable and that the tibial and femoral components are working smoothly.

The final femoral and tibial components may be inserted simultaneously.

If a tourniquet has been used, it is now removed and any bleeding is appropriately controlled. The wound is again carefully and thoroughly irrigated and closure is begun. If the synovial membrane is still present, it is closed with continuous 3-0 chromic catgut. The medial and all lateral expansions are closed with No. 1 interrupted chromic catgut sutures, the subcutaneous tissue is closed with 3-0 plain catgut, and the skin is closed with 3-0 black silk. The entire leg is wrapped in wadding and a posterior long leg plaster splint is applied. A Hemovac is inserted prior to closure, to be removed 24 to 48 hours later.

Postoperative care

The patient is returned to his room with instructions for the leg to be elevated. Intravenous cephalothin is continued for the next 3 days in an average dosage of 4 gm in 24 hours. When the intravenous cephalothin is discontinued the patient is given cephalothin by mouth for an additional 5 to 6 days. He is encouraged to do straight leg raising and quadriceps exercises as soon after the operation as pain permits. The plaster splint is removed 3 to 4 days following the operation and the patient is encouraged to continue the exercises that he learned preoperatively. On the fourth or fifth day the patient begins to try to bend and straighten the knee. On the fifth or sixth day the patient is allowed to stand with full weight bearing with the help of an assistant or a walker. On the sixth or seventh day he begins walking and continues to try to bend and straighten his knee. Thereafter he is sent to the physical therapy department for intensive physical therapy. The sutures are removed 10 to 14 days following the surgery. The patient is discharged with full weight bearing using Canadian or conventional crutches on or about the fourteenth day postoperatively.

The following is a statistical analysis of our first 100 successive cases, excluding only 13 done on the opposite knee at the request of the patient. All of the cases presented were done at least six months prior to evaluation. Of the total number of operations, 56 were done by one of us (A. A. S.), 35 by the other (V. A. Z.), and 9 by residents.

STATISTICAL ANALYSIS

Number of cases

Private	91
Service	9

Indications for replacement

Osteoarthritis	77
Rheumatoid arthritis	17
Traumatic arthritis (fractures)	1
Mixed arthritis	1
Failed MacIntosh prosthesis	2
Failed McKeever prosthesis	2

Patient population

	Female	Male
Number of patients	84	16
Age		
Oldest	82	69
Youngest	55	51
Mean	70.26	57.12
Knee affected		
Left	38	8
Right	46	8

Side of knee affected

	Female	Male
Lateral	30	0
Medial	54	16

Use of supports

	Preoperative	Postoperative
1 cane	38	2
2 canes	10	2 (1 cane)
Canadian crutches	6	2 (1 cane)
Walkerette	6	3 (1 cane)
No support	40	No support

Previous surgery

Previous internal meniscectomies	5
Previous house cleaning procedures	2

Complications

Wound seepage	1
Phlebitis	0
Embolism	0
Worn out tibial component	None in this series
Patellar impingement	0
Loosening or sagging	None so far
Deaths	2

Grading

Excellent: No pain, no crutches or canes, full exetnsion and with flexion to 90° or more, no residual deformity

Good: Mild pain on moderate activity, no canes or crutches, very mild varus or valgus deformity with flexion to 90° or better, extension complete

Fair: Mild, constant discomfort with use of cane, retained deformity, flexion less than 60° to 90°, extension complete

Poor: Severe pain, use of crutch or cane, flexion less than 60°, infection

Results

Excellent	40%
Good	50%
Fair	9%
Poor	1%

CASE REPORTS

Case 1. A 68-year-old woman sustained a comminuted depressed fracture of the outer tibial plateau of the left knee, which was treated with open reduction and internal fixation with a bar bolt 6 years prior to the unicondylar knee replacement operation. See Fig. 21-1.

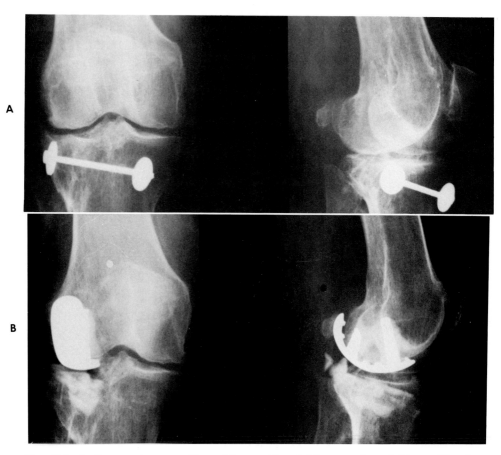

A

B

Fig. 21-1. A, Preoperative x-ray films of knee with painful traumatic arthritis resulting from comminuted depressed fracture of lateral tibial plateau treated with open reduction with fixation using Barr bolt. **B,** Postoperative x-ray films showing replacement components in place. **C,** Degree of active extension 9 months postoperatively. **D,** Degree of flexion 9 months postoperatively.

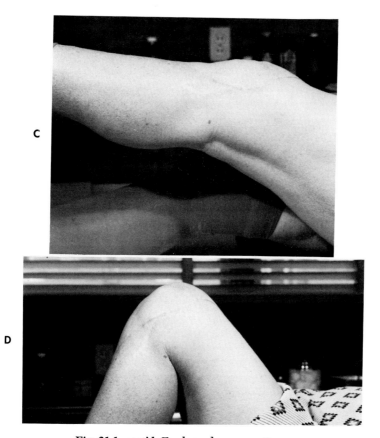

Fig. 21-1, cont'd. For legend see opposite page.

Case 2. A 69-year-old woman complained of pain in the right knee of 1½ years' duration. A unicondylar knee replacement operation was done on the medial half of the knee. See Fig. 21-2.

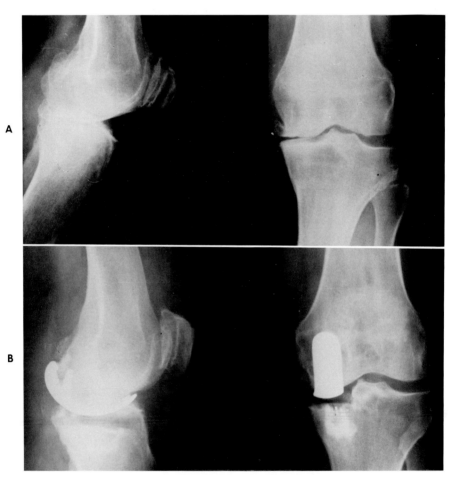

Fig. 21-2. **A,** Preoperative x-ray films showing narrowed painful osteoarthritis in medial half of knee joint. **B,** Postoperative x-ray films showing medial half replacement components in place. **C,** Degree of extension 4 months postoperatively. **D,** Degree of flexion 4 months postoperatively.

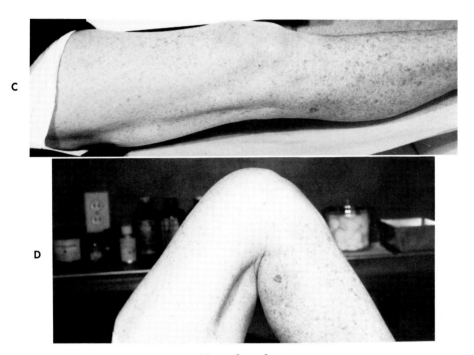

Fig. 21-2, cont'd. For legend see opposite page.

CONCLUSION

We think that unicompartmental replacement is definitely indicated when only one compartment of the knee joint is diseased. Thirteen of our patients were so pleased with the operation done in one compartment of one knee that they requested that the opposite knee also undergo the same procedure; results were equally good.

The principal features of the system that we use are that the tibial component rests on peripheral cortical bone, which renders the possibility of sagging quite remote. Other features include the preservation of rotation of the knee, correction to some degree of deformities of the knee, and versatility of the system.

References

1. Coventry, M. B., et al.: Geometric total knee arthroplasty. II. Patient data and complications, Clin. Orthop. **94**:177, 1973.
2. Peterson, L. F. A., Bryan, R. S., and Combs, J. J., Jr.: Surgery for arthritis of the knee, Bull. Rheum. Dis. **25**:794, 1974-75.
3. Potter, T. A.: Arthroplasty of the knee with tibial metallic implants of the McKeever and MacIntosh design, Surg. Clin. North Am. **49**:903, 1969.
4. Shoji, H., and Insall, J.: High tibial osteotomy for osteoarthritis with valgus deformity, J. Bone Joint Surg. **55-A**:963, 1973.
5. Walker, P. S., Insall, J., Ranawat, C. S., and Shoji, H.: Total knee prosthesis: bio-engineering principles and clinical applications, scientific exhibit of annual meeting, American Academy of Orthopaedic Surgeons, Las Vegas, January, 1973.
6. Walldius, B.: Arthroplasty of the knee using an endoprosthesis: 8 years' experience, Acta Orthop. Scand. **30**:137, 1960.
7. Wilson, F. C.: Total replacement of the knee in rheumatoid arthritis: part II of a prospective study, Clin. Orthop. **94**:58, 1973.
8. Young, H. H.: Use of a hinged Vitallium prosthesis for arthroplasty of the knee: a preliminary report, J. Bone Joint Surg. **45-A**:1627, 1963.

22. Variable axis total knee prosthesis: design considerations, testing, and clinical experience

David G. Murray
James A. Shaw

DESIGN

Of the total knee prostheses currently available from orthopaedic suppliers, most can be classified as either a hinge or a condylar replacement. Although satisfactory results have been reported in the literature for reconstruction procedures incorporating both types of prostheses, compelling criticisms have been published as well. Two particularly cogent critiques are reprinted here:

> Hinge devices, Walldius, Young, Shiers, etc., replace both the femoral and tibial articular surface and possess great intrinsic stability. However, unlike a normal knee, mechanical hinges allow no motion in the frontal plane (abduction-adduction) and no torsional motion. Therefore, forces which tend to produce torsion or abduction-adduction, are transmitted, without damping, to the implant-bone interface where they contribute to loosening and bone resorption. The hinge knees all incorporate metal to metal stops which generate high peaking impact loads at the termination of flexion and extension. Impact loads significantly contribute to implant-bone interface breakdown which is likely a factor in postoperative implant failure, pain, limitation of motion, and infection. . . .

> [Condylar replacement] is used to describe the several designs of tibiofemoral replacement which reproduce, with varying closeness, the shapes of the femoral and tibial condyles and the menisci, and which enable both the collateral and the cruciate ligaments to be preserved. This approach was tried by the authors in 1969, but was discarded because (a) a prosthesis of this type does not lend itself to the use of alignment guides which are highly desirable, if not essential, if accurate alignment is to be obtained; (b) in many knees with flexion contractures the load bearing tibial condyles have collapsed, leaving the intercondylar eminence of the tibial interfering mechanically with the intercondylar notch of the femur in such a way as to require its removal before full extension can be obtained; (c) division of soft tissues in the intercondylar notch is frequently required to increase the range of flexion in a previously stiff knee; and (d) the cruciate ligaments, were frequently found to be of doubtful mechanical effectiveness.[*]

---

[*]From Freeman, M. A. R., Swanson, S. A. V., and Todd, R. C.: Clin. Orthop. 94:155, 1973.

In general agreement with these authors we have attempted to develop a total knee prosthesis that would provide a maximum capability for replacing severely impaired joints and at the same time minimize the incidence of failure through loosening.

Design objectives

The design characteristics of an ideal total knee prosthesis have been presented by many authors over the past few years. We have selected the following criteria as being most critical in a successful implant design.

1. A knee prosthesis should be designed so as not to exclude a salvage procedure. Since an arthrodesis appears to be the most viable way (short of amputation) of arresting a chronic infection secondary to prosthesis implantation, a knee prosthesis should require no more bone removal than would be acceptable for a primary arthrodesis.
2. Prosthesis materials should be compatible with the intra-articular environment, and debris production under physiologic loads should be minimal and innocuous.
3. The prosthesis should allow an unrestricted range of motion in the sagittal plane from full extension to at least 130° of flexion.
4. The axis of rotation in the sagittal plane should represent an anatomic average. This affords the appropriate mechanical advantage to the quadriceps muscles and allows physiologic gait patterns.
5. A wide range of abnormal knee joint configurations, including varus, valgus, and flexion deformities, should be correctable with the knee prosthesis.
6. Large, flat prosthesis-bone contact areas should be incorporated in the prosthesis design. In support of this concept, Walker and Shoji[7] cite a tenfold decrease in the compressive strength of trabecular bone during disease states. Since the forces carried by the articulating surfaces of the knee are large, even during normal activity,[4] one can predict sinking or shifting of the prosthesis components if large load-bearing areas are not provided.
7. Limitations to extension should ultimately be under muscular, ligamentous, and capsular control. Use of passive stops characteristic of hinge joints can generate high impact loads, leading to fatigue of metal components and breakdown of the bone-joint interface.
8. The prosthesis should exhibit inherent stability and should resist translational forces in the anteroposterior and lateral-medial directions. Dependence on the cruciate ligaments for anteroposterior stability or for correct functioning of the prosthesis should not be necessary. Cruciate ligaments in knees in which prosthetic replacement is justifiable are often absent or degenerated. Moreover, replacement of normal knee joint surfaces (which are characterized by changing radii of curvature) with surfaces of con-

stant curvature or "approximates" to normal curvature would significantly compromise the function of the cruciates.

9. The femoral and tibial components should be unconstrained relative to each other to the extent that excessive twisting or abduction-adduction forces are not transmitted to the interface between the cement and the bone.

10. In the interest of fixation, short intramedullary stems should be part of both femoral and tibial components. In addition to enhancing fixation, these stems provide some protection against subsequent fracture adjacent to the prosthesis during manipulation or incidental trauma.

11. Since significant symptoms are traceable to abnormalities in the patello-femoral articulation, the patellar surface of the femur should be resurfaced in addition to the tibial surface. This allows for patellar resurfacing concurrently or later if indicated.

12. The prosthesis should be compatible with a standard insertion procedure that can be performed reliably by general orthopaedic surgeons.

Prosthesis description

The variable axis prosthesis is shown in Figs. 22-1 and 22-2. As can be seen, the prosthesis is a three-component system, consisting of chromium-cobalt femoral and tibial components and a removable high-density polyethylene (HDP) tibial insert. One prosthesis is used for both left and right knees.

The prosthesis features a modified ball-and-socket joint, with the ball on the femoral component and the socket in the HDP insert on the tibial side. The axis of rotation in the sagittal plane is located at the center of the spheric portion of the femoral component, at what we consider an average anatomic position. This allws normal gait and good mechanical advantage for the quadriceps muscles. The posterior portion of the sphere has been removed to eliminate interference with the posterior capsule and to facilitate insertion of the tibial surface.

The articulation of the ball and socket provides the anteroposterior stability of the cruciate ligaments and the lateral-medial stability of the tibial spine. No constraint is provided to rotation about the long axis. Torsional loads are carried by the collateral ligaments, joint capsule, and surrounding musculature, not by the prosthesis. The probability of loosening of either component is therefore significantly reduced.

On either side of the spheric portion of the femoral component are intersecting cylindric surfaces. These surfaces articulate with the top of the polyethylene insert, providing inherent stability to the joint without recourse to mechanical linkages between the components. Anteriorly the cylindric surfaces blend into a flat surface to provide an intrinsically stable "stop" at 3° of hyperextension. Although the prosthesis provides some resistance to valgus-varus stress, it should be noted that ultimately forces of abduction-adduction or hyperextension are resisted

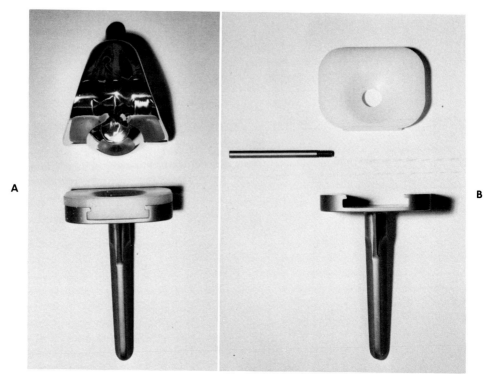

Fig. 22-1. A, Assembled prosthesis. B, Tibial components disassembled.

by the collateral ligaments, joint capsule, and surrounding musculature, not by the prosthesis.

The prosthesis features large, flat bearing surfaces to distribute loads over maximal areas of the tibia and femur. Insertion requires approximately 1.8 cm of bone removal and is therefore compatible with arthrodesis as a salvage procedure. (It should be noted that, as with other prostheses, the actual amount of bone removed depends not only on the thickness of the assembled device but also on such factors as fixed flexion contracture, ligament length, and previous surgery.) Short medullary stems on both the tibial and femoral components improve fixation and aid in insertion. A patellar flange on the femoral component is provided for resurfacing the patellofemoral articulation. Patellar resurfacing with an available prosthesis is optional.

As mentioned previously, the prosthesis is a three-component system having a removable HDP tibial insert that articulates with the femoral component. The insert fits into a T slot in the tibial component at the anterior edge and is pushed posteriorly until the anteroposterior taper of the slot prevents further posterior displacement. A transverse retaining screw pevents anterior motion of the insert following its insertion into the tibial component.

The tibial inserts are available in three thicknesses and in elevated right and

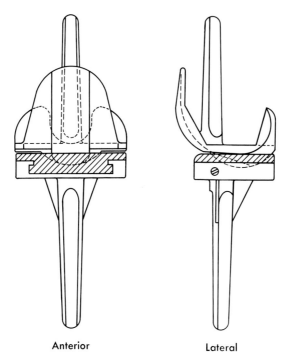

Anterior   Lateral

Fig. 22-2. Line drawing of variable axis prosthesis showing anterior, lateral-medial, and posterior views. Cross-hatched areas represent removable high-density polyethylene (HDP) insert.

elevated left models. This variety allows the prosthesis to be tailored to the individual after the metallic components are fixed in the tibia and femur. (Prescription inserts are, of course, a possibility if the standard inserts are not appropriate for the particular knee.) Moreover, in the event that postoperative adjustments are called for, or excessive wear of the polyethylene dictates reoperation, the tibial inserts can be removed and replaced without disturbing either metalic component. This obviously reduces potential trauma to the patient.

LABORATORY EVALUATION
Simulator testing

An extensive program of laboratory evaluation was carried out on the variable axis prosthesis prior to its clinical use. A knee joint simulator[6] was built to test the prosthesis as well as other prostheses currently available from orthopaedic suppliers. The simulator with its accompanying force measurement instrumentation is shown in Fig. 22-3.

The simulator was designed to test the knee prosthesis under dynamic conditions similar to the in vivo loading environment. The prostheses tested were implanted in cadaver joints, using the recommended jigs and fixtures, and

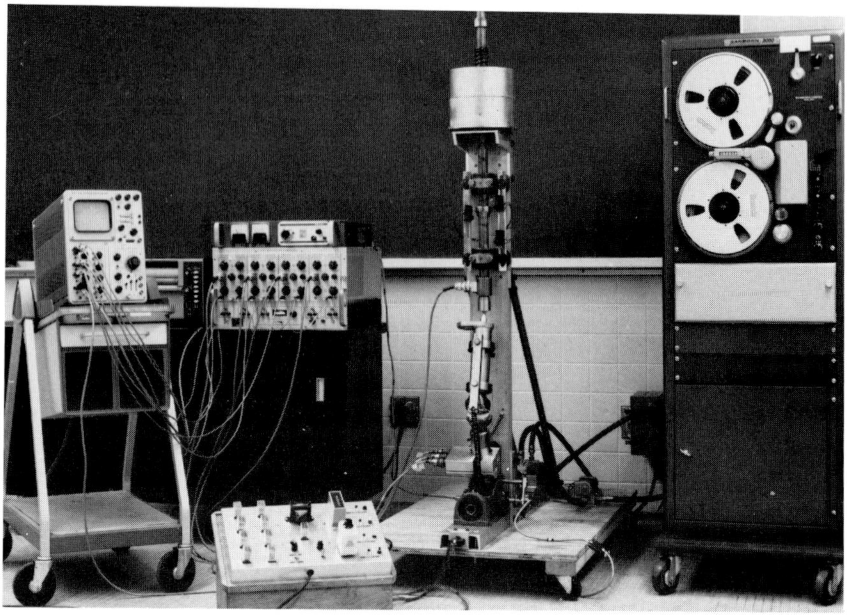

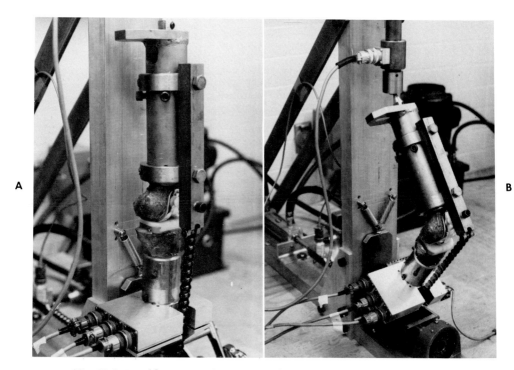

Fig. 22-3. Knee joint simulator with accompanying force measurement instrumentation.

A

B

Fig. 22-4. Variable axis prosthesis mounted in cylindric pots of knee simulator.

mounted in the cylindric pots of the simulator as shown in Fig. 22-4. Polymethyl methacrylate was used for prosthesis fixation in all cases. All joints were wrapped in a compress moistened with 2% phenol to keep the surrounding soft tissue pliable. No attempt was made to lubricate the bearing surfaces, although fluid accumulated on them from the moistened compresses and tissue leaching.

A hydraulic cylinder, simulating the quadriceps muscles, controlled extension and flexion of the test knees. Force was transmitted across the test joints by a roller chain attached to the femoral pot at one end and the cylinder at the other. Tightening of the chain by the cylinder extended the joints in a physiologic fashion. Similarly slackening of the chain allowed the knees to flex by gravity.

The active extension and flexion of the test knees raised and lowered a mass (150 pounds) located at the top of the simulator (Fig. 22-3). Depending on the test setup, this mass, representing the body weight, could be carried by the knee throughout the entire cycle of flexion and extension or any portion thereof. Since normal gait requires that the knee support the body mass during the stance phase only, and since the knee normally flexes up to 20° as the body moves over the supportive limb and then extends obliquely backward as the body moves forward, the laboratory evaluation was carried out with the test knees carrying the "body mass" through 20° of flexion and extension only. As flexion proceeded beyond 20°, the weights were unloaded on the supportive structure located at the top of the simulator and therefore did not contribute to joint loading. Con-

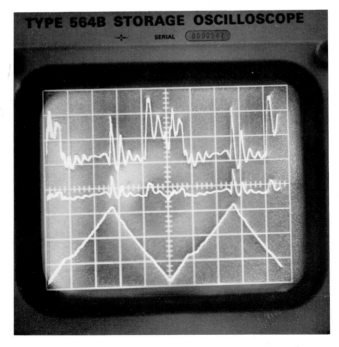

Fig. 22-5. Typical output from force transducers monitoring joint loading. See text for discussion.

tinued flexion to approximately 60° of flexion simulated the "swing" phase of the normal gait cycle.

Fig. 22-5 shows a typical output from the force transducers monitoring joint loading. The bottom tracing indicates the angle of flexion, with each major division representing approximately 20°. The top tracing indicates the compressive loads (normal to the tibial plateau) on the prosthesis, and the middle trace represents the anteroposterior directed loads. Peak compressive loads of approximately 300 pounds were found for most joints, although some variation was caused by the different joint geometries and the resulting differences in mechanical advantage offered to the quadriceps mechanism. The maximum compressive loads occurred during the stance phase (0° to 20° of flexion) when the knees were carrying the "body weight," with additional peaks occurring at the initiation of the swing phase. Peak posteriorly directed loads of approximately 100 pounds, occurring at the initiation of the swing phase, were also found for most prostheses.

Since the tibial pot was free to swing in a lateral or medial direction as well as in the sagittal plane and since the femoral pot was constrained only by a ball-and-socket joint at the proximal end, any instability that developed from material wear or loss of fixation could be readily observed. Instability, wear of articulating surfaces, loosening of components, and mechanical failure all represented modes of failure that were directly observable through the use of the simulator.

Results. In addition to the variable axis prosthesis, four other types of knee joint prostheses were tested: the geometric, Walldius, polycentric, and Herbert prostheses. Each represented a unique concept in knee joint design and, through a testing program incorporating such designs, we were able to substantiate the validity of most of the design criteria listed previously. A summary of the results is given in Table 22-1.

The geometric prosthesis was the first tested. It ran for a total of 4,600,000

Table 22-1. Knee joint simulator test results

Prosthesis	Cycles tested	Estimated life expectancy	Mode of failure
Geometric	4,600,000	4.2 years	Loss of fixation of tibial component at cement-bone interface
Walldius	2,800,000	2.5 years	Loss of fixation of femoral component at prosthesis-cement interface
Polycentric	200,000	0.2 years	Inherent instability
Variable axis	11,500,000	10+ years	No failure
Herbert			
No. 1	1,300,000	1.2 years	Wear-related instability
No. 2	900,000	0.8 years	Fracture of femoral component

*Based on an estimate by Seedham et al.[5] that a typical arthroplasty patient undertakes 3,000 walking cycles per day.

cycles before failing because of gross loosening of the tibial component at the bone-cement interface. No loosening at the prosthesis-cement interface or wear of articulating surfaces was noted. Based on an estimate by Seedham et al.[5] that a typical arthroplasty patient undertakes 3,000 walking cycles per day, this figure represents slightly more than 4 years of clinical use.

The Walldius prosthesis, representing the fixed-hinge type of knee joint prosthesis, failed at 2,800,000 cycles when the femoral component broke loose from the bone. As with the geometric knee, primary failure was at the bone-cement interface. The mass of cement surrounding the femoral stem loosened. With continued cycling a toggle developed, which eventually led to splitting of the distal femur.

A fixed-hinge prosthesis transmits all torsional, bending, and impact loads directly to the bone-cement interface. Considering the magnitude of the forces characteristic of normal activity,[4] it is not surprising to find this type of failure of a hinged prosthesis in spite of improved fixation with stems.

This cycle time for the Walldius prosthesis represents approximately 2.5 years of use. Evidence of wear on the pin joining the tibial and femoral component was present but minor. The total weight loss was insignificant and could not be determined with any precision.

Simulator testing of the polycentric prosthesis proved totally unsatisfactory, in part because of the extreme difficulty encountered in implanting the prosthesis correctly. Arranging the four components so that the loads were distributed equally on the lateral and medial sides, or so that excessive stresses were not imposed on ligamentous structures, was a formidable task.

Two polycentric prostheses were tested in the simulator. Both proved so unstable under the conditions of laboratory testing that within short periods of time they exceeded the capacity of the simulator to accommodate varus or valgus deformity (approximately 30° of varus or valgus deformity). At this point the tests were stopped.

The greatest cycle time achieved for the polycentric prosthesis was 200,000 cycles. During this short time, no wear or loosening of the components was noted, as might be expected with such small load-bearing areas.

The variable axis prosthesis proved to be quite durable under the conditions of simulator testing. The prosthesis ran for 11,500,000 cycles with no evidence of failure. At this point the prosthesis was removed from the simulator to allow continued testing of other prostheses. Over this testing period, representing almost 200 days of continuous simulator cycling, roughly equivalent to 10 years of projected clinical use, there was no evidence of fixation loss, no loosening of the tibial plateau retaining screw, and little evidence of wear.

Two Herbert prostheses were tested in the simulator. The Herbert prosthesis consists of a ball-and-socket joint constrained to swing in the sagittal plane by a trapezoidal neck on the tibial component and a mating femoral slot. The sides of the femoral slot serve as guiding walls for the tibial component, limiting undesired motion by impinging on the neck of the tibial component. Some lateral-medial motion and axial rotation is made possible, however, by built-in dimensional differences between the slot in the femoral component and the tibial neck. This feature is intended to make the range of motion more physiologic.

The first Herbert prosthesis was removed from the simulator after 1,300,000

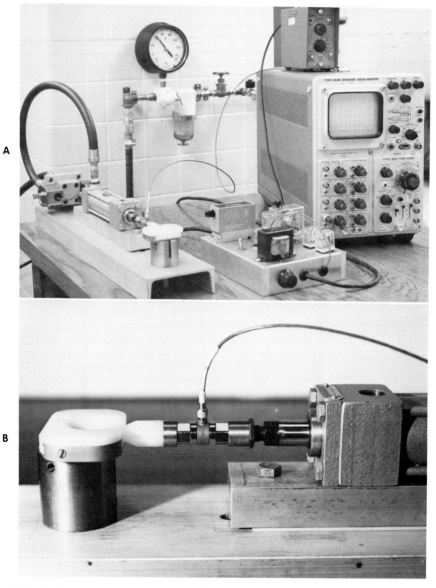

Fig. 22-6. A, Transverse retaining screw fatigue test apparatus and force measurement instrumentation. **B,** Transverse retaining screw fatigue test apparatus showing application of load to posterior edge of tibial insert.

cycles for inspection. The total lateral-medial laxity had increased markedly (from 6° to 17.5°) and fixation problems were suspected. On removal it was found that the decrease in the medial-lateral stability was caused primarily by major metallic wear along the inferior femoral slot and tibial neck.

A second Herbert prosthesis was tested for further examination of wear-related instability. The prosthesis ran for 900,000 cycles with continuously increasing instability and eventually failed because of fatigue fracture of the femoral component on the medial side. The fracture started at the top of the anterior recess and proceeded posteriorly toward the top of the posterior recess. The fracture was accompanied by considerable wear on the posteromedial post of the tibial component and medial wall of the femoral slot.

Although the Herbert prosthesis allows some lateral and torsional motion, these displacements are ultimately limited by the prosthesis itself, in part by gliding metal-to-metal restraint, not by soft tissue. Since limitation of these motions by the prosthesis must be done against large mechanical advantages (much like trying to lift a large weight with the short end of a long lever), enormous loads are carried by the prosthesis. As demonstrated by the simulator, the result may be excessive wear with the creation of metallic debris and joint instability, as well as early failure of metallic components.

Fatigue testing

In addition to the simulator testing program, an apparatus was built to fatigue test the transverse retaining screw of the variable axis prosthesis. This apparatus is shown in Fig. 22-6. The retaining screw prevents anterior displacement of the tibial insert after it has been inserted into the tibial component. Posteriorly directed loads are carried by the tapered walls of the tibial component T slot and therefore do not affect the retaining screw.

Based on the work of Morrison, Jones[2] has estimated that an anteriorly directed load of 35 pounds should be considered in the design of knee joint prostheses. Based on this estimate, a cyclic pulse load of 50 pounds magnitude and 0.5 second duration was applied to the tibial plateau in an anterior direction (Fig. 22-6, *B*). A Kistler load cell was used for force measurements. After 12,000,000 cycles the testing was discontinued with no evidence of loosening or fatigue failure of the retaining screw.

SURGICAL TECHNIQUE

The design of the variable axis prosthesis takes into consideration the desirability of simplified insertion. The basic steps are two parallel cuts, the first made across the tibial articular surface perpendicular to an imaginary line between the anterior tibial spine and the midpoint of the ankle joint. The second cut is made across the distal end of the femur parallel to the tibial cut with the knee in full extension and properly aligned. No more than 5 mm of bone should be removed from the proximal end of the tibia. The amount of bone to be removed from the distal femur is varied to accommodate the thickness of the prosthesis. All other cuts are developed from these two with the aid of jigs.

Instruments for insertion include the standard osteotomes, saws, etc. of the surgeon's choice. Special instruments consist of a spacing block notched anteriorly to accommodate a stem locator and drilled on the anterior face to accept an adjusting handle. A femoral shaping jig determines the final cuts on the femur and a rotational guide is used to assist with proper alignment of the jig about the longitudinal axis of the femur. The prosthetic components are seated with a standard femoral prosthesis driver and the slotted locking screw can be set with any screwdriver of the appropriate size and diameter.

The surgical procedure is performed through a medial parapatellar incision with tourniquet control of blood flow. The patella is displaced laterally and the joint flexed to 90°. Redundant soft tissue, infrapatellar fat pad, menisci, cruciate ligaments, and synovial tissue are debrided. As a rule, a limited rather than total synovectomy is carried out.

When the tibial plateau can be well visualized, and with the knee in 90° of flexion, the articular surface is removed by a saw cut perpendicular to the long axis of the tibia. The thickness of the bone removed should be no greater than 5 mm to ensure subsequent stability of the prosthesis in flexion. Existing bony deformities such as central or marginal depression of a plateau can be ignored and filled in later with cement under the tibial component.

After removal of the tibial articular surface, the knee is extended and proper alignment can generally be achieved by simple longitudinal traction on the foot. The spacing block is applied to the joint with the inferior edge parallel to the cut surface of the tibia. The superior edge is then used as a guide to mark the femur for the second cut. The distal end of the femur is removed by cutting along this line, parallel to the tibial cut with the knee in extension and properly aligned. (The cut can be made three quarters of the way through from front to back with the knee extended and completed by osteotome with the knee flexed to avoid damage to popliteal structures.) After removal of the distal articular surface of the femur in this manner, the spacing block should fit snugly into the interval between the femur and tibia with the leg in full extension, properly aligned, and stable. If these conditions are not met, the original cuts can be revised until they are. The success of the rest of the procedure depends on a satisfactory fit at this point. If it appears that the fit is unstable because of inadvertent removal of too much bone, this slack can be taken up later by the use of a thick tibial insert, providing that the other criteria are met.

The marker for the stem sites is inserted into the notch in the spacing block and tapped against the femur and tibia alternately to leave an indentation as an indicator for drilling holes for the stems. The spacing block is removed and the knee flexed to inspect the marks for placing stems. These should be centrally located from side to side, somewhat anteriorly placed on the tibia and more posteriorly oriented on the femur. Using these guidelines, holes are drilled in the respective bones, perpendicular to the cut surfaces. The hole in the tibia can be immediately enlarged to accommodate the stem and flanges of the tibial component. The hole in the femur is enlarged to accommodate the femoral shaping jig, which is seated at this point.

With the femoral shaping jig in place and the knee flexed, the posterior condyles are removed along the line indicated by the jig. The jig is removed, débridement of the posterior part of the joint is completed, and the tibial component is inserted provisionally without cement. A standard plateau insert is placed into the slot of the tibial component.

The appropriate orientation for the femoral component is determined by inserting the rotation guide into the femur and articulating the joint. This device can be adjusted until flexion and extension occur smoothly, at which point the anterior edges of the guide are marked on the femur. The guide is removed and the shaping jig reapplied with the anterior edges aligned with these marks. The remainder of the shaping of the distal femur is completed as indicated by the jig.

Once the distal end of the femur is shaped, the femoral component is seated provisionally and the joint articulated once again. The joint should be stable and should come easily to full extension. If a residual flexion contracture exists, this may be corrected by removal of more bone from the femur. The patellar flange of the femoral component should be flush against the anterior cortex of the femur (Fig. 22-7).

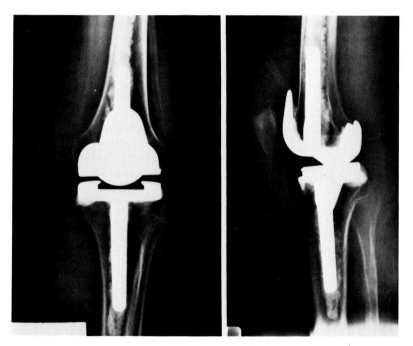

Fig. 22-7. X-ray films showing alignment of inserted prosthesis. Anterior flange is parallel to anterior cortical surface of femur. Ideally, flange should lie against cortical bone.

When the provisional seating is acceptable, all components are removed and reseated with cement, first the tibial component and then the femoral. Excess cement can easily be removed from posterior recesses prior to inserting the tibial articular surface.

If alignment or stability problems are encountered in this final phase, adjustments can be made by selecting a plateau of different thickness or one properly angled to compensate for valgus or varus deformity. The final step is insertion of the locking screw.

The patella may require trimming if there is an inferior beak that impinges on the central sphere of the femoral component in flexion. Alternatively the patella can be resurfaced using one of several commercially available prostheses.

The tourniquet may or may not be released prior to closure. A suction drain is left in the joint and a bulky compression dressing is applied with splints to limit motion.

Postoperatively the patient is encouraged to walk with as much weight as tolerated on the involved leg. The dressing is removed in 10 days and active and passive motion begun. If the range of flexion does not approach 70° by 1 week, the knee is manipulated.

RESULTS

The initial series of cases is composed of 67 patients who have had a total of 80 knee replacements. Thirty-eight patients (47 knees) had rheumatoid arthritis, 28 (32 knees) had degenerative arthritis, and 1 had posttraumatic arthritis. The indications used in determining the need for surgery and the contraindications that have emerged with experience in implanting the device are as follows:

Indications
1. Knee pain with the following diagnoses:
    a. Rheumatoid arthritis
    b. Degenerative arthritis
    c. Posttraumatic arthritis
    d. Hemophiliac arthritis
2. Limited motion
3. Flexion contractures with joint destruction

Contraindications
1. Septic arthritis
2. Surgical arthrodesis
3. Flexion contracture greater than 60°
4. Valgus or varus malalignment greater than 30°

The maximum length of follow-up has been 2 years and the minimum 2 months, with an average of 1 year. Results therefore are not long-term and must be considered as interim in nature. The following complications were noted:

Complication	Number
Deep infection	2
Peroneal palsy	1
Stiffness	1
Subluxation	2
Manipulation	10
Instability	1
Delayed wound healing	4
Patellar pain	4

Range of motion. The range of flexion as measured at the time of the most recent examination was between 40° and 110°, with an average ·between 80° and 90°. In one case the patient had significantly less motion than before the operation and was dissatisfied with the outcome on this basis. Review failed to reveal the cause of restriction other than dense scar tissue formation. The range of extension was from 5° hyperextension to 20° of residual flexion contracture (in one case), with an average of 5° flexion contracture. One patient was unhappy because of residual flexion contracture; review indicated that a preoperative contracture of 45° had been insufficiently corrected. Overall the average range of motion was 5° to 90°, and patients were generally satisfied with the degree of mobility.

Stability. With one exception the knees were stable in an extended weight-bearing state. The exception was a case in which a 60° valgus deformity was incompletely corrected and the residual 20° valgus deformity was unstable.

In two cases the knees were unstable in flexion. Both were characterized by a tendency for the tibia to sublux posteriorly on the femur when the patient contracted the hamstrings while the knee was flexed. This was not troublesome for one patient; the other required reoperation with insertion of a thicker tibial plateau to take up the slack; this corrected the problem.

Patellar pain. None of the cases in this series involved patellar resurfacing as an adjunct to knee replacement. Four patients complained spontaneously of postoperative retropatellar pain. Approximately half of the patients would admit to some retropatellar discomfort, which they did not find disabling or which they could at least accommodate to without limitation. Review of cases failed to reveal any consistent causes for persistent patellofemoral pain.

Loosening. There were no signs of loosening, either radiologic or clinical, encountered in this series.

Surgical complications. There were two cases of deep infection, which were manifest at approximately 3 months after surgery. One of these patients had a history of drainage from a staple site at a previous osteotomy. Both were treated by débridement and irrigation with antibiotics, leaving the prosthesis in place. One patient continues to do well; the other has persistent pain without drainage and with sterile joint aspirant. Delayed wound healing occurred in four patients, with no significant sequelae. Peroneal palsy occurred in one case on the second postoperative day, with incomplete recovery. No cases of clinically evident thrombophlebitis or pulmonary embolism were demonstrated.

Reoperation. In the series of 80 knees, seven secondary procedures were performed on 4 knees. The reasons for reoperation were as follows:

Reason	Number
Infection	2
Subluxation	1
Stiffness (1 patient)	3
Removal locking pin	1
Patellectomy	1

Summary of results. As of this report, all prostheses remain in place and all patients are ambulatory. Four procedures in four patients are considered failures. These include one patient with deep infection and persistent pain, one with a residual 20° flexion contracture and pain, one with flexion limited to 40°, and one with a residual 20° valgus deformity and instability. This represents a failure rate of 5%. None of these failures could be attributed to prosthetic design. The remainder of the results are classified as good on the basis of comfort, mobility, and level of activity achieved. The durability of these results has not been determined by this review, as the length of follow-up is insufficient.

SUMMARY

Beginning with an analysis of the desirable physical and mechanical features of a knee replacement prosthesis, a device has been designed to incorporate as many of these as possible. The resulting prosthesis was mounted in a specially constructed knee simulator and successfully completed 200 days of continuous cycling without failure. The validity of this machine as a testing device was supported by tests with other prostheses, which failed in the simulator in a manner consistent with clinical reports of failure. The surgical procedure for implanting the prosthesis has proved to be straightforward, and the entire operation can be completed in 60 to 90 minutes. The long-term results are not available at this time, but analysis of 80 cases with an average follow-up of 1 year reveals predominantly good results and no failures directly attributable to defects in prosthetic design or to failure of the prosthesis itself.

References

1. Freeman, M. A. R., Swanson, S. A. V., and Todd, R. C.: Total replacement of the knee using the Freeman-Swanson knee prosthesis, Clin. Orthop. 94:155, 1973.
2. Jones, G. B.: Total knee replacement—the Walldius hinge, Clin. Orthop. 94:51, 1973.
3. Matthews, L. S., Sonstegard, D. A., and Kauffer, H.: The spherocentric knee, Clin. Orthop. 94:234, 1973.
4. Morrison, J. B.: Function of the knee in various activities, Biomed. Eng. 4(12):573, 1969.
5. Seedham, B. B., Dowson, D., and Wright, V.: Wear of solid phase formed high density polyethylene in relation to the life of artificial hips and knees, Wear 24:35, 1973.
6. Shaw, J. A., and Murray, D. G.: Knee joint simulator, Clin. Orthop. 94:15, 1973.
7. Walker, P. S., and Shoji, H.: Developing a stabilizing knee prosthesis employing physiological principles, Clin. Orthop. 94:224, 1973.

23. The spherocentric knee: current developments and experiences

Larry S. Matthews
Herbert Kaufer
David A. Sonstegard

The spherocentric knee[1] is a new intrinsically stable knee joint replacement prosthesis (Fig. 23-1) for use in the treatment of severely damaged knee joints in which gross instability, severe deformity, or failure of a previous prosthesis contraindicate conventional resurfacing procedures. This prosthesis is based on a contained, or trapped ball-in-socket, articulation (Fig. 23-2), which resists all relative translational movements between the tibial and femoral components. Thus the joint cannot dislocate or sublux in the anteroposterior or the medial-lateral direction, and it cannot easily be pulled apart in axial tension.

At the same time, however, the ball-in-socket joint permits unrestricted rotational motions in any direction. To reasonably control this extensive rotational freedom, femoral and tibial projections were designed to resemble normal bony condyles. By selecting appropriate radii of curvature of the posterior portions of the femoral condylar projections and by locating the axis of rotation near that of the normal knee, it was possible to provide 120° of flexion and extension motion while eliminating all but very little medial-lateral (varus-valgus) motion. This assured medial-lateral rotational stability of the knee. Similarly, by choosing appropriate transverse radii of curvature of the femoral condylar runners and tibial bearing tracks and by selecting an appropriate free clearance between the femoral and tibial prosthetic condyles in flexion, it was possible to appropriately limit rotational freedom to a maximum of 20° of external and 20° of internal rotation of the tibia on the femur. Thus it is evident that optimal design of femoral condylar runners and tibial tracks allowed a limitation of rotational freedom to that resembling a normal knee. We had hoped to provide greater flexion than the total of 120° of motion allowed by the present design but could not do so if the strength and stability of the prosthesis were to be preserved.

The mating relationship of the tracks and runners limits extension end range of motion in a special way. In flexion there is a clearance between the femoral runners and the tibial tracks (Fig. 23-3). Attempts to rotate the components beyond a normal degree of extension cause the front parts of the femoral prosthetic

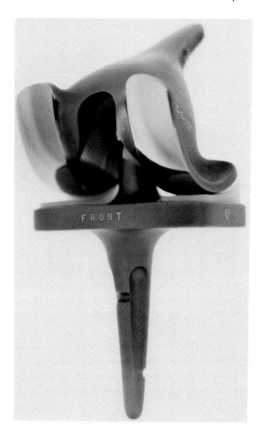

Fig. 23-1. Spherocentric knee.

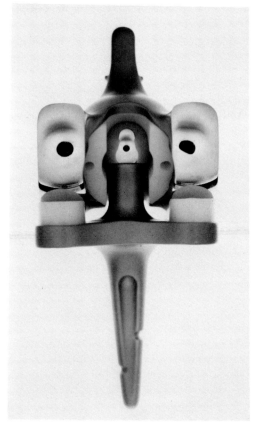

Fig. 23-2. Posterior view of extended spherocentric knee demonstrating contained or trapped ball-in-socket articulation.

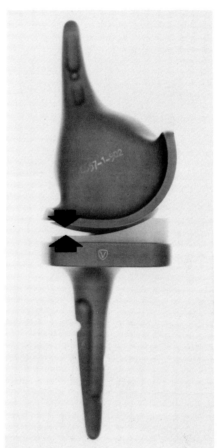

Fig. 23-3. Side view of spherocentric knee in flexion. Arrows demonstrate clearance between femoral runners and tibial tracks.

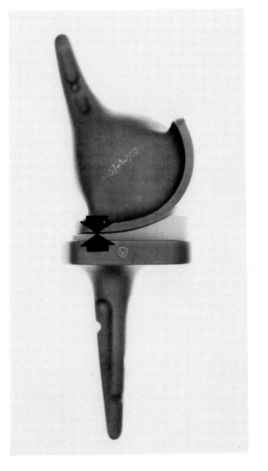

Fig. 23-4. Side view of spherocentric knee in full extension demonstrating closure of clearance and cam action, which minimizes impact effects at full extension.

condylar runners, which have a larger radius of curvature than the posterior regions, to press downward on the anterior regions of the contained plastic tibial tracks (Fig. 23-4). The knee rotates to a gentle stop. This cam deceleration at the end of extension prevents the "clunk" so familiar to hinged joint users. In fact, this cam deceleration greatly decreases the impact loading of the prosthesis-patient interface and may decrease the chances of prosthetic loosening.

Similarly the nearly mating femoral and tibial condylar projections prevent excessive rotation of the tibia on the femur. Although the prosthetic joint itself limits excessive rotation of the components, we believe that in the clinical use both hyperextension and excessive rotation of the tibia on the femur are in many cases prevented by the patient's own soft tissue. While this to some extent reduces the possible range of motion, it may partially protect the plastic components of the prosthesis from end range-of-motion stresses and thus increase the functional life span of the prosthetic joint. If the extremes of range of motion are in fact limited by the patient's soft tissues, then the femoral and tibial metallic components of the prosthesis should tend to be loaded more in compression, and any tendency to toggle from the cement bed would be greatly minimized.

DESIGN FEATURES

There are many important design features of the prosthesis that deserve independent consideration. All of the bearing surfaces are of polished metal (cobalt-chrome-molybdenum alloy) on ultrahigh molecular weight polyethylene, a combination that has proved satisfactory for years in total hip replacement arthroplasty. The central and dominant ball-in-socket articulation is relatively large, 21 mm, minimizing joint bearing contact stresses throughout the functional range of motion. This feature should minimize wear, particularly when compared to total knee prostheses in which point or line contact exists between metal convex femoral components and flat and largely unsupported plastic tibial components. The central socket is inverted, and thus wear particles as they occur may float free from this all-important bearing. All plastic bearing components are supported on at least three sides by metal, minimizing the likelihood of cold flow plastic deformation and protecting the prosthesis-cement-bone interface from shear forces generated when plastic spreads as it is compressed. All patient-prosthesis interfaces are of a metal-cement-bone configuration, again tending to minimize shear loading on the trabecular metaphyseal bone. The prosthesis is designed with relatively short stems to maximize the surface interface with trabecular bone, which we believe has the functional potential to respond to forces and to rapidly remodel in such a way as to physiologically support a prosthesis with the lowest possible incidence of loosening.

BIOMECHANICAL TESTS

Prior to the initiation of clinical trials, a great many biomechanical tests were done to identify weak points in the design, to evaluate the value of design modifications made to increase the strength of the prototype prosthesis, and to document the functional behavior of the final spherocentric knee. These tests were done on the metal and plastic prosthesis itself and on fresh human cadaver knees used as controls and prepared with hinged and spherocentric prostheses. The first series of tests simply demonstrated in cadaver limbs that the operation was reasonable and that the desired functional characteristics were in fact present. The range of motion was as expected and the knee did not "clunk." In a second series of experiments, human cadaver knees were cleared of all soft tissues except for the ligaments and the joint capsule. The midfemurs and midtibias were supported on iron brackets and a testing machine ram was directed downward onto the central portion of the knee until failure. Throughout this test on an Instron machine, the downward force and the amount of hyperextension were recorded. After failure, usually of the posterior capsule and the cruciate ligaments, a spherocentric or Walldius hinged arthroplasty was performed on the specimen using methyl methacrylate bone cement. The same test was then repeated on the same specimen with the prosthesis in place.

These tests indicated that the specimens prepared with the spherocentric knee supported a higher load at failure, reversibly deformed more before failure, and absorbed more energy before failure than did the normal knees. These results were all statistically significant. A second and perhaps more important observation was that the low-slope, low-stiffness recordings obtained from specimens treated with the spherocentric knees paralleled curves representing the behaviors of normal knees. This effect is different from the results obtained from specimens with hinged-joint prostheses treated similarly. The hinged-joint specimens supported great loads with little deflection and produced curves of an impact character. These "hinged" curves documented the "clunk" behavior characteristic of all of the hinged prostheses at the end of the extension range.

The same types of tests were performed in varus and valgus directions with the prepared knee specimens locked in full extension. In every case the strength characteristics of the spherocentric knees was at least equal to the values obtained for normal knee specimens. Since normal people during normal activities rarely encounter mechanical stresses that cause structural failure, we thought that these tests provided some appropriate and affirmative evidence that the prosthesis should be safe for use in patients. We were pleased that the experiments had tested not only the device but also the prosthesis-cement-bone interfaces of the representative specimens.

Although the normal knee joint is usually loaded in compression, we were concerned that in the unexpected event of tension on the limb the tibial or femoral components might be pulled from the bone or the prosthesis might be pulled apart. A series of tension tests demonstrated that a pulling force in excess of 300 pounds was necessary to cause damage to the implanted prosthesis. Failure always occurred at the prosthetic socket. The tibial or femoral components were never pulled from the bone at this critical load level. The important clinical implication is that, should a tension incident occur, a failure would likely be through the replaceable plastic socket and not by catastrophic fracture of the metaphyseal implant site. Finally, since pure compression is the most functional stress mode for normal and prosthetic knees, we tested normal and human cadaver knees with a spherocentric prosthesis in pure axial compression. No significant differences were found. Interestingly, specimens from a young individual were able to support in excess of a ton prior to failure.

All of these tests gave some indication that the implanted spherocentric prosthesis system should be able to withstand the immediate stresses of normal usage in normal individuals, but we still had no knowledge regarding the anticipated cyclic load or fatigue life of the implanted prosthesis. Fatigue failure is a frequently encountered clinical implant problem. Hip nails are noted to fatigue at the nail-plate junction. Stem fracture of total hip replacements is usually caused by fatigue. Accordingly, implanted spherocentric knee specimens were coated with Tens-lac,* a brittle lacquer, and were loaded to normal knee failure levels. This allowed us to measure surface strains. Areas of maximum surface strain were instrumented with strain gauges. The resulting data directed many modifications of the design, and ultimately these types of tests indicated that it would be reasonable to expect an infinite fatigue life from metal components of the final prosthetic design used for normal activities in normal individuals. It must be recognized, however, that all of the possible stress locations and directions or modes of stress may not have been identified by these preclinical trial tests, and only after long-term clinical trials will we know whether the hoped-for fatigue safety factor will have been accomplished.

CLINICAL TRIALS

The first clinical trials included 25 spherocentric arthroplasties performed on 23 patients with severely destructive knee joint disease who could not reasonably be treated except by hinge arthroplasty or knee joint arthrodesis. Hinge arthroplasty has not proved to be dependably successful, and loosening of the hinge prosthesis appears to be a nearly universal end result of its impact at hyperextension and lack of multiaxial rotation freedom. Joint fusion would have been intolerable to most of our population of severely disabled individuals. The 23 patients and their families were informed of the experimental aspects of the use of the newly designed and tested prosthesis. A protocol approved by the University of Michigan Medical Center Human Subject Review Committee was followed. The specific indications for spherocentric arthroplasty were and still remain gross deformity, gross instability, and failure of a previous prosthetic arthroplasty. Our average patient was able to walk little and required considerable support, usually crutches or a walker. In most cases pain was described as severe, being present throughout the day and increasing with any knee joint activity. It usually ex-

---

*Photolastic, Inc., Malvern, Penn.

tended through the night, and most patients had difficulty sleeping. The average patient could not attend social affairs or purchase food independently.

We now have followed all of this group of patients at 4-month intervals for an average of more than 3 years and for a maximum follow-up of more than 48 months for our first patients. All patients have been greatly relieved of their pain. The average patient at this time has little or no pain and none requires pain medication other than salicylates. At this time 18 of the 23 patients are walking without cane or crutches. All but two patients are able to walk into and use the bathroom facilities in their homes and are able to shop for themselves and to attend out-of-house social affairs. The increase in knee joint stability obtained at surgery with the intrinsically stable knee joint prosthesis has been maintained. The patients' ranges of flexion-extension have continued to improve, with an average of 18° of increased motion recorded so far.

In this early experience we have recognized a number of problems and complications. One patient had a complete peroneal nerve palsy that resolved completely within 3 weeks after her surgery. Rehabilitation of another was delayed 6 weeks by a large hemarthrosis. A midshaft femoral fracture spontaneously resulted from unprotected activity in one patient who had been virtually at bedrest for the 2 years prior to surgery. Another patient tripped in her home and fractured the femoral component from the metaphyseal bone. These two patients with femoral fractures required surgical treatment, with eventual good results in both cases. One patient's femoral condyle was fractured at surgery. It was cemented back into place and did not affect the postoperative course. Recently a diagnosis of delayed joint infection has been made in one of our early patients. Presently she has only moderate symptoms at the knee and many other serious systemic problems. Consequently we have not removed the prosthesis. In total we have performed or have personally assisted in the procedure approximately 80 times since 1973. One hundred twenty-six spherocentric arthroplasties have been performed at the University of Michigan and affiliated hospitals.

TECHNICAL PROBLEMS

Although a complete description of the surgical technique will be presented elsewhere, a number of recurrent technical problems warrant consideration and further comment here. A few physicians have reported postoperative recurvatum or excessive hyperextension requiring brace support. The most common cause of this problem has been surgical malalignment of the prosthetic components. The key to accurate alignment of the prosthetic parts is an accurate transverse tibial saw cut that is perpendicular to the long axis of the tibia in all directions. A new femoral positioning tool allows the femoral component to be implanted more dependably into the appropriate position. To provide the recommended full extension at surgery, the stem of the femoral component should usually point toward the femoral head and be inclined at about 10°, with the tip of the femoral stem directed slightly toward the anterior femoral cortex.

Although the prosthesis was designed with its outer dimensions two standard deviations smaller than the average for 50 adult knees, several arthritic patients have had insufficient metaphyseal bone for the standard prosthesis. Templates are presently being provided to help the physician estimate whether the standard size components can be used. A new smaller prosthesis is presently being developed. It should, when available, be used only in patients with bones that cannot accept the standard size components. Even then, considering long-term fatigue as well as short-term mechanical stresses, caution is recommended in its use. The patient's size, weight, and activity levels should be considered before selection of the small prosthesis.

Operative assembly of the prosthesis has been difficult for some. After a careful but strong push has snapped the socket over the polished metal ball, it should be accurately rotationally oriented with the front forward and the flat directed exactly backward. The slots in the plastic skirts should be aligned perfectly with the corresponding anterior and posterior slots in the femoral component. The tip of the socket should be manually placed into the femoral component with the knee in nearly full flexion. The knee is then extended until the metal stem supporting the central ball is directly centered within the opened area in the base of the socket. With the limb in this position (usually about 30° of flexion) the foot is secured to the table and the prosthetic joint components are pressed firmly together. When the socket has snapped into place, its base is inspected with the knee in flexion, and the impacting tool is used to impact the socket securely into position. Both socket skirts should be visibly located under the appropriate femoral component overhanging metallic ledges. On occasion it has been difficult to initiate penetration of the socket into its receptacle. Under these circumstances the socket skirt–compressing instrument can be used advantageously to assist in inserting the socket.

Great care must be exercised when using the socket skirt–compressing tool to prevent deformation of the holes in the base of the skirts and consequent difficulty with later disassembly. The instrument should always be positioned so that its pins are fully inserted into the socket skirt holes. No attempt should be made to use the socket skirt–compressing tool to manipulate the position of the socket within the femoral component. When the socket skirt–compressing tool is used for joint disassembly, all of the above cautions apply. In addition, the tool should not be used to lever or pull the socket from the femoral component but only to compress the skirts; care must be taken that the supporting stem is directly in the center of the opening in the base of the socket. With the skirts compressed and freed from the overhanging femoral ledges, traction is applied to the tibia. A dull elevator applied as a lever between the dome of the socket and the femoral component at this stage often helps in disassembly. If in spite of all of these precautions (we have disassembled the prosthesis more than 50 times without damage) the socket skirt holes are deformed, a small, thin osteotome may be used to destructively remove the socket.

SUMMARY

The spherocentric knee has been designed to duplicate as nearly as possible, the functions of the normal knee. It has features (tibial rotational freedom and cam deceleration at end range hyperextension) that should decrease the incidence of loosening of the components from bone. Efforts have been made to minimize wear and to control the chances of fatigue failure. Biomechanical tests have indicated that the prosthesis appears to function as planned. Carefully controlled early clinical trials in a select population of patients with severely damaged knees have demonstrated the usefulness of the implant in the treatment of patients with gross instability, severe deformity, or failure of other prosthetic arthroplasty of the knee.

Reference

1. Matthews, L. S., Sonstegard, D. A., and Kaufer, H.: The spherocentric knee, Clin. Orthop. **94:**234, 1973.

24. Total knee replacement by intramedullary adjustable prosthesis

Nas S. Eftekhar

HISTORIC BACKGROUND

Recent interest in total knee replacement by resurfacing of the knee joint is only a natural course of events following successful results obtained by total hip replacement. The choice of materials, chromium-cobalt alloy or stainless steel against high-density polyethylene, and the method of fixation of the components into the bone by acrylic cement are now established through the experiences with total hip replacement. There are, however, numerous problems inherent in the knee joint that obviously complicate the matter of replacement as compared with a simple ball-and-socket replacement in the hip joint. Among these differences are the subcutaneous nature of the knee joint; multicompartmental anatomy; complex stability mechanism, with principal reliance on ligaments and capsule; complex rotational and axial motion; as well as complex geometry of the articulating bones of the knee. Early experiences with the knee replacement suggest a definite biologic role of the soft tissue in limiting gain in mobility unrelated to the features of the prosthetic design. The surgical technique itself appeared to be extremely "exacting" and, unlike total hip replacement in which early results still could be gratifying in regard to relief of pain despite a compromised technique, in total knee replacement minor deviations from a "perfect" fixation and alignment would lead to failure.

It is of historic interest that, since 1861, many attempts for arthroplasty of the knee joint have been made using autogenous soft tissue as interpositioning materials. There are also extensive reports on the use of nonmetallic substances for arthroplasty of this joint. Development of metallic hemiarthroplasty was a natural course of development following the work of Smith-Peterson and led to the MacIntosh prosthesis, which was widely used with beneficial results in certain cases. MacIntosh's major contribution was the idea of building up the space within the joint to provide stability via restoration of musculofascial structures of the thigh and ligaments of the knee joint. However, hemiarthroplasties, such as the MacIntosh prosthesis or MGH femoral replacement resurfacing, were doomed to failure because of (1) bicompartmental involvement of the joint

272

replacement and (2) inadequate fixation of prosthetic devices in the bone. In general the results of these unipolar prostheses were somewhat comparable to the results of hemiarthroplasty of the hip, such as with the Austin-Moore prosthesis or cup arthroplasties used in osteoarthrosis or rheumatoid arthritis of the hip joint.

A mechanical replacement of the knee joint by the so-called hinged prosthesis introduced and popularized by Waldius and others did not receive wide acceptance despite their extensive modification of the prosthesis through the years. The prosthesis was considered bulky and constrained, thus likely to fail by loosening or fractures. Extensive tissue reaction as the result of metallic wear debris and

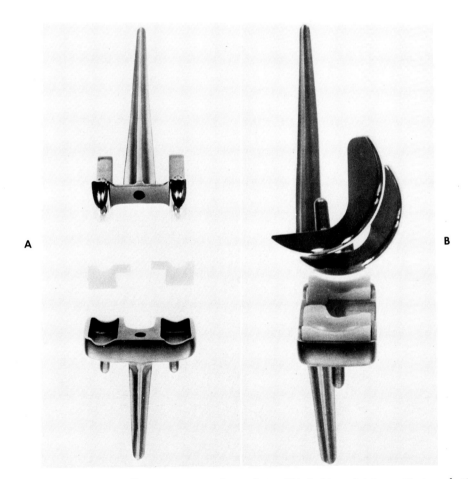

Fig. 24-1. A, Two metallic components of prosthesis (Mark 1) and interpositioning plastic pads. Differential heights of plastic pieces were conceived to provide spacing and adjustability at surgery. **B,** Profile of prosthetic component (Mark 1) with plastic components press fitted in place. Note elements of fixation consisting of intramedullary stem and studs to produce cement injection into bone and prevent rotary forces.

occasional catastrophic results forced surgeons to continue to use arthrodesis of the knee joint as the only reliable surgical procedure in extreme conditions. At this joint procedures such as osteotomies and synovectomies continue to be temporizing procedures in many instances.

Gunston is responsible for development of a bicompartmental prosthesis for resurfacing of the tibia and femur, which he termed polycentric knee arthroplasty, at Wrightington Hospital in Great Britain. Since his initial work utilizing the principal materials and concept of total hip arthroplasty, numerous modifications of this concept have developed in both Europe and the United States.

We designed our total knee prosthesis at the New York Orthopaedic Hospital in late 1969. Laboratory investigations on wear, stability, and anatomic features of ligaments in relation to the design of the prosthesis were done prior to human implantation. The first implantation was in February, 1970. The prosthesis was designed on the polycentric concept (Fig. 24-1) and was to allow the surgeon to implant the two components independently with accuracy and ease, the components being inserted following a geometric resection of bone perpendicular to the axis of the femur and tibia without any effort to build up the bone with a layer of cement. The principal fixation mechanism is to be achieved by intramedullary fixation to distribute the load through the endosteum of the femur and the tibia in addition to the weight-bearing segments of the platforms of the tibial and femoral components. Additional elements were added in both components to resist rotary forces. Plastic pads of variable thickness were press fitted into the metallic component of the tibia to prevent cold flow of the plastic, thus preventing loosening at the interface by deformation of plastic under the load. By selecting the appropriate thickness of plastic to be interposed between the metallic tibial and femoral components, optimal tension could be produced across the knee joint for stability through the fascioligamentous-capsular sleeve of the knee joint. Therefore severe varus or valgus deformity of the knee could be corrected along with extreme degrees of flexion. The main concern was to release the deforming soft tissue prior to implantation of the prosthesis.

DESCRIPTION OF PROSTHESIS

The femoral component consists of two polycentric runners connected by a web, which is in turn bisected by a tapered stem. The articular runners are circular in cross section in the frontal plane, and each has a small stud sagittally to resist rotary forces. The walls of cavities in the runners are aimed to retain cement. The tibial component is a T-shaped piece consisting of a socket containing the plastic component. The socket with verticular walls accommodates the ultrahigh molecular weight polyethylene plateau, which can be press fitted into its cavities at surgery. There are also two studs symmetrically placed on each side of the tibial component to resist rotary forces. The ultrahigh-density polyethylene tibial pieces are available in 6, 10, 14, and 20 mm thicknesses, which are selected at surgery by testing a trial prosthesis and press fitted into the tibial

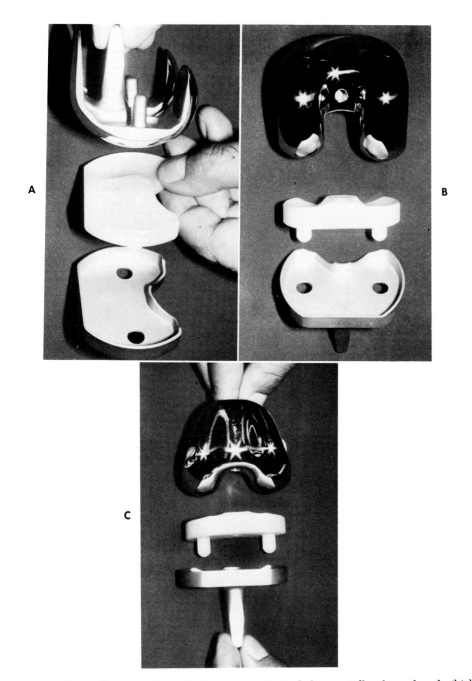

Fig. 24-2. A, Profile view of prosthetic components including metallic femoral and tibial components. In Mark 2 (present design), plastic was designed in a single piece, thus allowing broadening of bearing surface. **B,** Femoral and tibial metallic components in frontal plane with femoral component demonstrating patellar flange on femoral component. Concavity of surface of femoral flange does not produce any constraint for patellar prosthesis (large radius). **C,** Components shown in **B** with femoral component in extension. In both **B** and **C** threads can be seen at center of femoral component for use of holder for insertion of prosthesis.

piece just prior to cementing of the tibial component (Fig. 24-2). The plastic runner has double radii, which provide complete freedom of movement in flexion but allow 40° of rotation without disengagement. The prosthesis is completely stable in translational movements (side to side movements) (Fig. 24-3).

INDICATIONS AND PREPARATIONS

Regardless of underlying conditions, the patient must accept the subsequent arthrodesis if replacement surgery fails at a future date. Advanced rheumatoid arthritis, panarthrosis of osteoarthritis and rheumatoid arthritis, and previous unsuccessful operations are primary indications for this procedure. Unicompartmental osteoarthritis with mild degrees of varus or valgus deformity usually is suitable for osteotomy and is not treated by replacement. History or presence of infection, especially in a previously failed operation, is an absolute contraindication for surgery in our series. As a preoperative requirement, an anteroposterior standing x-ray film (14 × 17 inches) is obtained in addition to conventional x-ray views of the knee. A knee evaluation proforma ("yellow card") is com-

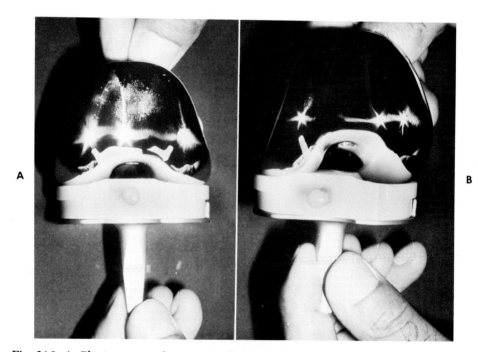

Fig. 24-3. **A,** Plastic test prosthesis 6 mm thick interposing metallic femoral and tibial components (note open front of test tibial component), demonstrating compliance of femoral runners in tibial tract in neutral rotation. **B,** Compliance of components with femoral component in maximum medial rotation (40°) without subluxation or disengagement of components. **C,** Femoral component is rotated 40° laterally, illustrating same compliance without dislodgement. **D,** Top surface of tibial component and its double radii arrangement. Center hole is designed for positive hold for insertion of prosthesis.

pleted preoperatively (Fig. 24-4) and a similar assessment is done postoperatively. Preoperative systemic antibiotics are administered routinely, starting 12 hours prior to surgery; one dose is given as an intravenous bolus just prior to surgery and the application of a tourniquet. A continuous antibiotic infusion is started during surgery and continued after the operation for 3 days. Ether and 2% tincture of iodine in 70% alcohol are routinely used for preparation of the skin in addition to routine surgical preparation.

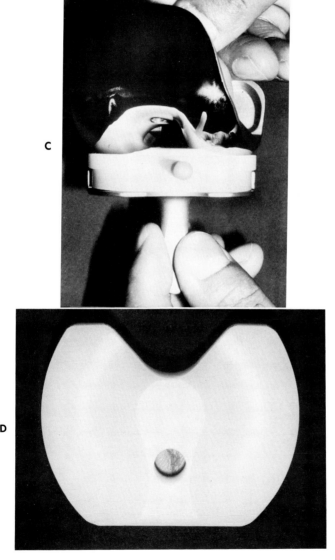

C

D

Fig. 24-3, cont'd. For legend see opposite page.

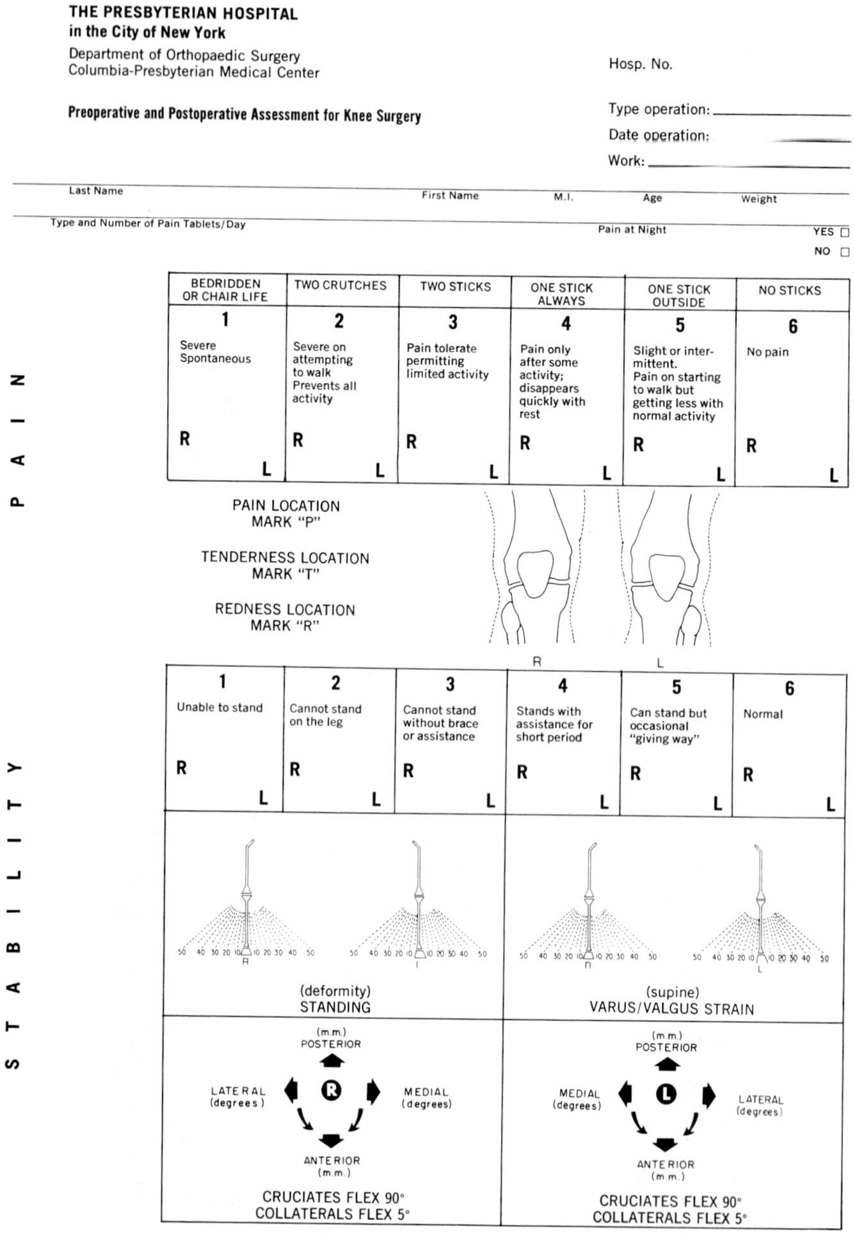

THE PRESBYTERIAN HOSPITAL
in the City of New York
Department of Orthopaedic Surgery
Columbia-Presbyterian Medical Center

Hosp. No.

Preoperative and Postoperative Assessment for Knee Surgery

Type operation: _____

Date operation: _____

Work: _____

Last Name		First Name	M.I.	Age	Weight

Type and Number of Pain Tablets/Day			Pain at Night	YES ☐
				NO ☐

PAIN

BEDRIDDEN OR CHAIR LIFE	TWO CRUTCHES	TWO STICKS	ONE STICK ALWAYS	ONE STICK OUTSIDE	NO STICKS
1	**2**	**3**	**4**	**5**	**6**
Severe Spontaneous	Severe on attempting to walk Prevents all activity	Pain tolerate permitting limited activity	Pain only after some activity; disappears quickly with rest	Slight or intermittent. Pain on starting to walk but getting less with normal activity	No pain
R L	R L	R L	R L	R L	R L

PAIN LOCATION
MARK "P"

TENDERNESS LOCATION
MARK "T"

REDNESS LOCATION
MARK "R"

R   L

STABILITY

1	**2**	**3**	**4**	**5**	**6**
Unable to stand	Cannot stand on the leg	Cannot stand without brace or assistance	Stands with assistance for short period	Can stand but occasional "giving way"	Normal
R L	R L	R L	R L	R L	R L

50 40 30 20 10 ⌂ 10 20 30 40 50
R

50 40 30 20 10 ⌂ 10 20 30 40 50
l

(deformity)
STANDING

50 40 30 20 10 ⌂ 10 20 30 40 50
n

50 40 30 20 10 ⌂ 10 20 30 40 50
L

(supine)
VARUS/VALGUS STRAIN

(m.m.)
POSTERIOR

LATERAL (degrees) ◄ **R** ► MEDIAL (degrees)

ANTERIOR (m.m.)

CRUCIATES FLEX 90°
COLLATERALS FLEX 5°

(m.m.)
POSTERIOR

MEDIAL (degrees) ◄ **L** ► LATERAL (degrees)

ANTERIOR (m.m.)

CRUCIATES FLEX 90°
COLLATERALS FLEX 5°

A

Fig. 24-4. A, "Yellow card," preoperative and postoperative assessment to evaluate pain and stability. **B,** Reverse side of card for evaluation of function and mobility in addition to classification of function.

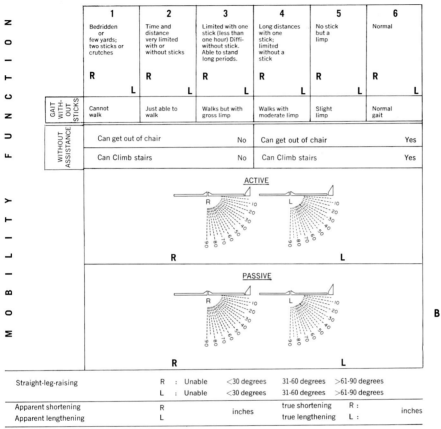

		1	2	3	4	5	6
		Bedridden or few yards; two sticks or crutches	Time and distance very limited with or without sticks	Limited with one stick (less than one hour) Difficult without stick. Able to stand long periods.	Long distances with one stick; limited without a stick	No stick but a limp	Normal
		R	R	R	R	R	R
		L	L	L	L	L	L
GAIT WITH-OUT STICKS		Cannot walk	Just able to walk	Walks but with gross limp	Walks with moderate limp	Slight limp	Normal gait
WITHOUT ASSISTANCE		Can get out of chair		No	Can get out of chair		Yes
		Can Climb stairs		No	Can Climb stairs		Yes

FUNCTION (vertical label, left)

MOBILITY (vertical label, left)

ACTIVE

R ─ 10 ─ 20 ─ 30 ─ 40 ─ 50 ─ 60 ─ 70 ─ 80 ─ 90

L ─ 10 ─ 20 ─ 30 ─ 40 ─ 50 ─ 60 ─ 70 ─ 80 ─ 90

R   L

PASSIVE

R ─ 10 ─ 20 ─ 30 ─ 40 ─ 50 ─ 60 ─ 70 ─ 80 ─ 90

L ─ 10 ─ 20 ─ 30 ─ 40 ─ 50 ─ 60 ─ 70 ─ 80 ─ 90

R   L   B

| Straight-leg-raising | R | : Unable | <30 degrees | 31-60 degrees | >61-90 degrees | |
| | L | : Unable | <30 degrees | 31-60 degrees | >61-90 degrees | |

| Apparent shortening | R | | | true shortening | R : | |
| Apparent lengthening | L | inches | | true lengthening | L : | inches |

COMMENTS:

Date   Examiner

CATEGORICAL CLASSIFICATION FOR FUNCTION

A) Unilateral knee: no other functional disability
B) Bilateral knee: no other functional disability
C) Unilateral or bilateral WITH other joints or medical condition affecting function

SUMMARY:

Category "C" Cases
☐ CVS
☐ RS
☐ CNS
☐ Senility
☐ Obesity
☐ Psychiatric
☐ Other

☐ orthopaedics

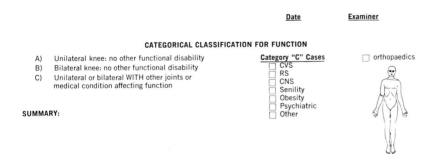

Fig. 24-4, cont'd. For legend see opposite page.

SURGICAL TECHNIQUE

Surgical technique consists of three steps:

A. Soft tissue operation: exposure of the knee joint and correction of soft tissue deformity, including removal of cruciates and posterior capsular release

B. Preparation of bone and trial of test prosthesis

C. Cementing of the components

Soft tissue operation

The patient is placed under spinal, epidural, or general anesthesia and a pneumatic tourniquet is applied to the limb. Preparation of the lower extremity is done in the usual fashion, utilizing ether and 2% tincture of iodine, which is left on the skin. The pneumatic tourniquet must be applied as high as possible on the thigh and the edges of the tourniquet insulated from the skin to avoid running of preparation solution underneath the tourniquet.

A double stockinette is applied, and a perforation is made to reveal the knee joint. An adhesive plastic drape is then applied from approximately 4 inches proximal to 4 inches distal to the level of the knee joint, and a straight incision is made through an adhesive drape (Steri-Drape). The incision begins at the junction of the vastus medialis and rectus femoris, approximately 2 inches (5 cm)

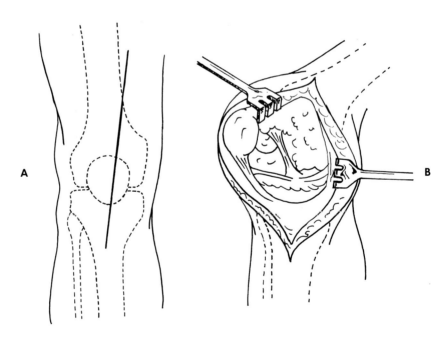

Fig. 24-5. A, Incision is begun at interval vastus medialis and rectus femoris approximately 2 to 3 inches proximal to upper border of patella extending toward tibial tubercle. Straight incision is located over patellar border, but fascia is incised medial to patellar border for subsequent repair. **B,** Exposure of knee through medial approach. Patella is everted and remnants of cruciates are excised.

proximal to the upper pole of the patella, and extends just beyond the tibial tubercle (Fig. 24-5, A). The subcutaneous layer is incised along the same line, avoiding undercutting of the skin. The fascia and quadriceps expansion are incised by a slightly curved line to allow 3 to 5 mm of quadriceps expansion to remain on the patellar border for subsequent closure. Proximally, the incision must split the rectus femoris tendon longitudinally along its fibers, leaving ¼ inch lateral to the vastus medialis muscle without disturbing the fibers of this muscle. The incision of the capsule and synovium now is completed, and a routine culture of the synovial fluid is obtained. In knees with rheumatoid arthritis a synovectomy is performed as indicated. With the knee at 90° and the patella everted (Fig. 24-5, B), two knee retractors are placed on either side of the knee joint. Remnants of menisci, loose bodies, synovial tags, and cruciates are removed. Excision of the cruciates is best accomplished by the use of a rongeur and flexion of the knee to a maximum degree to allow visibility of its fibers from the medial femoral condyle. A complete posterior capsular release must be performed to allow full extension of the knee joint (Fig. 24-6, A and B), which also allows the flexed knee to be displaced forward in relation to distal femur. (Fig. 24-6, C). With the knee at 90° the top of the tibia must be visible from corner to corner. Exposure may be maximized by partial or total removal of prepatellar fat pad and further synovial membrane and lateral meniscus removal from the joint.

The main concern is to provide a balanced medial-lateral tension on the capsular ligamentous complex of the knee when the knee is placed in full extension and no more than 5° of valgus (anatomic angle). This correction cannot be achieved if any varus or valgus deformity of more than 15° is present. In a severe varus deformity the medial collateral ligament and capsule of the joint are contracted, and the lateral collateral ligament and the lateral capsule are lax. The reverse situation exists in a valgus deformity in which the lateral collateral ligament and lateral capsule of the joint are contracted and the medial collateral ligament and medial capsule are lax. In either condition posterolateral or posteromedial capsular contracture may also be present, placing the knee in a varus internal rotation or a valgus external rotation deformity. To correct a varus deformity of more than 15° it is often necessary to release the deep and superficial medial collateral ligament; at times even the insertion of pes tendons are released, which allows correction of severe deformities. However, in a valgus deformity a careful release of the lateral collateral ligament from the lateral condyle or resection of the iliotibial tract just proximal to the knee joint level or both are indicated to correct a severe valgus deformity. Care must be taken to avoid peroneal nerve damage by overstretching of the knee joint into a varus position. Resection of bone must not be attempted prior to complete soft tissue release, including posterior capsular release from the distal end of the femur. Soft tissue release is considered the most fundamental step toward a successful replacement. Although it is true that a relatively unstable knee has been made at this stage into a more unstable knee, as will be discussed later, the tension on the ligaments is adjusted by spacing the joint by the prosthesis to overcome the

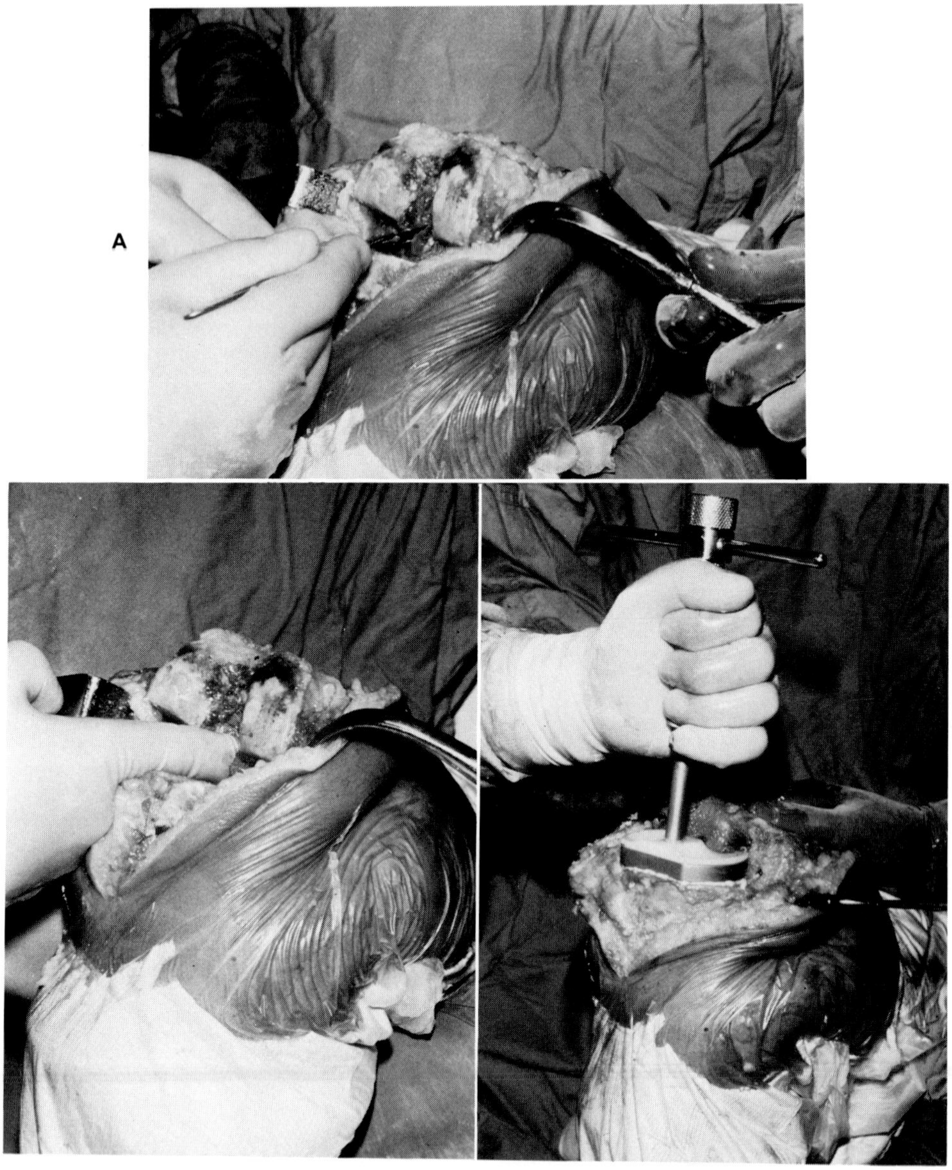

Fig. 24-6. A, Operative photograph illustrates maximum exposure, accompanied by extreme flexion of knee and facilitated by complete posterior capsular release following excision of cruciates. B, Following capsular release and complete excision of cruciates, along with re-section of posterior condyles, index finger introduced into posterior capsular region ascertains complete mobilization of posterior capsule. Any taut bands or residual contractures are re-leased at this point. C, Only following complete mobilization of posterior capsule and release of soft tissue is opportunity provided to have entire top of tibia at surgeon's disposal for optimal insertion of tibial component. Line of insertion of force onto cement is perpendicular to top surface of tibia.

"balanced laxity" of the joint produced by removal of the cruciates and release of the posterior capsule and collateral ligaments.

Preparation of bone and trial of test prosthesis

The second phase involves (1) preparation of bone of the distal femur, upper tibia, and articular surface of the patella and (2) the test rehearsal for spacing of the joint by the prosthesis.

Preparation of the bone is begun by using the tibiofemoral jig (Fig. 24-7, A). With the knee at a right angle, three cuts are made with an oscillating saw. Removal of bone is done by parallel cuts corresponding to three bars of the instrument, while the main member (handle) is applied onto the tibial crest. The point of reference is the lowest bar, which should indicate a *minimum removal* of bone from the top of the tibia. Conservation of the bone of the tibia is essential to provide adequate fixation for the prosthetic device. The posterior condyles (aligned with the middle bar) and the anterior femur (the top bar), which automatically are lined up with the top of the tibia, are cut. It is of extreme importance to remove a minimum of bone from the tibial plateau. Following resection the cut tibial surface should be perpendicular to the axis of the tibia in both planes. In other words, if adjustment is needed (because of depression of the medial or lateral plateau), then more bone may be removed from one side of the tibial plateau than the opposite. It must be noted that if laxity is present in the knee joint at 90°, the knee joint must be pulled apart with a blunt instrument (periosteal elevator) to maximize the space between the condyles of the femur and the top of the tibia. Likewise, medial-lateral shifts of the tibia in relation to the femur with the knee at 90° may be needed to align the distal femur with the middle and top bars. Once the optimal level of tibial cut is determined, the pins of the instrument are secured into the bone and the osteotomies are completed.

With removal of three segments of the bone from the femur (anterior surface and two posterior condyles) and one segment from the tibia, the instrument is removed and the knee is extended following removal of the tibiofemoral jig. The femoral jig spacer is now inserted, and the maximum spacing of the joint is accomplished by elevating the center bar of the instrument via the thumb knob of the instrument (Fig. 24-7, B and C). Maximum spacing also allows the surgeon to feel the balance of medial and lateral capsular, ligamentous, fascial structures and enable him to place the knee in desired valgus alignment and mark the top of the instrument corresponding with the level of the cut of the distal femur. Following completion of the cut, the third instrument, the spacer-aligner template is inserted (Fig. 24-7, D and E) to ensure that (1) adequate bone is removed from the tibia and femur and (2) varus or valgus deformity is adequately corrected, allowing no more than 5° of valgus, (3) optimal tension is present both medially and laterally, and (4) no recurvatum occurs if the leg is lifted up by the heels, with the surgeon observing the knee from a profile view.

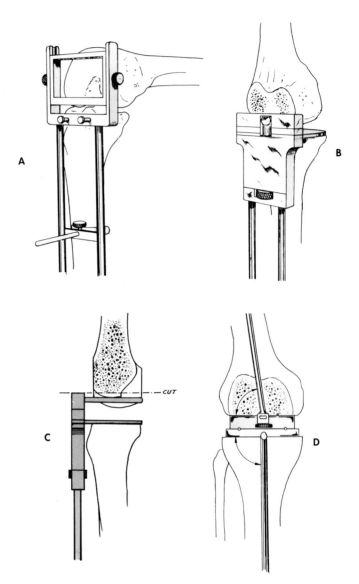

Fig. 24-7. A, With knee at right angle, tibial-femoral jig is applied so that only minimum bone is resected from tibial articular surface. To provide surface perpendicular to axis of tibia, knee must be carefully positioned at *right angle* to avoid error of too much backward or forward slope. **B,** Femoral spacer jig in position with knee fully extended to determine level of femoral cut by maximizing space between tibia and femur. Resection of bone as well as spacing must be done after complete soft tissue mobilization as described in text. **C,** Lateral view of instrument spacing joint. **D,** With knee extended, tibiofemoral spacer-aligner is placed, and alignment of knee and its stability are verified.

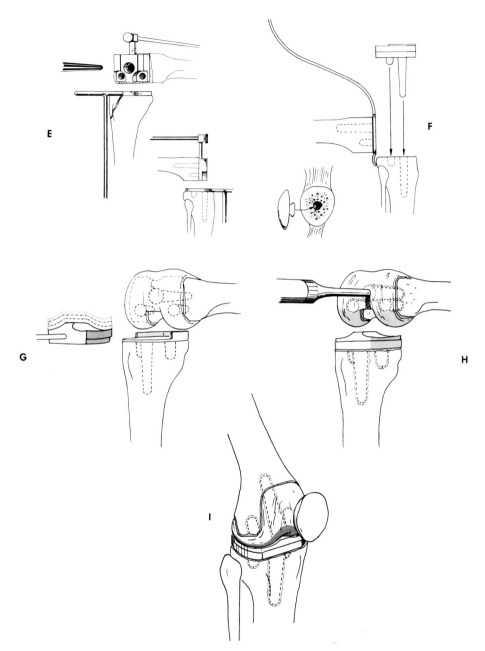

Fig. 24-7, cont'd. E, Same instrument used to prepare medullary cavities of upper tibia and distal end of femur. Tapered reamer is used to prepare medullary canals. **F,** Tibial component being inserted (following selection of appropriate thickness). Tibial retractor has displaced tibia forward as it is engaged onto posterior rim of tibia, which allows tibial component to be driven onto upper tibia unimpeded. Inset shows patellar surface prepared to receive patellar prosthesis. **G,** Tibial and femoral test prostheses in place ready to receive variety of thicknesses of plastic pieces to verify appropriate thickness to be inserted. **H,** Insertion of prosthesis cemented in place using special holder attached to femoral component of prosthesis. **I,** Forty-five degree angle of components in place illustrating intramedullary fixation elements and patellar resurfacing.

If adjustments are needed, they must be done prior to testing by trial prosthesis. The spacer-aligner template is now used for marking and drilling of the intramedullary canal and holes for the studs of the prosthetic components.

Preparation of the articulating surface of the patella is now done by removal of its articular surface to a flat surface and by drilling of the center to its anterior cortex to accommodate the stem of the patellar prosthesis. Undercutting of the patellar hole would allow an improved cement fixation into the patella (Fig. 24-7, *F*).

Test prostheses are inserted (Fig. 24-7, *G*), and different thicknesses of plastic pads are tried (through the opening of the tibial test component). The test must prove that (1) all deformities are corrected, (2) alignment of the knee is perfect (allowing 5° of valgus), (3) no recurvatum exists, and (4) the patellar prosthesis can be centered over the femoral flange of the femoral component.

Cementing of components

After removal of the test prosthesis, the bone fragments, debris and redundant tissue are removed to ensure a clean surface for fixation with cement. The tibial component is cemented first. A specially designed tibial retractor should facilitate a forward displacement of the tibia in relation to the femur (Fig. 24-7, *F*), which conveniently produces the entire surface of the tibia for a direct and positive fixation of the prosthesis. The surgeon must be able to forcefully drive the tibial component into the cement bed and be able to remove the excess cement from posterior, medial, and lateral aspects of the knee without impediment. This can only be achieved (1) if adequate posterior capsular release has been achieved and (2) if the tibial retractor is properly applied and the knee is hyperflexed (beyond 90°). Following insertion of the tibial prosthetic component (carrying a properly selected high density polyethylene pad), the patellar prosthesis is cemented to hold in the patellar holding clamp. Both tibial and patellar components may be cemented simultaneously using one packet of cement. Excess cement must be removed prior to full polymerization.

With the knee kept at a right angle and the prosthesis held in the prosthetic holder, the femoral component is cemented, and the excess cement is removed in the same manner as for the tibial component. It is essential to have the medullary canal and perforations of the distal end of the femur identified prior to insertion of the femoral component, which is inserted parallel with the axis of the shaft and perpendicular to the cut surface of the femur. The prosthetic device is hammered home, as indicated, ensuring its full penetration. The prosthetic holder is now released, and excess cement is removed (Fig. 24-7, *H*).

At the completion of the cementing of the components, the patellar component must be centered over the femoral component (Fig. 24-7, *I*). In a knee with persistent valgus deformity the patella is usually displaced laterally, which can be corrected by release of the quadriceps expansion and capsule through the knee joint.

POSTOPERATIVE COURSE

1. Quadriceps exercises are begun after the removal of the drain at 24 to 48 hours; straight leg raising is encouraged immediately following removal of drains.

2. The bulky dressing (Jones-type bandage supplemented by a posterior splint) applied at surgery is removed on the fifth day postoperatively.

Walking is begun and weight bearing as tolerated is initiated at about the tenth day postoperatively, which generally coincides with the patient's ability to do straight leg raising. A light posterior splint may be worn in bed or at night during the first 2 weeks. The exercise program includes active assisted range-of-motion exercises with a knee sling and the knee exerciser, with special emphasis on quadriceps control and improved maximum extension at the knee.

CLINICAL RESULTS AND COMPLICATIONS

Between 1970 and 1974, 71 patients (31 men and 40 women) underwent knee replacement with Mark 1 of our design. Both knees were replaced in nine patients, bringing the total number of knees operated on to 80. Age of patients ranged from 41 to 80 years. This series provided a follow-up of a maximum of 6 years and a minimum of 2 years, with an average of 3.4 years for this study. Thirty-six patients had rheumatoid arthritis, 33 had osteoarthritis, 10 operations were done for previous unsuccessful operations, and one patient had a Charcot knee. The method of assessment, as cited before, was based on a pro forma evaluation of pain, stability, function, and mobility (Fig. 24-4). In each category the disability was rated from 1 to 6, grade 1 indicating severe pain, instability, functional disability, and stiffness and grade 6 indicating normality. Using this system of numeric grading, pain was relieved in 80% of the cases, functional improvement of grade 5 or 6 was achieved in 80%, stability improved in 70%, and

Table 24-1. Systemic and local complications

Complication	Number	Number of reoperations	Comments
Pulmonary embolism	1	0	
Deep vein thrombosis	1	0	
Urinary tract infection	1	0	
Delayed wound healing	3	0	Treated by excision and secondary closure
Hematoma	2	0	Evacuated surgically
Deep wound infection	0	0	
Peroneal nerve palsy	0	0	
Death	0	0	
Complications at prosthesis site			
Fracture of prosthesis	2	2	Converted to nonhinged Mark 2 prosthesis
Dislocation	1	1	Converted to hinged-type prosthesis
Loosening	0		
Subluxation	1	0	
Patellofemoral pain	4	1	One converted to Mark 2 prosthesis

mobility improved in 60% of the cases. The overall assessment indicated that in the absence of complications, the operation was beneficial to the patient and no patient's postoperative condition was worse than his or her preoperative condition.

Local and systemic complications are listed in Table 24-1. Thromboembolism was not a problem in this series as compared with its prevalence in total hip replacement. On the other hand, delayed wound healing and hematomas (in five patients) were of special concern because of fear of the possibility of deep infection. Two hematomas that developed were evacuated surgically, and all three delayed wound healings were treated by excision of the wound and secondary wound closure.

Of complications at the prosthesis site, two femoral components fractured and required replacement. In both prostheses a defective segment at the junction of the intramedullary stem and the runners led to fatigue fracture. One knee in a patient with suspected Charcot joint and bilateral knee disability dislocated postoperatively, and conversion to a constrained (hinged-type) knee prosthesis was required. One patient experienced a subluxation in the extreme range of flexion. He has achieved 140° of flexion. At this range of motion a feeling of a click demonstrates subluxation of the knee. It is presumed to be related to disengagement of the runners from the tibial tract. Four patients in this series developed considerable patellofemoral pain; in one revision surgery became necessary. Reoperation was necessary in a total of four patients. One hinged prosthesis

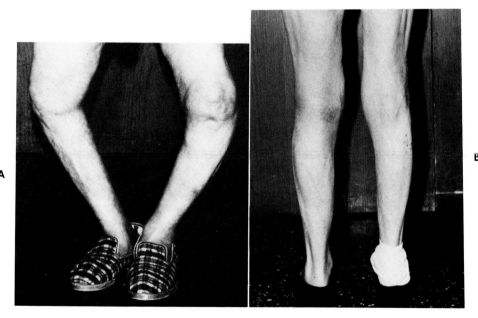

Fig. 24-8. For legend see opposite page.

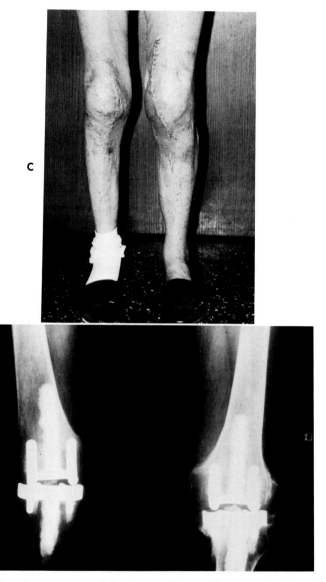

Fig. 24-8. A, Bilateral severe varus deformity in 68-year-old man with advanced rheumatoid arthritis. Prior to surgery ambulation was possible only by assistance and limited to a few yards (pain 2, stability 2, function 2, mobility 5). **B,** Posterior view of both knees following bilateral knee surgery. **C,** Both knees were operated on within 2-week intervals. Note original incision of curved medial parapatellar type, which is now obsolete. Fully corrected extremity must preserve 5° of valgus. **D,** Anteroposterior view of both knees, 4½ years following surgery. Patient's overall improvement has been significant. Postoperative grades: pain 5, stability 5, function 5, and mobility 5.

was inserted for dislocation, two broken prostheses required replacement by Mark 2 of the nonhinged prosthesis, and patellofemoral pain necessitated revision in another patient.

CASE REPORTS

Case 1. A 68-year-old man with bilateral *varus* deformity secondary to rheumatoid arthritis and advanced steroid treatment was bedridden at the time of the operation. He could only stand holding onto objects. He had 40° of varus deformity in each knee with marked medial-lateral instability (Fig. 24-8, *A*).

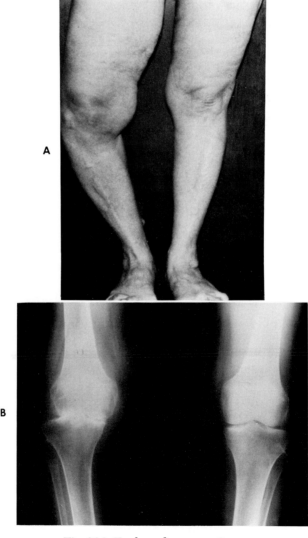

Fig. 24-9. For legend see opposite page.

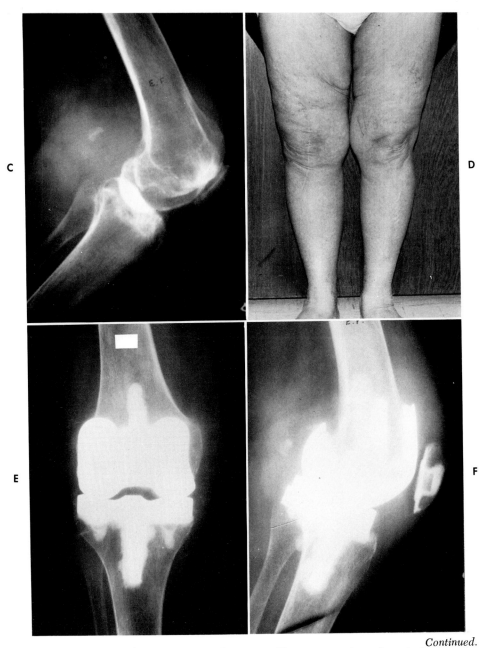

Continued.

Fig. 24-9. A, Anterior standing view of 64-year-old woman with unilateral degenerative osteoarthritis of right knee demonstrating weight-bearing varus deformity. Left knee is normal. **B,** Anteroposterior x-ray view of both knees (standing). Marked joint narrowing and lateral subluxation accompanied by severe varus deformity were contraindications to osteotomy. **C,** Panarthrosis as demonstrated by lateral view of same knee to indicate patellofemoral involvement as well. **D,** Three years following surgery of right knee, illustrating excellent correction of varus deformity. **E,** Anteroposterior view of knee with correction of varus deformity. **F,** Lateral view of knee illustrating optimal position of components, including patellar replacement. **G,** Flexion of right knee in sitting position is 20° less than normal left knee. **H,** Active extension of right knee demonstrated excellent power of quadriceps mechanism. Preoperative grading was pain 4, stability 3, function 4, and mobility 2. Postoperative improvement was scored pain 6, stability 6, function 6, and mobility 5.

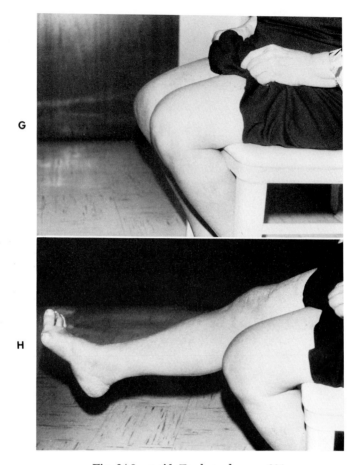

Fig. 24-9, cont'd. For legend see p. 291.

Following bilateral total knee replacement (Fig. 24-8, B to D) the patient achieved an excellent range of motion and walked with one cane for support. Preoperative grading of the knee was 2, 2, 2, 5 and postoperative results were graded as 5, 5, 5, 5.

Case 2. A 64-year-old woman had unilateral degenerative osteoarthritis of the right knee that was considered too advanced for an upper tibial osteotomy (Fig. 24-9, A to C). Treatment was by a nonhinged intramedullary adjustable prosthesis (Fig. 24-9, D to H). Postoperative recovery was remarkable, and now the patient is walking without a walking aid for limited distances. Preoperative grading was 4, 3, 4, 2. Postoperative grading is 6, 6, 6, 5. This patient works as a sales clerk in a department store.

DISCUSSION

From the surgeon's point of view, three major principles are emphasized in this technique: (1) understanding of the soft tissue operation involved in total knee replacement to provide accurate balance between the medial and lateral structures, fascioligamentous structures, and the capsule, (2) removing all deforming forces from the knee joint prior to actual replacement surgery, and (3) precise replacement of the knee joint by a prosthesis, aided by instrumentation that can only adequately be performed if the soft tissue operation has been adequately handled. From the prosthetic design point of view, several theoretical advantages are attributed to design of this prosthesis. Although only time can evaluate its merits or disadvantages, the following are considered advantages of the design of the prosthesis and the surgical technique.

1. This prosthesis and design of surgery call for *minimum bone removal* from the top of the tibia, therefore conserving the maximum bone of the tibia for fixation and principal correction of the deformity through the soft tissue and the distal end of the femur.

2. Because of the double radii of the design, there is *no constrainment* in the prosthetic articulating surfaces. However, the design of the runners mating with the tibial segment provides a translational (side to side movement) constraint under load conditions.

3. The *principal fixation* of the component is achieved by intramedullary fixation, which places acrylic cement under constant compression and minimizes the shear-tension forces from the cement-bone bond. The design of the prosthesis and operative technique provide an excellent opportunity for the surgeon to anchor the tibial component onto the top of the tibia using a perpendicular force in relation to the top surface of the tibia. The tapered stem of the prosthesis provides injection pressure via the stem into the cancellous bone of the medullar canal. Rotary forces are resisted by four studs, two on each component, as well as the design of the stem of the components.

4. *Improved technique of insertion* is accomplished by a simple geometric resection of bone (perpendicular to the axis of the femur and tibia) using special jigs and spacer devices to ensure accuracy of replacement. Correct alignment and perfect fixation are the sine qua non of the technique of knee arthroplasty.

5. *Adjustability and replaceability* are provided by the different thicknesses of plastic tibial plateaus available at surgery (selection is based on the test prosthesis), which enable the surgeon to (1) maximize the tension across the ligaments and (2) observe the correct angle of valgus alignment during the testing of the prosthetic device which does not require removal from the femur and tibia. Replacement of the tibial plastic piece may be considered if undue wear takes place. This can be simply achieved without disturbing the fixation of the metallic tibial component.

6. *Cold flow of plastic* is prevented. Because the tibial plateau of the prosthetic component is subjected to abnormal loads and the possibility of plastic flow exists, especially in the use of a thin plastic piece, the plastic component is press fitted into a metallic base for support. In later surgical exploration of four knees, no cold flow was observed in the plastic contained within the metallic segment.

The articulating surfaces provide no constraint in the axial plane and the runners are polycentric with decreasing radii from the front.

The original design (Mark 1) called for retention of cruciate ligaments if they were present. During that period, several tibial spines were fractured inadvertently during surgery, but the results of these cases were similar to those in knees with a good cruciate ligament. Because cruciate ligaments, particularly in the presence of any deformity, become a great handicap in correcting the deformity, their removal now is considered essential to correct the deformity and space the joint maximally for stability from the ligaments and the fascial capsular layer of the joint. Almost any severe degree of varus or valgus deformity (with the exception of grotesque valgus deformity) may be corrected with this type of knee joint prosthesis provided that adequate soft tissue adjustment is made and the joint is maximally spaced. A minimum bone resection from the top of the tibia and the distal end of the femur is possible only when the soft tissue allows maximum spacing for insertion of the prosthesis. This, of course, is of fundamental importance should arthrodesis become necessary at a later date.

PATELLOFEMORAL JOINT

The patellofemoral joint was not considered an important feature in the early design (Mark 1); therefore the femoral component had no extension to include this joint. However, with further experience we have concluded that this joint should be considered a significant cause of failure when it is not replaced. Quick recovery and good quadriceps strength during the postoperative course following patellofemoral replacement indicate the absence of feedback pain. The patellar replacement is, of course, a new and experimental procedure that awaits long-term follow-up prior to a final appraisal.

SUMMARY

The total knee replacement developed at the New York Orthopaedic Hospital since 1969 is a nonhinged unit designed to replace articulating surfaces of the tibia and femur (Mark 1) and to include the patellofemoral joint as well (Mark 2). The principal fixation mechanism is via the intramedullary stems of the tibial and femoral components, as well as the platform and studs that are incorporated in the design of the prosthesis. The operative technique calls for conservation of the bone of the proximal tibia by a minimum bone resection and a complete soft tissue correction prior to implantation of the prosthetic device. Accuracy of replacement becomes possible if the cruciate ligaments are excised and the space between the tibia and femur is maximized following posterior capsular release as indicated. With patellar replacement and routine excision of the cruciates, the operation has become more predictable than it was in our earlier experience.

ACKNOWLEDGMENT

I wish to thank Mr. Rudy Gand for his assistance in execution of design of the prosthesis and instruments and Mr. Marvin Alpern for the mechanical drawings used in this chapter.

25. Wear and fixation of condylar replacement knee prostheses

Peter S. Walker

Condylar replacement knee prostheses using metal on plastic have only been in use since about 1970, with the introduction of the polycentric and the geometric designs. There are now many others, but with the common features that the femoral condyles are replaced with metal runners, generally convex in two planes; the tibial surfaces are replaced with plastic blocks, generally concave in one or two planes; and methyl methacrylate cement is used for fixation. Probably every design has suffered from one or more of the following mechanical problems:

1. Wear of the polyethylene
2. Localized distortion of the polyethylene
3. Gross distortion of the tibial component
4. Loosening of the tibial or femoral component
5. Instability or dislocation

Some of these factors are interrelated. Instability can result in high forces being applied at the periphery of the plastic components, leading to local distortion and possibly loosening. Any degree of instability or loosening is likely to result in the production of acrylic fragments, which will increase the wear and release both polyethylene and acrylic particles into the joint.

WEAR

In total hip prostheses, wear of the plastic over the long term is regarded by some as a serious problem in that the accumulation of particles may contribute to bone resorption as well as to capsule thickening. In the knee joint, however, the follow-ups have been insufficiently long for wear to have emerged as a significant clinical problem as compared with the more immediate problem of loosening. However, Bullough et al.[1] reported that the count of polyethylene and acrylic particles in the tissue around the joint, particularly in knees in which loosening had occurred, was far in excess of that seen in the hip joint.

A number of authors have studied the wear on removed knee prostheses. Reckling et al.[3] studied a removed geometric prosthesis, noting score marks in the direction of motion, as well as pits that were probably caused by the loose fragments of acrylic cement that were found. Shoji et al.[4] found considerable distortion and wear of the plastic in four failed polycentric knees. They also noted loose fragments of acrylic cement. In a study of eleven removed prostheses, Trent and Walker[6] attempted to correlate the type of wear with the conformity between the femoral and tibial components. Consistent with the findings of the other authors, score marks in the sliding direction and pits caused by entrapped acrylic particles were commonly found. In prostheses with low conformity, such as the modular and the duo-condylar, surface cracks and pits were seen and were thought to be a result of repetitive high shear stresses beneath the small areas of contact. A series of wear experiments suggested that if the initial Hertzian contact stress exceeded somewhere in the region of 10 to 20 N/mm², the wear rate was increased. In prostheses in which the tibial surfaces are close to flat, the stresses can readily exceed this under the peak loads encountered in walking.

Surface contact stresses

An example of the wear pattern on a nonconforming modular prosthesis is shown in Fig. 25-1. The sliding surfaces are polished, but there are numerous dimples and pits superimposed, representing fatigue pitting. Nonetheless, the depth of wear was small, with the depths of pits being around 0.25 mm. Sections seen in the light microscope and the scanning electron microscope showed the pits to be shallow with sloping sides. It appeared that the pits were formed by the coalescing of surface cracks, which were seen extensively over the surface (Fig. 25-2).

Table 25-1. Sizes of areas of contact and contact stresses for knee prostheses with different radii of curvature

Component	Extension (femoral radius 35 mm)		Flexion (femoral radius 22 mm)	
	Contact diameter or width (mm)	Average contact stress (N/mm²)	Contact diameter or width (mm)	Average contact stress (N/mm²)
Point contact				
Dished tibial component (R = 38 mm)	12.6	8.0	6.2	33.6
Flat tibial component (R = ∞)	5.4	43.7	4.6	59.7
Line contact				
Curved tibial component (R = 38 mm)	10.3	6.1	3.5	17.8
Flat tibial component (R = ∞)	2.9	21.7	2.3	27.3

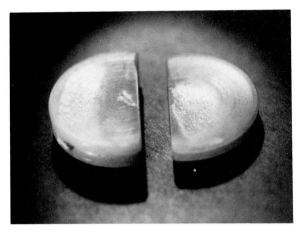

Fig. 25-1. Areas of sliding on modular plateaus show burnishing and pitting.

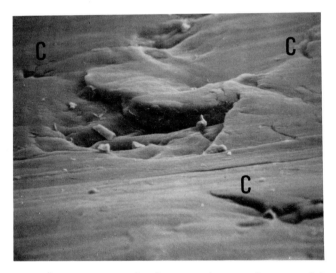

Fig. 25-2. Scanning electron micrograph of pit on plastic surface caused by coalescing of surface cracks (C).

Calculations* using Hertzian equations give an approximation of the contact stresses that occur in the plastic in different types of prostheses (Table 25-1). The assumptions made are as follows:

1. Correct alignment between the femoral and tibial condyles
2. Modulus of elasticity of the polyethylene of 1214 N/mm² (176,000 lbf/in²)
3. Poisson's ratio of 0.3

---

*The SI system (International System of Units) has been used: 1 Newton (N) = 0.102 kilogram force (kgf); 1 kgf = 9.81 N; = 2.205 lbf; 1 N/mm² = 10.197 kgf/cm² = 145 lbf/in².

4. Load on each condyle one and one-half times body weight, 1000 N (225 lbf).

For two spheric surfaces with radii R_1 and R_2, a load W, a modulus of elasticity E, and a Poisson ratio V, the radius of the area of contact a is:

$$a = \left(\frac{3}{2} \frac{WR^1}{E^1} \right)^{\frac{1}{3}}$$

where R^1 = relative radius of curvature given by

$$\frac{1}{R^1} = \frac{1}{R_1} - \frac{1}{R_2}$$

and E^1 = equivalent elasticity given by

$$\frac{1}{E^1} = \frac{1 - V^2}{2E}$$

The area of contact is πa^2 and the average contact stress is $W/\pi a^2$. In the case of cylindric surfaces, where W is the transverse width, half the contact width b is:

$$b = \left(\frac{8WR^1}{\pi LE^1} \right)^{\frac{1}{2}}$$

The area of contact is 2wb and the average contact stress is W/2wb.

Several inferences can be made from the results in Table 25-1. For a doubly convex femoral component running on a flat or nearly flat plateau, the diameter of the contact is only about 5 mm and the stresses are exceedingly high, particularly in flexion. Dishing the tibial plateaus reduces the stresses considerably to what might be considered acceptable. A cylindric femoral runner on a flat plateau produces twice the contact area and half the stresses of a doubly convex runner. If, in addition, the plastic component is dished, the stresses are reduced to a range of about one to two times that in a Charnley total hip. Of course, the greater the width of the runners, the less the stress, but this does not apply when the femoral surfaces are spheric.

It seems, then, that cylindric surfaces would be better than spheric surfaces. For cylindric surfaces, alignment in the frontal plane would be critical, so a slight curvature in the frontal plane is required to alleviate this problem. Also, if a cylindric femoral component is rotated on a cylindric tibial component (of larger radius of curvature) about the long axis of the tibia, the contact ceases to be a line across the full width and becomes localized on the medial and lateral edges. Hence for this reason also the femoral runners have to be curved in the frontal plane.

Entrapped particles of acrylic cement

If acrylic particles enter the bearing surfaces and a load is applied, the particles indent the polyethylene surface (Fig. 25-3). The dents vary considerably

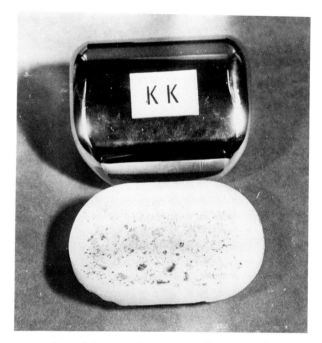

Fig. 25-3. Craters on surface of Freeman-Swanson prosthesis caused by entrapment of acrylic fragments.

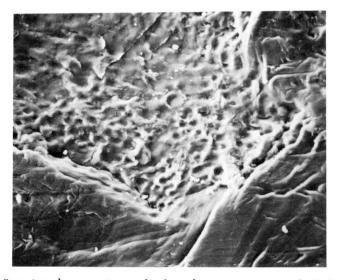

Fig. 25-4. Scanning electron micrograph of acrylic crater seen on polyethylene surface.

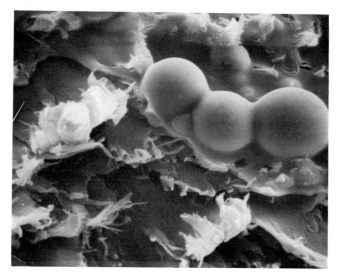

Fig. 25-5. Scanning electron micrograph of acrylic spheres, about 30 μm in diameter, and shredding of polyethylene that they cause.

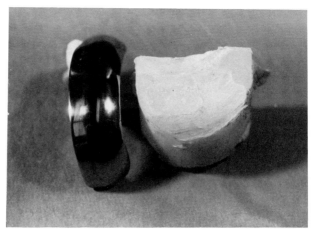

Fig. 25-6. Early unicondylar knee, removed after approximately 2 years for unsatisfactory performance. Gross wear was caused by abrasion from bone.

in size, but they can be several millimeters across and greater than a millimeter in depth.

Typically the craters show imprints of acrylic spheres at the base while the periphery is crumbling (Fig. 25-4), which can lead to the release of polyethylene fragments in the same way as a pothole in a road expands. In some cases a fragment of acrylic is seen to be firmly embedded in the surface. Surrounding the craters one sees smaller fragments of acrylic, broken from the initial piece, while observation in the scanning electron microscope shows numerous groups of spheric particles representing finely ground up acrylic cement (Fig. 25-5). The

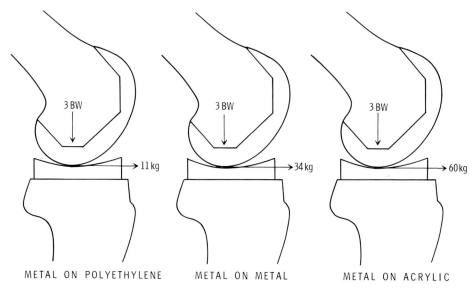

Fig. 25-7. Horizontal frictional forces imposed on tibial component if knee slides forward when there is compressive load of 3 times body weight acting.

surface of the polyethylene in the vicinity is shredded, from which numerous sheets and threads would be likely released.

Abrasion by bone

The type of wear just described, in which a third material ingresses between two other materials, is called three-body abrasion. Two-body abrasion occurs when roughnesses on the surface of a harder material directly abrade the surface of a softer material. This can occur severely if bone is allowed to rub against the polyethylene. The surface of bone is extremely rough when compared with the microfinish of a femoral runner. The result is a great deal of wear, as evidenced by the unicondylar knee (Fig. 25-6) in which the femoral runner was too narrow and there was misalignment and instability in the joint.

FIXATION

If components were to be designed and inserted so that reasonably normal compressive stresses were transmitted across the implant-bone interface, long-term fixation would probably be achieved. However, loosening is undoubtedly a problem in present knee prostheses,[5] which is likely to be mainly caused by the shear and tensile stresses that occur, which the interface is poorly able to withstand. All of the stresses are a direct result of the external and internal forces acting on the prosthesis. Before a discussion of the various external forces and moments, the internal frictional forces acting between the metal and plastic surfaces will be considered.

If the load between the two surfaces is W and the coefficient of friction is μ, the frictional force F is sliding or incipient sliding: $F = \mu W$. Fig. 25-7 depicts the femur pushing forward on the tibia with a force of three times body weight. For metal on polyethylene, μ is 0.05 and the frictional force is low. Metal on metal has a μ of 0.15, giving three times the friction. However, if the acrylic particles are trapped between the metal and the polyethylene surfaces, the friction of metal on acrylic applies. Since this is 0.25, the frictional force is so large as to adversely affect the fixation.

Cement-bone interface

A radiolucent line surrounding the cement of the tibial component, occurring with greater frequency in the conforming types of knee such as the geometric, has been frequently reported.[2] Around this radiolucency, however, there is usually a line of radiopacity. From examinations of a number of removed specimens, this has been found to consist of a layer of bone, equivalent to a new subchondral plate, as it were; the radiolucent zone is filled with fibrous tissue (Fig. 25-8). When a prosthesis is originally inserted, the cement interdigitates to some extent with numerous free ends of trabecular struts and sheets. Bone remodeling then presumably occurs, as a result of either the initial damage of the exposed ends or the subsequent localized high stresses that are imposed. Whatever the reason, the result is a substantial reduction of any cement-bone interdigitation that once occurred, reducing the load-carrying capacity in shear and in tension. In fact, the latter may be close to zero in many cases.

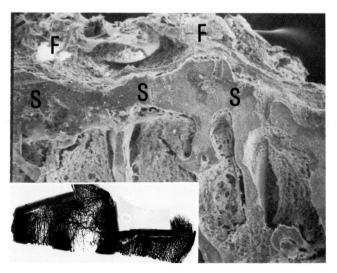

Fig. 25-8. New subchondral layer (S) and fibrous tissue above it (F) at cement-bone interface. (Cement is above, not shown.)

Walker[7] measured the shear strength of a laboratory-prepared cement to trabecular bone interface under different conditions. The strength was proportional to the compressive load, as expected. For a freshly prepared cement-bone interface, shear strength was 1.6 N/mm.[2] Once movement occurred, this reduced to 0.9, and when the acrylic was smoothed (to simulate the conditions of a new subchondral plate), the strength was only 0.5 N/mm.[2] The conclusion is that reliance can only really be placed on the compressive stresses between the cement and the bone, because the shear and tensile capacities, even if they exist initially, reduce or disappear with time.

Bending of plastic plateaus

Loosening could occur if the plastic component distorted so much under load that the cement underneath fractured or if lifting of the component-cement composite occurred in some areas. Bending of plastic plateaus was tested[9] by cementing parallel-sided plastic tibial plateaus 8 mm, 10 mm, and 12 mm thick onto the prepared surfaces of tibias. No cement keyholes were made, the cement being simply used to obtain a close fit. Loads were applied by a metal cylinder across the center, the line of contact being in the transverse direction. The bowing of the plastic in the sagittal plane was measured relative to a horizontal reference line on the metal cylinder. For the three thicknesses of plastic, there was little difference in the deformations measured. When the plateaus were mounted onto a rigid base or onto hard bone (compressive stiffness 3080 kg/cm²/cm), there was parallel sinkage to within 0.02 mm. On soft bone (stiffness 1125 kg/cm²/cm),

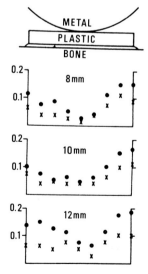

Fig. 25-9. Deflection of plastic plateaus (vertical axis in millimeters) of 8 mm, 10 mm, and 12 mm thickness, when mounted on soft bone and loaded to 122 kg (dots) and 85 kg (crosses).

however, U-shaped bending occurred where the center bowed about 0.07 mm relative to the front and the back (Fig. 25-9). Even this value is small, and hence it is expected that if the plastic thickness is 8 mm or more, deformation under load should not cause a problem unless long-term creep of the plastic occurred.

Tilting of tibial plateaus

If a tibial plateau that is convex in one or two planes is subjected to an antero-posterior force, there is a tendency for tilting to occur. To what extent this happens depends on the strength and type of the anchorage. However, tilting can occur even if the plateau is flat and a compressive force is applied within the boundaries of the upper surface. This was demonstrated in the following experiment.[9]

A tibial specimen was prepared by resecting the condylar surfaces a few millimeters below the subchondral bone. The upper trabecular spaces were cleaned and a metal tibial plateau (similar to a MacIntosh prosthesis) was cemented in place. Rods were affixed at the anterior and posterior of the plateau and the bone. Loads were applied at points along the upper surface on a line running from front to back down the center of the plateau. The relative movements between the plateau and the bone were measured across the rods. Two medial and two lateral sides were tested. In all cases tilting occurred for some positions of the load. In particular, the anterior tilted upward, separating from the bone by as much as 0.5 mm when the load was only about one third from the back. There was more tendency for tilting on the medial side than on the lateral side. Although it was not tested, if a plateau were placed covering the whole surface (such as a Freeman-Swanson prosthesis), tilting could occur as a result of the center of pressure in the frontal plane being toward one side or the other (Fig.

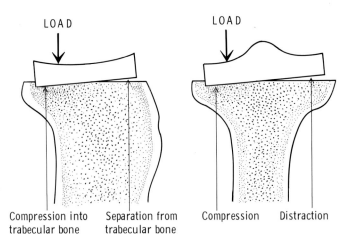

Fig. 25-10. Depiction of tilting phenomenon, whereby loads within boundary of plateau can cause compression on one side and distraction on other.

25-10). It may be reasonable to suggest that the majority of the radiolucency seen around tibial components is a direct result of repeated tilting movements, which are a reflection of elastic deformations within the trabecular bone and perhaps the entire shell of the upper tibia itself.

Methods of anchoring

Femoral components have the great advantage that they can be shaped to wrap around the bone. All of the forces tend to compress the components directly onto the bone, although in a strict sense this is not necessarily true. For example, a force on the posterior condyle with the knee in flexion produces shear stress along the distal interface and even tensile stresses at the patellar flange. From the clinical evidence, however, these effects are not nearly so pronounced as in tibial components. With flat plateaus, resistance to tilting can be achieved by drilling keyholes for cement anchorage. The pull-out strength of a hole 10 mm in diameter and 16 mm in length is about 1000 N, a considerable force. When the tibial component is a one-piece unit, the choices of anchoring configuration are greater. Although there are various possibilities, one method that has met with some success to date is to use a short central peg (Fig. 25-11). The rationale is as follows:

1. The strong trabecular bone on each side is preserved.
2. Anteroposterior tilting is resisted by the anterior and posterior cortices.
3. Medial-lateral tilting is resisted by the trabecular bone at each side.
4. Torque is resisted by the faces of the peg and by shear resistance across the upper cement-bone interface.
5. The compressive force is transmitted in an approximately normal manner over a wide area of bone.

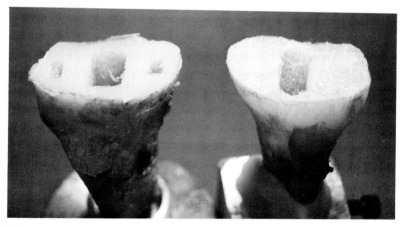

Fig. 25-11. Preparation of upper tibia for one-piece component with short central peg (total condylar). Small holes at each side help to resist rotation.

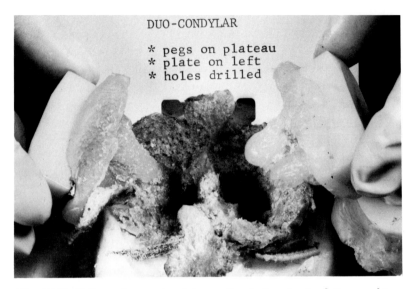

Fig. 25-12. Failure of separate plateaus after testing in simulating machine.

Disadvantages of the peg are as follows:

1. Cement sometimes balloons out into the upper intramedullary canal and beneath the medial and lateral trabecular bone.
2. Much of the tibial eminence must be removed.

Using a nine-channel machine, which flexed and extended the knee specimens and applied a pulsating load of three times body weight, different types of anchorage were compared.[8] For the test duration, none of the one-piece plateaus with a peg failed, whereas several failures of the separate plateaus occurred. This was thought to be a result of the stress concentrations caused by making the cuts and by drilling the cement keyholes (Fig. 25-12). In other words, islands of bone were created, destroying the integrity of the trabecular structure. There are still many unanswered questions as to the best design of tibial component for long-term fixation. A metal tray can be used to support the plastic, and pegs can be placed at each side, anteriorly or in combination. There have been suggestions for using screws or bolts through the cortex into the component. A further point is that most designs of tibial components (with the exception of Charnley's load angle inlay) require resection of several millimeters of bone from the upper tibia. It is this bone that is the strongest of all.

BALANCING WEAR, FIXATION, AND STABILITY

To avoid high local stresses on the plastic, there must be some degree of conformity. The more the conformity, the more restriction there is on the motion and the greater the forces on the fixation. At the present time a solution that appears to work satisfactorily is the compromise of using partially conforming surfaces and achieving strong fixation by use of a short central peg.

References

1. Bullough, P. G., Insall, J. N., Ranawat, C. S., and Walker, P. S.: Wear and tissue reaction in failed knee arthroplasty, J. Bone Joint Surg. **58-B**:366, 1976. (Abstract.)
2. Insall, J. N., Ranawat, C. S., and Shine, J.: A comparison of four models of total knee replacement prostheses, J. Bone Joint Surg. **58-A**:754, 1976.
3. Reckling, F. W., Asher, M. C., Mantz, F. A., and Helton, D. O.: Performance analysis of an ex vivo geometric total knee prosthesis, J. Bone Joint Surg. **57-A**:108, 1975.
4. Shoji, H., D'Ambrosia, R. D., and Lipscomb, P. R.: Failed polycentric total knee prostheses, J. Bone Joint Surg. **58-A**:772, 1976.
5. Skolnick, M. D., Coventry, M. B., and Ilstrup, D. M.: Geometric total knee arthroplasty. A two-year follow-up study, J. Bone Joint Surg. **58-A**:749, 1976.
6. Trent, P. S., and Walker, P. S.: Wear and conformity in total knee replacement, Wear **36**:175, 1976.
7. Walker, P. S.: Tibial fixation in condylar replacement knee prostheses. In Williams, D., editor: Biocompatability of implant materials, London, 1976, Sector Publishing Co. Ltd.
8. Walker, P. S., and Hsieh, H. H.: The conformity in condylar replacement knee prostheses, J. Bone Joint Surg., 1977. (In press.)
9. Walker, P. S., Ranawat, C. S., and Insall, J. N.: Fixation of the tibial components of condylar replacement knee prostheses, J. Biomech. **9**:269, 1976.

26. Total knee loosening

Herbert Kaufer
Larry S. Matthews
David A. Sonstegard

Although total knee replacement is a relatively new operative procedure, 2-year follow-up clinical studies on appreciable numbers of patients have recently become available and make it clear that total replacement yields early symptomatic and functional results far superior to other techniques of knee arthroplasty.* However, these studies show a complication rate of 7% to 25%. Of the reported complications, the early appearance of loosening severe enough to require revision surgery is especially distressing, approaching 10% of cases in some series of nonarticulated total knees.[17,18] Experience with hinged prostheses is even more ominous.[38,39,41] In spite of generally excellent early results, reports of 7- to 10-year follow-ups of these devices show an ultimate failure rate of nearly 100%, primarily caused by loosening.[38,41]

In all total joint replacements the incidence of loosening increases with the length of follow-up†; however, compared to total hips, loosening in total knees is more common, appears sooner, progresses more rapidly, and is more likely to compromise the clinical results.[2,31,34,35,40] Loosening of nonarticulated total knees is far more common on the tibial, or polyethylene, side of the joint.‡ Interestingly, loosening of total hip prostheses also appears most frequently on the polyethylene (acetabular) side of the joint.§ Although articulated total knees loosen more frequently, they show less tibial loosening and in one type (Herbert) loosening occurs most frequently on the femoral side.‖ The frequency and severity of loosening increases with the patient's activity level.[2,16-18,21] Total knees in patients with osteoarthritis have a greater loosening hazard than those in patients with rheumatoid arthritis.[7,16-18] Contrary to what one might expect, osteoporosis does not seem to favor loosening.[2,16-18,21]

A roentgenographic zone of lucency surrounding the methacrylate mass is

---

*References 2, 7, 10, 11, 14, 16-18, 21, 23, 24, 26, 32, 38, 39.
†References 2, 16-18, 31, 34, 35, 38-41.
‡References 10, 11, 14, 16, 21, 26, 32.
§References 1, 2, 31, 34, 35, 40.
‖References 7, 10, 18, 38, 39, 41.

308

the earliest sign of loosening and has been reported in up to 80% of cases followed for 3 years or more.[17,18] The lucent zone may be 3 mm or more wide and is usually bordered by a definite line of sclerotic bone. Most knees with lucency on x-ray films are asymptomatic and are doing well clinically.[17,18] Since many orthopaedists erroneously equate loosening with failure, they are reluctant to make a diagnosis of loosening unless the roentgenographic lucency is progressive, is associated with symptoms, or shows evidence of gross relative motion between implant and bone. This is a mistaken point of view. It is entirely possible for an implant to be loose and remain functional, asymptomatic, and clinically satisfactory.* The cup in a hip cup arthroplasty is, after all, always at least a little loose, but many of them are clinically successful and remain so for years.

Our laboratory recently performed a postmortem evaluation of a geometric total knee that had been inserted 3 years previously; it was functioning well, without symptoms or clinically apparent relative motion between implant and bone (Fig. 26-1). However, under laboratory conditions this prosthesis was shown to be markedly loose. One degree of angular displacement per 9 footpounds of torque was observed between the tibia and the tibial component of this prosthesis. Subsequent dissection and histologic examination showed a continuous fibrous membrane separating bone from the methacrylate mass (Fig. 26-1). This clinically successful asymptomatic total knee was certainly loose.

If, because of a surrounding lucent zone, an implant looks loose on x-ray films, it is probably loose, even if the joint is not symptomatic. The lucent zone need not surround the entire methacrylate mass, and relative motion between implant and bone may not be demonstrable by clinical means such as stress views or arthrography.[8,34,35] Lucent zones on x-ray films and physical loosening need not be progressive; they may remain static for long periods of time and may even regress.[35]

There are at least four categories of loosening. The types and criteria are as follows:

Simple loosening
1. Partial or complete radiolucent zone between implant and bone
2. Painless
3. Clinically satisfactory
4. Physical loosening may or may not be demonstrable by stress views, push-pull films, or arthrography

Symptomatic loosening
1. Radiolucent zone
2. Discomfort aggravated by activity and relieved by rest
3. Absence of other symptom-producing abnormalities: fracture, contusion, infection, etc. (Symptoms and loosening need not be causally related.)

---

*References 11, 14, 16-18, 21, 26, 32.

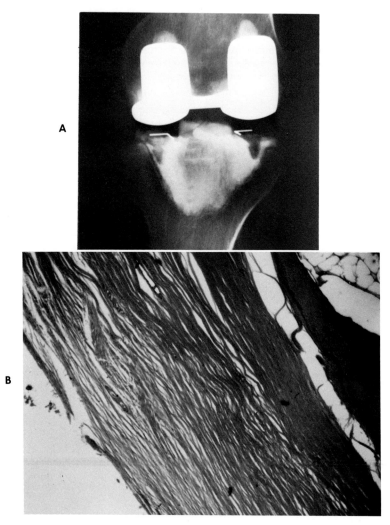

Fig. 26-1. A, Anteroposterior roentgenogram of geometric total knee in severely disabled rheumatoid patient shows radiolucent zone around tibial methacrylate mass and thin sclerotic line between lucent zone and adjacent cancellous bone. Prosthesis had been "in service" for 3 years and was asymptomatic. Patient walked without aids and was delighted with functional restoration. Postmortem studies of this knee showed gross loosening of tibial component. (See text.) **B,** Photomicrograph at implant-bone junction of tibial component shown in **A.** Methyl methacrylate dissolved out by fixative solutions is represented by clear space, which is separated from bone by continuous layer of mature, loose, fibrous tissue. Adjacent bone is viable. Marrow spaces are histologically normal. There is no inflammation.

Progressive loosening
1. Documented increasing length or width of the radiolucent zone
2. May or may not be painful
3. Clinically satisfactory

Functional loosening
1. Radiolucent zone
2. Progressive displacement of the implant relative to bone, leading to malalignment of the limb, instability or other malfunction of the implant
3. May or may not be painful

We urge adoption of this or some other acceptable classification of loosening so that we can arrive at relevant data for the frequency and severity of loosening and be better able to make meaningful comparisons between implants as regards their loosening hazard.

LOOSENING FACTORS
Infection

In all cases of progressive, functional, or symptomatic loosening of a prosthetic knee, the physician is obligated to rule out the possibility of infection. The roentgenogram can be of some assistance in this regard. If the loosening is secondary to infection, the adjacent bone tends to be much more osteoporotic than in cases of noninfectious loosening, and the sclerotic line surrounding the lucent zone tends to be less prominent or even be absent.

A positive bacteriologic culture is, of course, the best way to prove the infectious etiology of loosening. In addition to the usual pyogens, it is important to culture for fungi, anaerobes, and other atypical organisms, since they are relatively common causative agents in infection of prosthetic joints.[12] These organisms can be difficult to culture, and one may have to obtain tissue specimens for culture to be certain about the presence of infection. A frozen section for histologic examination may be useful in determining the presence or absence of infection. Although collections of histiocytes, foreign body giant cells, and other histologic evidence of chronic inflammation may be present, acute inflammatory cells are seldom seen in tissue adjacent to a loose prosthesis that is not infected.[4,5,15,20]

Fracture

The sudden onset of activity-related pain in a total knee that previously showed only simple loosening may be caused by a fracture through adjacent bone, even if there is no clear history of trauma. The fracture may be difficult or impossible to demonstrate by x-ray film. Laminagrams can be helpful (Fig. 26-2). Treatment of the fracture with a suitable period of immobilization and restricted weight bearing can achieve fracture healing and control of symptoms in many cases. Even if a fracture cannot be demonstrated, it is probably wise to assume that fracture may be the cause of symptoms in patients with simple loosening who suddenly develop activity-related pain. These patients should receive closed

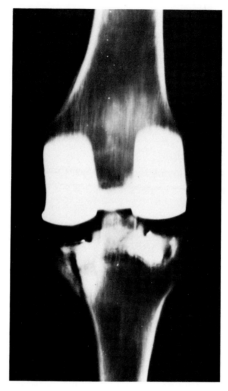

Fig. 26-2. Laminagram of geometric total knee demonstrates fracture of tibial metaphysis as well as lucency around methacrylate and methacrylate crack.

fracture treatment empirically. Revision of the total knee arthroplasty should be reserved for those patients who fail to get adequate symptom relief from a suitable period of nonoperative fracture treatment.

Load direction

Under static conditions the articular surfaces of a knee joint are either loaded in compression or not loaded at all.[22,29] It might therefore seem reasonable to assume that the implant-bone junction of a total knee is never exposed to appreciable stress in tension. It would be desirable if this were true because the major deficiencies of polymethyl methacrylate as a grouting material are that it has poor tensile strength, has poor shear resistance, and is rather brittle.[3,9]

Postmortem evaluation of a total knee specimen in our laboratory, using instrumentation capable of sensing and recording a 0.0001 inch displacement between implant and bone, showed that the implant-bone junction probably experiences very large loads in *tension* (Fig. 26-3). If loaded asymmetrically, the prosthesis behaves much like a boat in water; it tends to sink under an applied load and rise on the opposite side. In a specimen with no evidence of loosening,

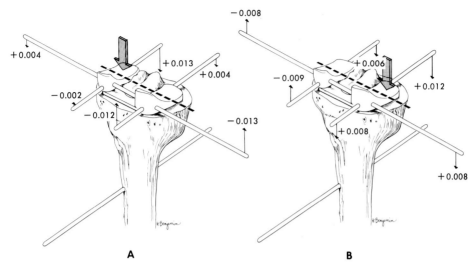

Fig. 26-3. Composite representation of instrumented tibial component of geometric total knee. Dashed line is anteroposterior midline of tibial component. Large shaded arrow indicates site of load application. **A,** Magnitude and direction of deflection in inches at sites shown, produced by load of three times body weight applied on posterior half of lateral tibial plateau. This loading configuration corresponds to moderate valgus strain applied to extended knee during midstance. **B,** Magnitude and direction of deflection in inches produced by load of three times body weight applied on posterior portion of medial tibial plateau. This loading configuration corresponds to moderate varus strain applied to extended knee during midstance. Direct measurement showed negative deflection of approximately 0.010 inch between prosthesis and bone at anterior aspect of prosthetic tibial component opposite from site of loading.

under a physiologic load of three times body weight, the measured difference between maximum positive deflection and maximum negative deflection of the prosthesis relative to bone was 0.0020 inch. The observed deflection is a composite measurement of the compliance of the bone-methacrylate-prosthesis assembly. Stress in tension generated by the relatively large negative deflection must contribute significantly to loosening at the methacrylate-bone junction because both methacrylate and bone have relatively poor tensile strength.

Coefficient of friction

Coefficient of friction is a numeric value that represents resistance to relative motion between objects in contact.[13] A free body in a vacuum has neither static nor dynamic friction acting on it. The coefficient of friction is determined by the nature of the materials in contact and by the geometry and finish of their contacting surfaces.[9,13] In general, metal-on-metal total knees have a higher coefficient of friction than metal–on–high molecular weight polyethylene total knees.[9] For both types of total knees, wear may produce irregularity of the articulating surfaces and therefore a gradually increasing coefficient of friction.[37] As the coefficient of friction increases, frictional torque exerted on the implant, and force at the bone-implant interface with each loaded movement also increase. The prostheses that have small areas of contact between articular surfaces (that is, modular, polycentric, ICLH, and condylar) generate relatively large surface contact stresses (surface load per unit area). This accelerates surface wear and thereby tends to accelerate the rate of increase of the coefficient of friction.

Malalignment

Malalignment of the lower extremity produces dramatic changes in the pattern of articular surface loading, leading to excessive local force concentrations (Fig. 26-4). Clinical experience with osteotomy about the knee for painful deformity has demonstrated that this is a reversible phenomenon.[6,25] Although it has not received as much recent attention, correction of flexion or hyperextension deformity is as important as correction of varus or valgus deformity. Ideal limb alignment minimizes the joint reaction force and results in more nearly uniform distribution of that force.[6,25]

Ideal alignment may not be the same for all total knee prostheses. Recent studies indicate that, for the geometric total knee, the minimal loosening moment is seen if the knee has 7° of valgus alignment with the tibial component at a right angle to the long axis of the tibia in the frontal plane and tilted forward 10° in the sagittal plane.[30]

These data suggest that total knee components might be more resistant to

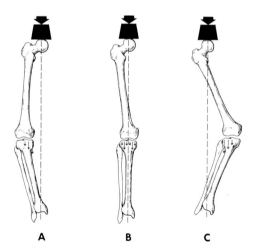

A   **B**   **C**

Fig. 26-4. Varus deformity, **A,** concentrates compressive stress on medial side of knee, producing large local loads. Valgus deformity, **C,** results in similar load concentration on lateral side of knee. In knee free of deformity, **B,** weight-bearing line passes through center of knee. There is more nearly uniform distribution of load.

loosening if they had stems that could minimize the "boat-in-water" deflection that occurs as a result of asymmetric loading. Medullary stems would also resist the loosening moment generated by friction and/or malalignment of the limb and prosthesis.

Load distribution

Polymethyl methacrylate surrounding the polyethylene component of a total joint is subjected to a uniform distribution of load if the polyethylene is uniformly loaded via total surface contact with the articulating metal component (Fig. 26-5, A), as is the case with the geometric total knee prosthesis. However, in most total knees (modular, polycentric, condylar, ICLH, etc.) the polyethylene component is loaded over a small area (Fig. 26-5, B). Methacrylate supporting a point-loaded polyethylene component experiences nonuniform loading with stress concentrations that could approach the compressive breaking limits of methacrylate and thereby accelerate the loosening process. This effect is most marked in thin polyethylene components.[36]

Poisson's ratio

All materials deform under load. Poisson's ratio is the number derived if one divides the change in length by the change in width, that occur when a material is loaded (Fig. 26-6). All materials have a specific and unique Poisson ratio.[13] If a structure composed of materials with dissimilar Poisson ratios is loaded, each material in the composite structure undergoes a dissimilar change in width rela-

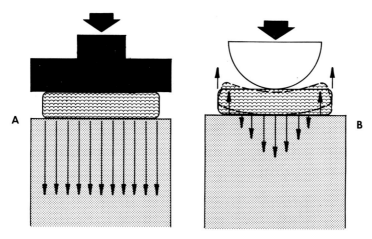

Fig. 26-5. A, If polyethylene (horizontal wavy lines) is uniformly loaded over its entire surface, supporting methacrylate (stippled) is subjected to even distribution of load. **B,** If polyethylene (horizontal wavy lines) is loaded at a central point, compressive stress will be concentrated in small region of adjacent methacrylate (stippled). With this loading configuration, unloaded edges of polyethylene tend to lift away from methacrylate, thus producing tensile stress at these sites.

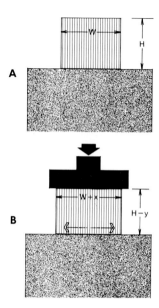

Fig. 26-6. A, Object free of load has height *H* and width W. **B,** When object is loaded, height is decreased *(H-Y)* and width is increased *(W+X).* Poisson's ratio is ratio of length change relative to width change of material when loaded. If square (vertical lines) and rectangle (stippled) are composed of dissimilar materials with different Poisson's ratios, then shear stress occurs at interface between these materials when they are loaded.

tive to its change in length, thus generating shear stress at each interface between dissimilar materials.

The magnitude of stress is proportional to the magnitude of the load and proportional to the the magnitude of the difference between Poisson's ratios of the loaded materials. Shear stress caused by dissimilar Poisson's ratios is of appreciable magnitude in total knees because physiologic loads are large[29] (three to four times body weight) and because Poisson's ratios of the materials used in total knees (steel, cobalt-based alloy, polymethyl methacrylate, and high molecular weight polyethylene) and bone are all markedly dissimilar.[9]

Elastic modulus

Elastic modulus is a specific numeric constant unique for each material and describes that material's linear deformation under load. It is proportional to the change in length per unit length of the material when loaded.[13] If a composite structure made of materials with dissimilar elastic moduli is loaded, the stiff materials deform less than the more elastic material (Fig. 26-7), thus generating shear stress at each interface between dissimilar materials. The magnitude of stress is proportional to the load and proportional to the difference between elastic moduli of the loaded materials in the composite structure. Here again, the shear stress is of considerable magnitude because the load is large,[29] and the

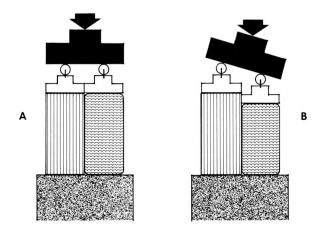

Fig. 26-7. A, Assembly composed of stiff material (vertical lines) bonded to more elastic material (horizontal wavy lines). **B,** When composite structure is loaded, elastic material deforms more than stiff material, thus generating shear stress at bond between the two materials.

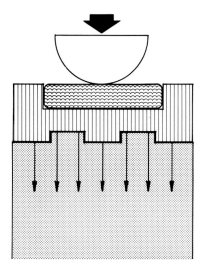

Fig. 26-8. Polyethylene (horizontal wavy lines) loaded at a central point is supported by and contained within metal (vertical lines), which rests on methacrylate (stippled). This arrangement transmits more nearly uniform load to methacrylate (see Fig. 26-5, *B*) and is better able to withstand shear at interfaces between dissimilar materials.

elactic modulus of commonly used total knee prosthetic materials (steel, cobalt-based alloy, polymethyl methacrylate, and high molecular weight polyethylene) and bone are all markedly dissimilar.[9] One way to minimize the problems created by dissimilar Poisson's ratios, dissimilar elastic moduli, and nonuniform loading would be to support and surround the polyethylene with metal as shown in Fig. 26-8.

Bone fixation

Although it may seem reasonable to assume that prosthetic fixation to cortical bone is stronger than fixation to cancellous bone, clinical experience shows that knee prostheses with long medullary stems that make cortical contact are at least as prone to loosening as the prostheses that rest only on spongy bone, and bone resorption is often most marked at sites where prostheses and cortex are in contact.[10,11,14,38,41] Experience with total hips also shows more clinically sig-

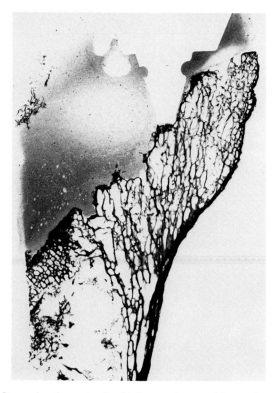

Fig. 26-9. Microradiograph of proximal tibial metaphysis of knee that has had geometric prosthesis "in service" for more than 2 years. There is no loosening. Methacrylate has penetrated many cancellous spaces and is in intimate contact with trabecular bone, resulting in large contact area.

nificant loosening of the femoral component, which often has appreciable cortical contact, than the acetabular component, which more often makes contact only with spongy bone.[31,35,40]

Penetration of methacrylate into the spaces surrounding trabeculae of cancellous bone provides a large surface area of contact between cement and bone (Fig. 26-9), thus assuring minimal contact stress. Determination of the strength of methacrylate to fresh human bone fixation in our laboratory (single compressive load to failure) indicates that fixation to cancellous bone is significantly stronger than fixation to cortical bone. With cyclic loading (fatigue testing) the superiority of methacrylate–cancellous bone fixation should be even greater because cyclic loading conditions would emphasize the superior energy and shock absorbing capacity of cancellous bone compared to cortical bone. It seems clear that at this time methacrylate in *cancellous* bone is the preferred method for fixation of prosthetic knee components. Close approximation of methacrylate to cortical bone should be minimized.

Bone strength

Most determinations of bone strength have been made on cortical bone.[9] These data are readily available but not relevant to the problem of prosthetic knee component loosening, because most total knee components rest on cancellous

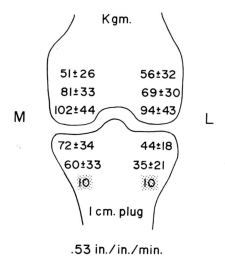

Fig. 26-10. Average compressive breaking strength of 1 cm cancellous bone cylinders taken from indicated opposing areas of fresh human knees when tested at strain rate of 0.53 inch/inch/minute. Strength differences between various areas are statistically significant (P <0.05). Compressive breaking strength values for bone at level 3 cm below articular surface of tibia (stippled) are not reliable, because bone at this site is so weak that most cylinders were destroyed by plug cutter and relatively few could actually be tested. (*M*, Medial; *L*, lateral.)

bone and make little or no contact with the cortex. Measurement of the strength of fresh human cancellous bone in our laboratory and others reveals that cancellous bone is highly variable in its material characteristics. Cancellous bone varies widely not only from individual to individual, but also from bone to bone within the same individual, and it even shows marked variation between different areas in the same bone (Fig. 26-10). The strongest cancellous bone is closest to the joint surface. Cancellous bone strength drops off progressively as the distance between the bone sample and the joint surface increases. In general, cancellous bone from the medial side of the knee joint is stronger than bone samples from the lateral side, and femoral bone is much stronger than tibial bone. These data correlate well with the clinically observed preponderance of tibial component loosening as well as the frequency of tibial plateau fracture compared to the relative rarity of femoral condylar fracture.

The observed variance in strength of cancellous bone adjacent to the knee suggests that to utilize the best quality cancellous bone for fixation, the prosthetic components should be implanted as close to the joint surface as possible. Less length of bone should be resected from the tibial side of the joint than from the femoral side. Whenever possible, the tibial component of a total knee ought to be as thin as possible, certainly thinner than the femoral component.

Methacrylate properties

Polymerization of polymethyl methacrylate is an intensely exothermic reaction.[3] Heat generated within the methacrylate mass and high temperature at the cement-bone interface are often indicted as causative factors for implant loosening. Although the thermal effects of polymerization are certainly somewhat injurious to local bone, in vivo measurements of temperature at the cement-bone interface show it to be at least 10° C less than the 56° C temperature at which protein is thought to be irreversibly damaged.[19,33] If any bone necrosis occurs adjacent to methacrylate, it is most likely caused by cytotoxic effects of the monomer or mechanical trauma from preparation of the bone bed rather than the thermal effect of polymerization.[19,33]

Recent studies have shown that polymethyl methacrylate shrinks after polymerization.[28] The shrinkage is probably the result of thermal contraction, which occurs as the methacrylate mass cools from the relatively high temperatures reached during polymerization. In all cases of cement fixation, postpolymerization methacrylate shrinkage (plus the inevitable interposition of small bits of tissue debris, clots, and tissue fluid between methacrylate and bone) results in less than a perfect fit between cement and bone[28] (Fig. 26-11). Micromotion may occur as a result of this less than perfect fit at the bone interface.[27] Because polymethyl methacrylate is relatively brittle and has poor shear resistance,[9] small spikes of methacrylate may fracture from strain produced by the micromotions and lead to progressive loosening, which in turn exposes adjacent living bone to excessive stress, thus triggering its active resorption.

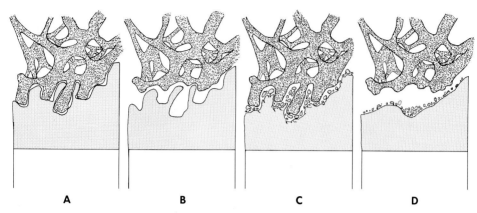

Fig. 26-11. Schematic representation of methacrylate–cancellous bone interface. **A,** Because of postpolymerization methacrylate shrinkage, as well as interposed bits of clot and tissue debris, fit between methacrylate (stippled) and bony trabeculae is never quite perfect. **B,** Active resorption of trabeculae would result in increasingly poor fit between methacrylate and bone. **C,** Fragmentation of methacrylate also contributes to increasingly poor fit between methacrylate and bone. One cannot be certain if methacrylate fragmentation and trabecular resorption occur simultaneously or if one precedes the other. In any event, the end stage of the loosening process is a very poor fit between methacrylate and bone, **D,** produced by combined effects of bone resorption and methacrylate fragmentation. Space that develops between the two is occupied by combination of fibrous connective tissue and fibrocartilage.

BIOLOGIC RESPONSE

Studies of cyclically loaded fresh human cadaver bone in our laboratory have shown that methacrylate–cancellous bone interfaces can be subjected to the laboratory equivalent of more than 10 years of patient use at physiologic load without any loosening. However, in actual clinical use in living patients, definite tibial component loosening has been reported in 50% to 80% of cases after 2 or 3 years.[17,18,38] Our own clinical experience includes several cases of noninfectious total knee loosening sufficiently severe to require revision surgery less than 1 year after the original total knee arthroplasty (Fig. 26-12). These observations force one to the inescapable conclusion that noninfectious loosening is a biologic response. Under proper conditions, living bone actively resorbs and retreats from contact with a cyclically loaded prosthesis. Dead bone (our laboratory tested cadaver specimens) seems clearly superior to living bone in its ability to withstand multiple weight-bearing cycles at physiologic load without loosening.

One is tempted to assume that active bone resorption is simply a response to toxins associated with the methacrylate mass, but this is certainly not the case. The width of the resorption zone surrounding a loosened prosthesis is seldom uniform and is not proportional to the mass of methacrylate. The resorption zone is often largest at sites of heaviest loading (Fig. 26-12).

Miller et al.[27] in Montreal have recently shown that in dogs the loosening

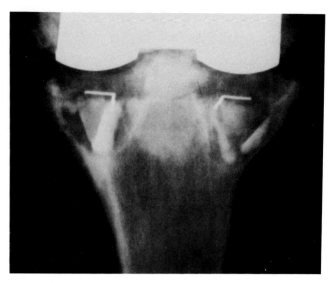

Fig. 26-12. Symptomatic geometric total knee 10 months after insertion with prominent lucent zones under both prosthetic plateaus. There is no lucency adjacent to relatively unloaded central portion of tibial prosthesis. Gross loosening was confirmed at revision operation. Multiple negative cultures and tissue specimens ruled out infection.

response occurs and progresses only if the prosthesis is a little loose to start with. His observations suggest that micromotion may be the stimulus for biologic loosening, presumably mediated through piezoelectric responses or similar phenomena. Although micromotion is certainly an important causative factor, it is not the only factor, since loosening is not always progressive.[35] Some prostheses that start out loose may stimulate hypertrophy rather than resorption of bone and often do.

Tissue sections of material adjacent to loosened prostheses show both mature (Fig. 26-1, *B*) and immature fibrous tissue as well as areas of fibrocartilage (Fig. 26-13).[4,5,8,15,20] Since the cement when initially inserted was in direct contact with bone, the interposed fibrous tissue must be the result of bone resorption and replacement.[3] It is therefore surprising that osteoclasts are quite rare in these tissues, even in areas where fibroblastic activity is quite intense. Although one may see collections of histiocytes and an occasional foreign body giant cell, acute inflammatory cells are quite rare and marrow spaces show normal fat with little fibrosis or infiltration. Necrotic trabeculae are quite uncommon.[4,5,8,15,20]

Sections taken from prostheses that have not loosened show direct contact between trabeculae and cement at many sites. Areas of interposed fibrous tissue or fibrocartilage are rare.[3,4] The marrow spaces look normal and the trabeculae are alive. There are virtually no histologic signs of inflammation. One gets the impression that the histologic changes adjacent to loose prostheses may be the effect rather than the cause of loosening.

Loosening has emerged as the single most important long-term problem asso-

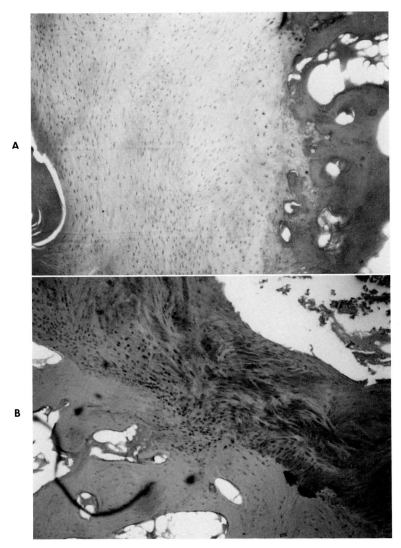

Fig. 26-13. Additional sections taken from lucent zone adjacent to tibial component of geometric knee shown in Fig. 26-1, A. **A,** Broad band of fibrocartilage. **B,** Intense fibroblastic cellular activity adjacent to viable bone. Methacrylate has been dissolved out of clear area in upper right corner.

ciated with total knee replacement. The pathogenesis of loosening is clearly multi-factorial. This chapter has briefly and superficially considered some of the known factors. A solution to the complex problem of prosthetic component loosening is beyond our grasp at this time. However, there is great hope for the future; improved designs, new prosthetic materials, and a better bone cement or perhaps porous metals should minimize many of our current mechanical problems. Laboratory research, some of which is already in progress, holds promise for ultimate understanding of the biologic response of bone to cyclically loaded prostheses and its ultimate control. For the time being, however, the prudent orthopaedist should recognize the frequency and severity of the loosening problem and use total knee arthroplasty only for those patients who, because of advanced age, systemic disease, or multiarticular involvement, are unable to place large functional demands on their artificial knee.

References

1. Andersson, G. B. J., Freeman, M. A. R., and Swanson, S. A. V.: Loosening of the cemented acetabular cup in total hip replacement, J. Bone Joint Surg. **54-B:**590, 1972.
2. Bargren, J. H., Freeman, M. A. R., Swanson, S. A. V., and Todd, R. C.: ICLH (Freeman, Swanson) arthroplasty in treatment of arthritic knee, Clin. Orthop. **120:**65, 1976.
3. Charnley, J.: Acrylic cement in orthopedic surgery, Baltimore, 1970, The Williams & Wilkins Co.
4. Charnley, J.: The reaction of bone to self-curing acrylic cement, J. Bone Joint Surg. **52-B:**340, 1970.
5. Charnley, J.: The histology of loosening between acrylic cement and bone, J. Bone Joint Surg. **57-B:**245, 1976.
6. Coventry, M. B.: Osteotomy about the knee, J. Bone Joint Surg. **55-A:**23, 1973.
7. Deburge, A.: Guepar hinge prosthesis, Clin. Orthop. **120:**47, 1976.
8. DeLee, J. G., and Charnley, J.: Radiological demarcation of cemented sockets in total hip replacement, Clin. Orthop. **121:**20, 1976.
9. Dumbleton, J. H., and Black, J.: An introduction to orthopaedic materials, Springfield, Ill., 1975, Charles C Thomas, Publisher.
10. Engelbrecht, E., Siegel, A., Rottger, J., and Bucholz, H. W.: Statistics of total knee replacement: partial and total knee replacement design St. Georg, Clin. Orthop. **120:**54, 1976.
11. Evanski, P. M., Waugh, T. R., Orofino, C. F., and Anzel, S. H.: UCI knee replacement, Clin. Orthop. **120:**33, 1976.
12. Fitzgerald, R. H., Peterson, L. F. A., Washington, J. A., Van Scoy, R. E., and Coventry, M. B.: Bacterial colonization of wounds and sepsis in total hip arthroplasty, J. Bone Joint Surg. **55-A:**1242, 1973.
13. Frankel, V. H., and Burstein, A. H.: Orthopaedic biomechanics, Philadelphia, 1970, Lea & Febiger.
14. Gunston, F. H., and MacKenzie, R. I.: Complications of polycentric knee arthroplasty, Clin. Orthop. **120:**11, 1976.
15. Harris, W. H., Schiller, A. L., Scholler, J. M., Frieberg, R. A., and Scott, R.: Extensive localized bone resorption in the femur following total hip replacement, J. Bone Joint Surg. **58-A:**612, 1976.
16. Ilstrup, D. M., Coombs, J. J., Jr., Bryan, R. S., Peterson, L. F. A., and Skolnick, M. D.: A statistical evaluation of polycentric total knee arthroplasties, Clin. Orthop. **120:**18, 1976.
17. Ilstrup, D. M., Coventry, M. B., and Skolnick, M. D.: A statistical evaluation of geometric total knee arthroplasties, Clin. Orthop. **120:**27, 1976.
18. Insall, J. N., Ranawat, C. S., Aglietti, P., and Shine, J.: A comparison of four models of total knee-replacement prosthesis, J. Bone Joint Surg. **58-A:**754, 1976.
19. Jefferiss, C. D., Lee, A. J. C., and Ling, R. M. S.: Thermal aspects of self-curing polymethylmethacrylate, J. Bone Joint Surg. **57-B:**511, 1975.
20. Johnson, K. D., Dunn, H. K., and Daniels, A. V.: Wear debris and bacteriologic findings in joint prosthesis removal, Trans. Orthop. Res. Soc. p. 225, 1977.
21. Kaushal, S. P., Galante, J. O., McKenna, M. D., and Bachmann, F.: Complications following total knee replacement, Clin. Orthop. **121:**181, 1976.
22. Kettelkamp, D. B., and Chao, E. Y.: A quantitative analysis of medial and lateral com-

pression forces at the knee during standing. In Proceedings of the Orthopaedic Research Society, J. Bone Joint Surg. **53-A**:804, 1971.

23. Laskin, R. S.: Modular total knee-replacement arthroplasty, J. Bone Joint Surg. **58-A**: 766, 1976.

24. Lotke, P. A., Ecker, M. L., McCloskey, J., and Steinberg, M. E.: Early experience with total knee arthroplasty, J.A.M.A. **236**:2403, 1976.

25. Maquet, P.: Biomechanique du genou et gonarthrose, Rev. Med. Liege **24**:170, 1969.

26. Marmor, L.: The modular (Marmor) knee, Clin. Orthop. **120**:86, 1976.

27. Miller, J., Burke, D. L., Stachniewicz, J., and Kelebay, L.: The fixation of major load-bearing metal prostheses to bone. An experimental study comparing smooth to porous surfaces in a weight bearing mode, Trans. Orthop. Res. Soc. p. 54, 1976.

28. Miller, J., Burke, D. L., Stachniewicz, J. W., and Kelebay, L.: A study of the interface between cortical bone under conditions of load bearing, Trans. Orthop. Res. Soc. p. 191, 1976.

29. Morrison, J. B.: The mechanics of the knee joint in relation to normal walking, J. Biomechanics **3**:51, 1970.

30. Mullen, J. O., Chao, E. Y., and Coventry, M. B.: Analysis of mechanical failure in the geometric total knee, Trans. Orthop. Res. Soc. p. 7, 1976.

31. Murray, W. R., and Rodrigo, J. J.: Arthrography for the assessment of pain after total hip replacement, J. Bone Joint Surg. **57-A**:1060, 1975.

32. Ranawat, C. S., Insall, J., and Shine, J.: Duocondylar knee arthroplasty, Clin. Orthop. **120**:76, 1976.

33. Reckling, F. W.: The measurement of the bone-cement interface temperature during total joint replacement procedures, Trans. Orthop. Res. Soc. 61, 1976.

34. Salenius, P., and Laurent, L. E.: Experience with the McKee-Farrar total hip replacement, Acta Orthop. Scand. **44**:451, 1973.

35. Salvati, E. A., Cheum, I. M., Virat, S., and Aglietti, P.: Radiology of total hip replacement, Clin. Orthop. **121**:76, 1976.

36. Walker, P. S., Ranawat, C., and Insall, J.: Fixation of the tibial components of condylar replacement knee prostheses, J. Biomech. **9**:269, 1976.

37. Walker, P. S., and Salvati, E.: The measurement and effects of friction and wear in artificial hip joints, J. Biomed. Mater. Res. Symp. **4**:327, 1973.

38. Watson, J. R., Wood, H., and Hill, R. C. J.: The Shiers arthroplasty of the knee, J. Bone Joint Surg. **58-B**:300, 1976.

39. Wilson, F. C., and Venters, G. C.: Results of knee replacement with the Walldius prosthesis, Clin. Orthop. **120**:39, 1976.

40. Wilson, J. N., and Scales, J. T.: Loosening of total hip replacements with cement fixation. Clinical findings and laboratory studies, Clin. Orthop. **72**:145, 1970.

41. Young, H. H.: Use of a hinged vitallium prosthesis (Young type) for arthroplasty of the knee, J. Bone Joint Surg. **53-A**:1658, 1971.

27. Prevention of sepsis in orthopaedic implant surgery

Carl L. Nelson

The problem of infection is not the only concern of the orthopaedist; however, continued implant surgery makes the preoccupation with infection indeed realistic. In all surgery, infection is one of the most ravishing consequences; the end result of infection is in vivid contrast to the usually expected result and certainly is in contrast to the result expected by the patient.

The problem of sepsis is common to all types of surgery and there is wide variation in reported ranges of incidence. Infections after surgery of the back, the hip, or the knee are often considered the most significant. These areas are often completely ravished by infection, and the Scandinavians have reported that these areas account for 50% of their serious infections.[22] It is of interest that 60% of their "serious" infections were about the hip. Implants are sensitive indicators of bacterial contamination, and in fact the milieu provided by implant surgery may be a more sensitive indicator of bacterial contamination than most standard bacteriologic testing systems. Consequently the emphasis on prevention of infection in implant surgery has magnified the consequences of infection and placed the orthopaedist in the forefront of preventing sepsis.

NONOPERATIVE FACTORS

There are unique features of implant surgery, whether it is in the knee or the hip, that predicate a high risk of infection. The size of the implants used, the material, the hematoma, the lack of viable tissue in immediate contact with the implant, and avascular bone about the implant are all factors that theoretically influence the rate of infection. A prosthesis of the size used in implant surgery is a significant amount of material to be placed anywhere in the body. The trauma of dissection and placement is formidable even to the uninitiated. The wear products of high-density polyethylene and the reaction to the acrylic bone cement, as well as the wear products of metal, produce a reaction that may be more conducive to infection. Indeed, the type of inflammatory tissue present may be significant in the development of infection.

Dead space is always present in large implant surgery. Even the smallest

326

implant produces some degree of dead space and hematoma. A hematoma always occurs; the degree of hematoma is, of course, directly related to the amount of dead space produced by the operation. A hematoma is not only a nidus for infection, but if it becomes tense and taut, it may also devascularize the surrounding soft tissue and impede the natural defense mechanisms. Taut, tense hematomas are, of course, to be avoided in all orthopaedic surgery.

A normal vascular supply to bony areas is a key to prevention of infection and is in direct relation to the body's ability to combat infection. There is little living tissue to combat infection directly in contact with many large orthopaedic implants. It should be recalled that when a bone is reamed, hematoma is formed and there is death of the immediate surrounding tissue. Even when bone is centrally reamed and acrylic cement is centrally placed, there is death of the bony tissue in immediate contact. When cement and reaming are placed eccentrically, the cement or metal lies against the cortex; major devascularization of the immediately surrounding bony tissue may occur and remain for a prolonged period. It has been shown experimentally in reamed femurs with implanted metal and acrylic cement that there is adequate space for intramedullary blood supply through cancellous bone, the tissue becomes well vascularized, produces new bone, and is theoretically capable of combating the same infection as any other bony tissue.[13,36]

On the other hand, where there is impairment of intramedullary vascular penetration, new bone does not form and bone may be devascularized for at least 1 year after implantation of acrylic cement. The orthopaedic implant patient therefore may have large amounts of dead bone in immediate contact with foreign materials for prolonged periods. These areas, of course, have little vascular supply to combat bacterial contamination, and avascularity in these areas may be related to early and late infection.

Superimposed on high-risk implant surgery is the high-risk patient that the orthopaedist is often forced to treat. Because of the improved benefits of implant surgery, patients who would not have been considered surgical candidates are now operated on. These patients often have predisposing problems that alter their host defects mechanisms and predicate a high risk of infection. Age, trauma, malnutrition, obesity, steroid treatment, diabetes, and rheumatoid arthritis all have been implicated in increased infection rates.[31] Although controversy surrounds the rheumatoid patient and perhaps the diabetic, there is little question that aged patients have double the infection rate of younger patients. The patient with infections at other foci has three times the normal infection rate. These factors may be further influenced by prolonged surgery, prolonged hospitalization period before surgery, and increased numbers of persons in the operating room.[12,22,31]

One group of patients of concern are those that have foci of infections remote from the operative site prior to surgery. Three areas that may be infected prior to surgery are the skin, the lungs, and the genitourinary tract. These patients are reported to have three times the normal surgical infection rate. The patient with a urological infection, for example, may have benign prostatic hypertrophy and urinary tract infection, especially an older individual. These urologic problems should be treated and the infection eradicated prior to orthopaedic surgery whenever possible. It is far better to have eradicated a urinary tract infection prior to joint replacement surgery than to have an infected joint replacement.

It is clear that all patients undergoing implant surgery should have any foci of infection eradicated prior to surgery to prevent a high rate of surgical infection. It is also appropriate to discuss specific preventative postoperative plans for implant patients. It is suggested that patients with implants should be treated similarly to those patients who have undergone cardiac valvular replacements. If a patient with a successful orthopaedic implant needs instrumentation such as a tooth extraction or cystoscopy, he should be treated with antibiotics preventively. The patient should be clearly informed of this need and also informed that if he develops an infection, he should receive immediate care from a physician.

OPERATIVE FACTORS

All of the factors mentioned probably in some way influence the rate of infection. There are also operative factors that increase the patient's risk. It has been stated that duration of an operation for more than 1½ hours may be critical and increase the rate of infection. However, it is not clear whether an increased infection rate is related to prolonged surgery, the length of time the wound is exposed, or the difficulty of the operation and the amount of soft tissue destruction that occurs. The size of the wound and the all-important operative technique, including tissue handling and hemostasis, have traditionally been cited as critical and related to the problem of infection. Hematoma and tissue death, or at least some degree of soft tissue trauma, probably need to be present for an infection to occur. Bacterial showers often occur with instrumentation without producing an infection in the area of an orthopaedic implant or fractures; consequently there must be a milieu established at surgery that is conducive to infection. Avoiding hematomas and tissue death are logical and time-tested methods of maintaining a low infection rate.

ASEPTIC TECHNIQUES

Are there any other concepts that can be considered to reduce the rate of infection in a high-risk patient? To prevent surgical sepsis a clear understanding of the background of infection prevention is necessary. Infection is indeed not a new problem for the surgeon; in 1880 Moynihan stated that two thirds of his patients died of infection after he opened the belly, and as late as 1895 Brewer showed that clean operations were followed by approximately a 39% infection rate.[4,30] In the 1880s Joseph Lister proposed a revolutionary concept of surgical sepsis.[24] His concepts were ridiculed and interestingly were not originally adopted in England. His concepts were first used on the European continent and then later established in England. The principles he outlined were finally applied throughout the world, and infection rates decreased. His concepts have lead to our modern era of aseptic surgery, which consists of preoperative skin cleansing combined with sterile scrub by the operating room personnel; wearing of rubber gloves, masks, and sterile clothing; proper housekeeping; and, of course, sterilization.

How effective are the commonly used aseptic techniques and what can one expect from them in maintaining a low infection rate? The first principle that must be clearly understood and utilized is that there is no substitute for strict adherence to standard well-known aseptic surgical techniques.

Meleney[29] in 1933 showed that he could reduce a serious infection rate from 4% to 1.7%; McKissock et al.[27] reduced their infection rate from 15% to 1.1%; Henderson showed that the infection rate could be held at 1.7%; and Steel[42] reduced the infection rate from 5% to 0.5%.[30] The criteria for maintaining a lower infection rate are similar for all studies.

It appears that rigid regulation of persons passing in and out of the operating room (particularly inadvertent and unnecessary visitors) is important in reducing the infection rate. Second, careful preparation of the patient and the operating room personnel is of paramount importance in maintaining a low infection rate. It appears that it is a simple matter of attention to detail. In addition, tissue handling, careful dissection, prevention of tissue destruction, protection of the skin edge, prevention of hematoma, and proper wound closure are factors that influence the infection rate. Finally, it appears there is a part of infection prevention that is intangible. Education of all operating room personnel with regard to the problem of surgical infection has a salutory effect on the infection rate.

There is often discussion about proprietary soaps and antiseptics, and there is wide variation in the preparation used. Although there are few scientific data that support the contention, it appears that it is better to be a disciple of aseptic technique than a devotee of any particular commercial preparation.

Almost everyone agrees that the majority of surgical infections occur in surgery, but there is controversy as to whether the infections are endogenous or exogenous. Direct implantation from the patient may occur with faulty technique and inadvertent breaks in the technique; these can usually be avoided by attention to detail. One area that continues to be controversial is the role of exogenous airborne contamination. In a study done by Walter, it was shown that in their group 20% of the infections at surgery were caused by airborne contamination. However, there is considerable controversy and although many facts are known, little is agreed on. There is general agreement that wound infections are directly related to the type of organism that is in the wound, the host's ability to combat infection, and the chance deposition of bacteria in the wound. Although there would appear to be a relationship between the number of bacteria that are deposited in the wound and the infection, the relationship is not completely known.

It is known that an individual may shed as many as 10,000 particles per minute depending on how recently he or she has showered and the type of clothing worn. Conventional operating room air may contain 1050 bacteria per cubic foot of air; on occasions the content may be even higher. The activities of the surgeon and the operating room crew produces particulate matter with accompanying bacteria. Convection currents from the body of the surgeon and the operating room personnel allow passage of particulate matter through the fine text of cotton and then theoretically into the wound. There is little question that if one releases particulate particles with attached bacteria above the wound, they are often deposited into the wound.

Historically, although airborne contamination has been observed, there have been attempts to statistically evaluate whether eradication of airborne bacteria is beneficial to the patient.

Ultraviolet light has been used in attempts to reduce infection rates by reducing numbers of airborne bacteria. One study has shown that the ultraviolet light used in the operating room decreased the bacterial contamination and when this method was employed, such as in reconstructive surgery, there was a statistically significant decrease in infection in the group.[15]

There have also been recent studies to evaluate the clean air system. There have been substantial data produced throughout the United States and Europe that have conclusively shown that the clean air system is capable of reducing bacterial contamination in the air not only with the room empty but also at the time of surgery.[32-34] Charnley, who popularized the concept of reducing airborne contamination, has reported his statistics and concepts. In 85 infections and approximately 5800 total hip replacements done between 1960 and 1970, the incidence of infection fell from 7% to 0.5%.[11] He suggested that of all the precautions taken against the infection, the most important improvement was reduction of airborne contamination. However, it was his opinion that this measure alone did not reduce the infection rate below 1.5%. He stated that a reduction below 1.5% was a result of measures taken to avoid penetration of bacteria through the surgical drapes and gowns and to improve the wound closures. Ritter has also reported a statistically significant reduction in the infection rate for total joint replacement by the use of clean air flow systems. Others have implied such a change.[32,33]

Although there are few hard statistical data universally agreed on, it would appear that the reduction of airborne contamination is not detrimental, that it is probably salutory, and that the principle is acceptable. In fact, the reduction of contamination of the wound is a listerian principle known to surgery since the 1800s. Although the conclusions from the data are not agreed on, the prin-

ciples that asepsis is better than antisepsis and that reduction of bacterial contamination of the wound is worthwhile will probably stand the test of time.

PREVENTIVE ANTIBIOTICS

The attempt to prevent sepsis has prompted the use of preventive antibiotics.
The use of antibiotics to prevent infection has been a controversy since the early
development of antimicrobial agents; in fact, early studies showed that antibiotic
prophylaxis in elective surgery served no useful purpose. Prophylactic antibiotics
were associated with the concept that the ill-informed, technically poor surgeon
used them to mask his mistakes. During the past 5 to 10 years there has been
a quiet scientific interest in the use of antibiotics in a different surgical sense.[1,14,44]
Initially interest was directed at the strict antibiotic-bacterial relationship. The
present interest focuses on the host, the bacteria, the antibiotics, and their inter-
relationships. Burke[9] has presented a clearer focus on the patient's ability to deal
with bacterial contamination when exposed to potentially dangerous surgical
procedures and suggested preventive antibiotics in certain instances. These factors
and other studies have influenced orthopaedists to use preventive antibiotics. It
has been shown by Eftekhar that more than 80% of surgeons doing joint replacement surgery use preventive antibiotics.

Early studies that showed the ineffectiveness of antibiotics as prophylactic
agents had errors in proctocol, such as lack of controls, the use of multiple antibiotics, improper timing of administration of antibiotics, and inadequate dosage
regimes. More modern studies have been designed to give preventive antibiotics
during the time of bacterial contamination rather than after surgery and at
therapeutic rather than at low irregular dosages.* It has not been considered
necessary to eradicate all organisms, simply specific pathogens. These more
recent and explicit studies have shown the statistically significant decrease in
the incidence of postoperative infection. Despite available data there continues
to be an honest difference of opinion as to the interpretation of the data and
whether preventive antibiotics should be used in ultraclean surgical procedures.
Before preventive antibiotics are condoned or condemned, data that are available
should be reviewed and studied. The use of antibiotics in the United States has
cost millions of dollars each year. Death and a multitude of other complications
are associated with antibiotic use. Smith studied 900 patients who received antibiotics and found the overall incidence of adverse effects to be approximately
10%. The incidence was also found to be much higher in patients receiving
many drugs than in those receiving few. Complications that can occur are local
effects, directly toxicity, superinfections, hypersensitivity, and a miscellaneous
group comprising such problems as fetal injury.

If one chooses to use preventive antibiotics, it should be based on the principle that the most important factor in preventing infection is the natural anti-

---

*References 1, 3, 14, 22, 38, 39, 44.

microbial defense mechanism of the patient. On the basis of this principle, there is a group of patients who have altered natural antimicrobial mechanisms who are called high-risk surgical patients. These patients fall into major categories such as the congenitally defective defense mechanism, low defense mechanisms, patients taking corticosteroids, patients with large areas of damage tissue, patients undergoing large implants, etc. When surgery is performed on these patients, the skin is obviously broken, bacterial contamination occurs, as well as tissue damage, and the anesthetic has the capability of decreasing the body mechanisms to prevent the development of infection. The timing of the use of antibiotic to prevent and eradicate bacterial contamination appears to be critically related to the surgical period. Burk and Wilson have shown that an appropriate antibiotic given at the time of surgery can prevent an innoculum of bacteria from causing infection.[2,9] However, if the antibiotics are started 24 hours after surgery, infection cannot be prevented. If antibiotics are started 6 hours after surgery, although there is little sign of late infection, lesions cannot be sterilized.

These studies support in theory the clinical studies that demonstrate the benefits of preventive antibiotics. All clinical studies showing the effect of preventive antibiotics are those in which the drugs have been given immediately before and at the time of surgery. It appears that there is a definite period of time when incisional contamination may be controlled. This surgical period is the appropriate time to supplement the natural defense mechanisms of the patient; this period has been termed the decisive period by Burke.[9]

The type of antibiotic and the duration of preventive treatment are often debated. Prolonged administration of preventive antibiotics does not appear to be necessary and, in fact, may be detrimental. It has been historically suggested that if a preventive antibiotic is given, a narrow-spectrum antibiotic aimed at a specific organism is the most effective mechanism with the least chance of untoward reaction. Weinstein[47] has advised the prophylactic use of broad-spectrum antibiotics such as a cephalosporin derivative for joint replacement surgery. It is his contention that a broader spectrum antibiotic eradicates a wider variety of bacterial contaminants and, if given for a short period of time, does not cause the problems of secondary bacterial overgrowth or drug toxicity related to increased dosage.

It has been suggested that antibiotic administration started immediately prior to surgery, maintained during surgery, and discontinued 1 day after surgery should be an adequate regime. Others have implied that antibiotics should be maintained until drainage devices are removed from the wound or until the cultures taken at the time of surgery have returned. These are more personal preferences, and unfortunately none of these preferences is proved.

In summary, surgery disturbs the natural host defense mechanisms and creates a state in which invasion by a small number of organisms is enhanced. This enhancement occurs in the perioperative period. This is the decisive period when incisional bacteria may be killed. Antibiotics therefore should be present in the tissue when primary lodgement of bacteria occurs. Short-term administration of broad-spectrum antibiotics presently appears to be the preferred choice. If one chooses to use preventive antibiotics these concepts should be used. However, it should be equally clear that asepsis is always preferred to antisepsis.

Antibiotics in bones, joints, and hematomas

The question should naturally be asked by the orthopaedist whether antibiotics penetrate bones, joints, and hematomas. This is reasonable concern since the ability of an antimicrobial to penetrate these areas is related to its ability to eradicate infection. In the past few years information has become available for the orthopaedist to review; however, previously most antibiotic use was based on empirical judgments.

It has been shown that most commonly used antimicrobials produce bacterial concentrations within inflamed joints; however, each new drug should be evaluated for joint penetration.[37]

Antibiotic penetration of wound sites and hematoma is an area in which few data have been provided. The wound and hematoma individually or collectively provide an ideal milieu for bacterial growth, and there is always a delay in living tissue penetration. It appears from various clinical and experimental studies that antibiotics are capable of penetrating wound fluid and hematomas even into the depths of the hip.[35,47] It is not proved but appears that diffusion into a wound area may be inhibited by a taut hematoma, and antibiotics may not be able to saturate the depths of a large hematoma if they are administered after the hematoma is formed. Consequently it would appear wiser to attain high serum levels of antibiotic when the hematoma is forming.

Antibiotics in bone. Antibiotics normally penetrate bone through the serum via the vascular tree.[40] Levels of antibiotic in bone increase as the amount in serum increases, and although the amount of antibiotic in bone is generally lower, the bone-to-serum ratio is constant when the dosage is within therapeutic ranges.[18,19] There is a variation in serum and bone concentrations with different antibiotics, apparently as a result of the relationship to the lower protein in the intercellular fluid of bone.[11] There is a slight delay in the vascular phase of antibiotic diffusion into bone; that is, intravenous antibiotics pass quickly into bone but at a slower rate and to a lower level than into serum. Twenty to 30 minutes after intravenous administration of antibiotics, bactericidal levels are reached in bone. Practically, one can saturate normal bone within 30 minutes of intravenous administration and it is not necessary to give antibiotics several days in advance to penetrate normal bone. In fact, it is probably better to start antibiotics for preventative use in the surgical suite, as this allows sufficient time for antibiotic penetration of bone, and if an adverse effect occurs, the patient is in the most appropriate place for resuscitation or treatment of any acute complication. For accuracy, antibiotics should be administered on the basis of body weight.

Local antibiotics

There is little unequivocal evidence that the use of local antibiotics reduces the overall infection rate in orthopaedic surgery, and, in fact, there is controversy as to the time needed for local antibiotics to cause bacterial death. It is more apparent that local antibiotics as usually used at the time of surgery are indeed local and penetrate the surrounding tissue to a limited amount. It has been suggested that the most rational method of producing antibiotic levels in the wound is through the serum and that adequate levels are achieved in the wound when intravenous antibiotics are used. It is generally agreed that one of the most beneficial effects of local irrigation is débridement. The prolonged use of huge concentrations of local antibiotics may allow absorption into the vascular tree and therefore can be dangerous.

Antibiotic-acrylic composites

The use of acrylic-antibiotic composites as preventive and therapeutic agents in joint replacement surgery has been popularized in, although not limited to, Europe. Knight and Long[17] reported the use of antibiotic-impregnated cement in more than 1500 patients operated on in the United States. Buchholz has suggested the removal of an infected total hip prosthesis, wide débridement, and insertion of a new prosthesis using acrylic cement impregnated with antibiotics.[5-8] He and Lindberg reported a significant success rate using this technique and have implied that a reduction in the infection rate occurs when antibiotic-laden acrylic cement is used as a preventative measure in initial joint replacement surgery.[23] Although acrylic cement is a hard, brittle material that would not appear to allow the release of antibiotics, it in fact allows elution of antibiotics for relatively long periods.[*] Elution is effected by concentration gradients; material lodged within the available interstices of the cement is exposed to body fluids and, if not bound, passes into the surrounding fluids and tissues.

Mechanical tests show that mixtures of aqueous antibiotics in acrylic cement significantly decrease the compressive and diametrial strengths of the composite and that dry antibiotic does not affect these two parameters.[20,25]

PROSPECTUS

Areas of research and development of infection prevention may influence patient care in the future. There has been a continued interest in evaluation of the host's ability to combat infection and in enhancing host defense mechanisms. Investigators are scrutinizing neutrophil functions, complement, and opsonization as predictable measures of innate ability to combat bacterial contamination and resist infection. For example, patients with severe trauma, burns, and malnutrition

---

[*]References 6, 8, 10, 16, 21, 25, 26, 28, 45, 46.

may have depressed resistance that may be improved by hyperalimentation, immunoglobulin injection, and possibly immunization.

It is provocative to consider a future in which the defense mechanism level of a patient entering the hospital is evaluated and, if found to be lacking, supplemented. Certainly this concept is conjectural; however, it presents another approach to the prevention of infection, and perhaps in the future we will no longer need to discuss the concept of an "acceptable" rate of infection.

References

1. Bernard, H. R., and Cole, W. R.: The prophylaxis of surgical infection: the effect of prophylactic antimicrobial drugs on the incidence of infection following potentially contaminated operations, Surgery **56**:151, 1964.
2. Bower, W., Wilson, F., and Green, W. B.: Antibiotic prophylaxis in experimental bone infection, J. Bone Joint Surg. **55-A**:795, 1973.
3. Boyd, R. J., Burke, J. F., and Colton, I.: A double-blind clinical trial of prophylactic antibiotics in hip fractures, J. Bone Joint Surg. **55-A**:1251, 1973.
4. Brewer, G. E.: Studies in aseptic technique, J.A.M.A. **64**:1369, 1915.
5. Buchholz, H. W.: Die Tiefe Infektion, ein Zentrales Problem der Galenkersatz-Operationen, Mat. Med. Nordmark, **25**:1, 1972.
6. Buchholz, H. W., and Engelbrecht, H.: Uber ide Depotwirkung einiger Antibiotica bei Vermischung mit dem Kunstharz Palacos, Chirurg **41**:511, 1970.
7. Buchholz, H. W., and Gartman, H. D.: Infektionsprophylaze und Operative Behandlung der Schleichenden Tiefen Infektion bei der Totalen Endoprosthes, Chirurg **43**:446, 1972.
8. Buchholz, H. W., and Siefel, A.: Erfahrungen mit Refobacin-Palacos in der Prosthesenchirurgie, Acta Traumatol. **3**:233, 1973.
9. Burke, J. F.: The effective period of preventive antibiotic action in experimental incisions and dermal lesions, Surgery **50**:161, 1961.
10. Chapman, M. W., and Hadley, W. K.: Polymethylmethacrylate and antibiotic combinations, J. Bone Joint Surg. **58-A**:76, 1976.
11. Charnley, J.: Postoperative infection after total-hip replacement with special reference to air contamination in the operating room, Clin. Orthop. **87**:167, 1972.
12. Cruse, J. P. E., and Foord, R.: A five-year prospective study of 23,649 surgical wounds, Arch. Surg. **107**:206, 1973.
13. Feith, R.: Side-effects of acrylic cement implanted into bone, Acta Orthop. Scand. Suppl. 161, 1975.
14. Fogelberg, E. V., Zitzmann, E. K., and Stinchfield, F. E.: Prophylactic penicillin in orthopaedic surgery, J. Bone Joint Surg. **52-A**:95, 1970.
15. Hart, D., Postlewait, R. W., Brown, I. W., et al.: Post-operative wound infections: a further report on ultraviolet irradiation with comments on the recent (1964) national research cooperative report, Ann. Surg. **167**:728, 1968.
16. Hessert, G. R., and Ruchdeschel, G.: Antibiotishce Wirksamkeit von Mischungen des Polymethylmethacrylates mit Antibiotica, Arch. Orthop. Unfallchir. **68**:249, 1970.
17. Knight, W. E., and Long, J. W.: The use of antibiotic impregnated bone cement in total joint replacement, Paper presented at Clinical Orthopaedic meeting, Oklahoma City, 1975.
18. Kolczun, M. C., and Nelson, C. L.: Antibiotics in bone. In The hip: proceedings of the second open scientific meeting of The Hip Society, St. Louis, 1974, The C. V. Mosby Co.
19. Kolczun, M. C., Nelson, C. L., McHenry, M. C., Gavan, T. L., and Pinovich, P.: Antibiotic concentrations in human bone. Preliminary report, J. Bone Joint Surg. **56-A**:304-310, 1974.
20. Lautenschlager, E. P., Marshall, G. W., Markes, K. E., and Nelson, C. L.: Mechanical strength of acrylic bone cements impregnated with antibiotics. (Accepted for publication.)
21. Levin, P. D.: The effectiveness of various antibiotics in methylmethacrylate, J. Bone Joint Surg. **57-B**:234, 1975.

22. Lidgren, L., and Lindberg, L.: Post-operative wound infections in clean orthopaedic surgery. Review of a 5-year material, Acta Orthop. Scand. **45:**161, 1974.
23. Lindberg, L.: Personal communication, 1977.
24. Lister, J.: On the antiseptic principles in the practice of surgery, Lancet **2:**353, 1867.
25. Marks, K. E., Nelson, C. L., and Lautenschlager, E. P.: Antibiotic impregnated acrylic bone cement, J. Bone Joint Surg. **58-A:**358, 1976.
26. Marks, K. E., Nelson, C. L., and Schwartz, J.: Antibiotic impregnated acrylic bone cement, Surgical Forum **25:**493, 1974.
27. McKissock, W., Wright, J., Miles, A. A.: The reduction of hospital infections of wounds. A controlled experiment, Br. Med. J. **2:**375, 1941.
28. Medcraft, J. W., and Gardner, A. D. H.: The use of antibiotic bone cement combination as a different approach to the elimination of infection in total hip replacements, Lab. Tech. **31:**347, 1974.
29. Meleney, F. L.: The control of wound infections, Ann. Surg. **98:**151, 1933.
30. Moynihan, B. G.: Infection acquired in hospitals, Lancet **2:**885, 1880.
31. National Research Council, Postoperative Wound Infections: The influence of ultraviolet radiation of the operating room and of various other factors, Ann. Surg. **160**(Suppl.):1, 1964.
32. Nelson, C. L.: Experience with a wall-less horizontal clean air system during total hip replacement. In Symposium on Clean Room Technology in Surgical Suites, Cocoa Beach, Fla., 1971, NASA, Midwest Research Institute, pp. 107-114.
33. Nelson, C. L.: Clean air symposium. Part I, Cleve. Clin. Q. **40:**97, 1973.
34. Nelson, C. L.: Introposition arthroplasty, Orthopaedic Clinics.
35. Nelson, C. L., Bergfeld, J. A., Schwartz, J., and Kolczun, M.: Antibiotics in human hematoma and wound fluid, Clin. Orthop. **108:**138, 1975.
36. Nelson, C. L., Rhinelander, F. W., and Stewart, D.: Microvascular and histological responses to acrylic bone cement, Paper presented at SICOT Meeting, Copenhagen, June 1975.
37. Nelson, J. D.: Antibiotic concentrations in septic joint effusions, N. Engl. J. Med. **284:**349, 1971.
38. Pavel, A., Smith, R. L., Ballard, A., et al.: Prophylactic antibiotics in clean orthopaedic surgery, J. Bone Joint Surg. **56-A:**777, 1974.
39. Raahave, D.: Postoperative wound infection after implant and removal of osteosynthetic material, Acta Orthop. Scand. **47:**28, 1976.
40. Rhinelander, F. W.: Effects of medullary nailing on the normal blood supply of diaphyseal cortex, In American Academy of Orthopaedic Surgeons: Instructional course lectures, vol. 22, St. Louis, 1973, The C. V. Mosby Co.
41. Schurman, D. J., Johnson, B. L., Finerman, G., and Amstutz, H. C.: Antibiotic bone penetration, Clin. Orthop. **111:**142, Sept. 1975.
42. Steel, H. H.: Surgical infections—orthopaedic considerations. In American Academy of Orthopaedic Surgeons: Instructional course lectures, vol. 18, Ann Arbor, 1961, J. W. Edwards Co.
43. Stevens, D. B.: Postoperative orthopaedic infections. A study of etiological mechanisms, J. Bone Joint Surg. **46-A:**96, 1964.
44. Tachdjian, M. O., and Compere, E. L.: Postoperative wound infections in orthopaedic surgery. Evaluation of prophylactic antibiotics, J. Int. Coll. Surg. **28:**797, 1957.
45. Wahlig, H., Hameister, W., and Grieben, A.: Uber die Freisetzung von Gentamycin aus Polymethylmethacrylate. I. Experimentelle Untersuchungen in Vitro. Langenbeck's Arch. Klin. Chir. **331:**169, 1972.
46. Wahlig, H., Schliep, H. J., Bergmann, R., Hameister, W., and Greiben, A.: Uber die Freisentzung von Gentamycin aus Polymethylmethacrylate. II. Experimentelle Utersuchungen in Vivo. Langenbeck's Arch. Klin. Chir. **331:**193, 1972.
47. Weinstein, L.: Personal communication, 1975.
48. Wilson, F. C., Worchester, N. N., Coleman, P. D., and Byrd, W. E.: Antibiotic penetration of experimental bone hematomas, J. Bone Joint Surg. **53-A:**1622, 1971.

28. Thromboembolism following reconstructive surgery of the knee

C. McCollister Evarts

Thromboembolism is a common complication of total knee replacement. A study of patients after knee surgery demonstrated a high incidence (57%) of deep venous thrombosis; 99% of the patients had pulmonary emboli.[1] Following tibial osteotomy 10% of patients have been observed to develop pulmonary emboli. A venographic survey of patients with tibial fractures revealed that 13 of 15 patients demonstrated lower limb venographic abnormalities.[5]

Although the early reports of the complications of knee replacement contained a paucity of data regarding the incidence of thromboembolic disease, a recent study of patients undergoing total knee replacement using I 125 fibrinogen and venography for diagnosis demonstrated that 47% of the patients developed deep venous thrombosis and 10% developed pulmonary emboli.[4]

It is recognized that the thrombogenic process begins during surgery. It may be that a tourniquet causes stasis and endothelial injury, subsequently contributing to deep venous thrombosis. It is obvious that if a clot begins during surgery, greater attention should be given to the administration of prophylactic agents before and during the operative procedure. The prevention of thromboembolism is much preferred to treatment after the disease has occurred.

Prevention is the hallmark of the treatment of thromboembolic disease. It should begin before embolism has occurred, especially in the high-risk patient. With the recent emphasis placed on the prophylaxis of thromboembolic disease, several studies have shown that two agents, crystalline sodium warfarin and low molecular weight dextran, an antiplatelet agent, reduce the incidence of thromboembolic disease following total hip replacement.[2,3] Both regimes require meticulous attention in their administration. There are dangers associated with both.

The following regime applies to the use of warfarin (Coumadin). On the evening before the operation the patient receives 10 mg warfarin intramuscularly. On the day of surgery 5 mg is usually administered. The daily maintenance dose ranges from 5 to 7 mg per day, administered intramuscularly until the patient is able to take medication orally. The prothrombin time should be maintained at 1½ to 2 times the control value.

The use of sodium warfarin is contraindicated in patients with hemorrhagic disorders, peptic ulceration, active liver disease, hematuria, melena, hemoptysis, and cerebral insufficiency. Other drugs, including barbiturates, decrease the effectiveness of warfarin; aspirin increases its activity. The patient receiving warfarin requires stool guaiac examinations periodically, hematocrit determinations three times per week, and a test of prothrombin time daily during hospitalization. For long-term maintenance less frequent tests of prothrombin time are necessary. Hemorrhage at the wound site, gastrointestinal bleeding, and renal bleeding are complications following the use of sodium warfarin.

Emphasizing the primary role of the platelet in venous thromboembolic disease, certain investigators have used dextran as a prophylactic agent. The clinical dextrans are glucose polymers containing a broad molecular weight distribution; low molecular weight dextran has an average molecular weight of 40,000 and clinical dextran has an average molecular weight of 70,000. Low molecular weight dextran results in a reduction of platelet adhesiveness in part as a result of absorption on the platelets and alteration of their membranes, interaction with the plasma proteins, and a coating of the endothelial walls. There appears to be no difference between the antithrombotic effects of low molecular weight dextran and clinical dextran. The efficacy of low molecular weight dextran as a prophylactic agent to prevent thromboembolic disease has been demonstrated in clinical studies.

Low molecular weight dextran must be administered before surgery and continued during and after surgery. A suggested regime is to begin dextran administration prior to the operation, continue it at a rate of 50 to 75 ml per hour during the operation, and give a total of 1000 ml the day of surgery. This dosage is reduced to 500 ml per day given by continuous, slow intravenous infusion for a period of 5 to 6 days, until the patient is ambulatory. If the patient does not become ambulatory in this period of time, then warfarin anticoagulation is begun and dextran is discontinued until the patient is ambulatory.

The contraindications to the use of low molecular weight dextran include pulmonary edema, congestive heart failure, renal failure, severe dehydration, and allergic reactions. Hypersensitivity reactions have been reported but almost always develop in the first few minutes following initiation of therapy. The cardiac status of the patient should be carefully evaluated preoperatively and monitored during surgery and the postoperative period. Fluid and electrolyte balance must be carefully observed if an elderly patient is being given low molecular weight dextran. It is important to observe the renal profile, and if chronic renal dysfunction is suspected, dextran should not be used.

It is recognized that thromboembolic disease ranks among the most dangerous and common complications in the patient undergoing lower extremity surgery. The pathogenesis of the thromboembolic disease and the predictability of its occurrence remain elusive. On the basis of the evidence that suggests that the thromboembolic process begins during surgery, greater emphasis should be given to the use of prophylactic agents before and during the operative procedure. The orthopaedist has a responsibility and a commitment to his patient to help prevent thromboembolic disease.

References

1. Cohen, S. H., Ehrlich, G. E., Kauffman, M. S., and Cope, C.: Thrombophlebitis following knee surgery, J. Bone Joint Surg. **55-A:**106, 1973.
2. Evarts, C. M., and Feil, E. I.: Prevention of thromboembolic disease, J. Bone Joint Surg. **53-A:**1271, 1971.
3. Harris, W. H., Salzman, E. W., DeSanctis, R. W., and Coutts, R. D.: Prevention of venous thromboembolism following total hip replacement, J.A.M.A. **220:**1319, 1972.
4. McKenna, R., Bachmann, F., Kaushal, S. P., and Galente, J. O.: Thromboembolic disease in patients undergoing total knee replacement, J. Bone Joint Surg. **58-A:**928, 1976.
5. Nylander, G.: Phlebographic diagnosis of acute deep leg thrombosis, Acta Chir. Scand. **387**(Suppl.):30, 1968.

29. Preoperative and postoperative management of patients for total knee replacement

Alan H. Wilde

PREOPERATIVE CONSIDERATIONS

In evaluating a patient for the possibility of knee replacement, several considerations must be made. The surgeon must ascertain whether the knee disease is unilateral or bilateral and whether there is also associated disease of one or both hips. Ordinarily one should deal with the joint problem that is giving the patient the most difficulties from the standpoint of pain and/or disability. If both the hip and the knee are producing equal disability, then the hip should be done first, as correction of a knee flexion contracture is simpler following hip surgery. If both knee joints are the site of severe disease and are equally responsible for great difficulty in ambulation, both knee joints may need to be replaced. In this situation I prefer to replace the knees about 2 weeks apart. When there is less severe disability in both knees, the second knee may be replaced months later.

Evaluation of the skin of the leg, specifically the anterior aspect of the knee in the region where the incision will be made, is important. If there is severe atrophy of the skin secondary to prolonged steroid use and this area has been the site of previous breakdown with minor trauma, it will be likely to break down following knee replacement. Then, perhaps, consideration should be given to bracing the leg or arthrodesis of the knee. Any ulcerations on the leg should be healed prior to knee replacement to prevent development of sepsis in the knee joint. Similarly, psoriatic skin lesions over the anterior aspect of the knee in the region of the proposed incision should be treated and any scale removed prior to knee replacement. This may be often accomplished by a dermatologist within a few days. The location of previous incisions over the anterior aspect of the knee is important if skin slough is to be avoided postoperatively. If there is a previous medial parapatellar incision, this should be utilized for the operative approach. A second incision should not closely parallel a preexisting one and leave a narrow margin of skin between the two incisions because necrosis may occur. If a lateral parapatellar incision has been utilized previously, a medial parapatellar should not be utilized. The old lateral parapatellar incision should be utilized for the approach.[1] If a transverse incision has been employed previously, the usual straight anterior incision can be used and can cross the transverse incision at 90°. This has been done on several occasions in our series without difficulty.

The leg to be operated on should also be evaluated for the presence or absence of vascular disease. If the pedal pulses are absent or diminished, and the capillary beds do not fill properly, a peripheral vascular disease consultation should be obtained prior to the consideration of knee replacement. Occasionally a calcified popliteal artery is visible on the roentgenogram. This is usually not a contraindication for surgery, although the tourniquet may not be able to occlude the circulation. Knee replacement may then need to be done without tourniquet control. If the patient has a history of phlebitis, the surgeon may hesitate regarding knee surgery because of an increased risk of thromboembolism. Special precautions need to be taken with such patients.

We have been able to correct knee flexion contractures of up to 45° with a resurfacing prosthesis such as the geometric knee replacement.[5,6] If the knee flexion contracture is greater than 45°, the surgeon should consider preoperative correction by skin traction, if the skin is suitable for a short course of skin traction, or by skeletal traction with a pin through the tibial tubercle. An alternate means of correcting flexion contracture is by serial plaster cast changes. Knee flexion contractures of greater than 45° may require the use of prostheses other than a resurfacing prosthesis such as the geometric prosthesis.

POSTOPERATIVE REHABILITATION REGIME

The knee is bandaged in a Jones-type compression dressing at the time of surgery. The foot of the bed is elevated at the completion of the operation, as this has shown to decrease the incidence of thrombophlebitis. Exercise of both feet, ankles, knees, and hips are encouraged as soon as the patient can participate. The suction catheter inserted into the knee joint at the time of surgery is generally removed 48 hours postoperatively. Isometric quadriceps exercises are begun on the first postoperative day. The physical therapist visits the patient in the room at this point. As much flexion as the bandage will allow is encouraged after the first postoperative day. The Jones dressing is removed on approximately the fourth postoperative day and a simple nonrestricting dressing is placed over the incision. Knee flexion is actively assisted by the patient by use of the knee exerciser attached to the patient's bed. A rolled-up towel is placed beneath the calf and the active extension exercises of the knee are also begun. In this way the vastus medialis is brought into action and full active extension is sought. Manual resistance exercises are given to the quadriceps muscle and these are followed by progressive resistance exercises to rebuild the quadriceps muscle group in the manner prescribed by Delorme et al.[3]

Ambulation with partial weight bearing is allowed when the patient can perform straight leg raising. Ambulation is begun with the use of bilateral axillary crutches or walker or platform walker. Full weight bearing is ordinarily not allowed for a period of 6 weeks following surgery. This length of time is necessary to allow repair of tissue damage at the bone-cement interface.[4] Progressive resistance exercises are continued and the patient is encouraged to lift 25 pounds of weight. This can be accomplished in many patients, although in those with advanced age or severely atrophic quadriceps muscles, a compromise may have to be reached. After the patient can bear full weight on the operated extremity without the use of crutches, a cane is advised for at least an additional 6 week period of time. We instruct patients to continue exercises for at least 1 year postoperatively.

Manipulation of the knee is not performed routinely and should be avoided as long as the range of motion is increasing. If no progress in knee flexion occurs during the first 2 to 3 weeks postoperatively, then the knee should be manipulated under general anesthesia, with extreme gentleness. There occasionally arises the need to perform an open release of adhesions of the knee, usually several months postoperatively if a satisfactory range of motion is not obtained. In such a case adhesions must be released in the suprapatellar pouch and beneath the medial and lateral collateral ligaments.

Occasionally a large amount of fluid may be evacuated continuously through a small opening in the incision in the first 2 weeks after surgery. A sinogram may be done and reveal communication with the knee joint. These sinus tracts occurred in 4 of our first 100 cases of the original geometric knee replacements, when the knee was sutured in extension.[6] These were explored and it was found that the suture line in the quadriceps expansion had separated on the medial side. This complication may be avoided by closing the knee in flexion at the time of surgery. Should a sinus tract develop within the early postoperative period, it should be closed promptly; otherwise secondary infection may occur.

The complication of skin necrosis or skin slough may require débridement and split-thickness skin grafting. This should be accomplished as soon as it is recognized to obviate the real possibility of a deep wound infection.[2] Function need not be compromised by a split-thickness skin graft.

It should be noted that the foregoing material applies to knee replacements in general. We have had experience with hemiarthroplasties such as the MacIntosh tibial plateau prosthesis; resurfacing prostheses such as the geometric and geometric II, Townley, and Marmor prostheses; and hinge or hinge-like prostheses such as the Herbert, Waldius, and Guepar knee replacements.

References

1. Coventry, M. B., Upshaw, J. E., Riley, L. H., Finerman, G. A., and Turner, R. H.: Geometric total knee arthroplasty. I. Conception, design, indications, and surgical technic, Clin. Orthop. **94:**171, 1973.
2. Coventry, M. B., Upshaw, J. E., Riley, L. H., Finerman, G. A., and Turner, R. H.: Geometric total knee arthroplasty. II. Patient data and complications, Clin. Orthop. **94:** 177, 1973.

3. Delorme, T. L., West, F. E., and Shrober, W. J.: Influence of progressive resistance exercises on knee function following femoral fractures, J. Bone Joint Surg. 32-A:910, 1950.
4. Slooff, T. J. J. H.: The influence of acrylic cement, Acta Orthop. Scand. 42:465, 1971.
5. Wilde, A. H., Collins, H. R., Evarts, C. M., and Nelson, C. L.: Geometric knee replacement arthroplasty. Indications for operation and preliminary experience, Orthop. Clin. North Am. 4:547, 1973.
6. Wilde, A. H., Collins, H. R., DeHaven, K. E., Bergfeld, J. A., Evarts, C. M., and Nelson, C. L.: Geometric knee replacement arthroplasty, early results, J. Bone Joint Surg. 57-A: 134, 1975.

30. Hinge arthroplasty of the knee

Clement B. Sledge
William H. Thomas
Robert H. Arbuckle

For more than 100 years surgeons have attempted to restore motion to arthritic knees by a variety of techniques. Starting with the interposition of muscle in 1860 and progressing through a wide variety of common and exotic materials including fascia, skin, celluloid, rubber, and nylon, interposition arthroplasty produced limited success in fewer than 50% of the cases. Reasons for failure, in addition to sepsis and incompatible materials, were chiefly related to the difficulty of providing an adequate range of flexion and extension with maintenance of lateral stability. Patients function better with arthrodesed knees than with unstable knees.

It was inevitable therefore that a variety of hinged joint replacements would be developed. The first of these was the acrylic hinge developed in 1951 by Walldius[9] in Sweden. This uncemented hinge failed because of fracture of the acrylic, and in 1957 the prosthesis was manufactured of vitallium.[10] It remains virtually unchanged today and represents the prototype of the uncemented hinge.

Other similar prostheses were reported by d'Aubigne in 1953,[12] Moeys[6] in 1954, MacAusland[4] in 1957, Shiers[8] in 1960, and Young[12] in 1963. Except for the Shiers and Walldius prostheses, all of these attempted to supplement intramedullary fixation with cortical screws and bolts and all failed because of eventual loss of fixation.

Factual reporting of the failure rate in hinge arthroplasty of the knee by Young led to widespread distrust of the concept in this country until Wilson reported a series of uncemented Walldius arthroplasties in 30 patients in 1972.[11] He reported uniform loosening at the prosthesis-bone interface but "satisfactory" results in the majority.

Realizing the limitations of the Walldius in terms of (1) inadequate flexion, (2) loosening, and (3) excessive bone resection, and desiring a prosthesis to retain the patellofemoral joint, unlike the Shiers, a group of 11 French surgeons developed the Guepar hinge in 1970.[5]

344

CASE MATERIAL

Between February 1971 and December 1975, 144 hinge replacements of the knee were carried out in 113 patients. Of these 121 were for rheumatoid arthritis and 23 were for osteoarthritis. One hundred twenty-four replacements were in women and 20 in men. The average age of patients was 64, with a range from 21 to 85 years.

Indications

All patients were judged to be incapacitated by either pain or deformity and all were in the later stages of joint disease, with gross destruction of articular structures. When this series began, our alternative procedures were arthrodesis and hemiarthroplasty with McKeever tibial implants. In 1973 we began knee replacement using metal-to-plastic unconstrained components. Indications for a hinge replacement therefore became more stringent in the last part of this series. The prime indication throughout, however, was disabling pain. The few patients who did not have pain had knees ankylosed in positions that were functionally unacceptable. The case distribution by year indicates a combination of increasing therapeutic alternatives and a growing disenchantment with metallic hinges:

Year	Number of cases
1971	17
1972	40
1973	53
1974	24
1975	10

Choice of prosthesis

One hundred eleven Walldius hinges and two of the Shiers design were used. Theoretical considerations, including hinge location, range of motion, and patello-femoral groove, as well as early clinical failures with the Walldius, led to adoption of the Guepar design in January 1974. Since that time all of our hinge knee replacements have been of this type.

TECHNIQUE

Initially the technique described by Walldius—transpatellar approach, no methacrylate, and postoperative immobilization—was followed. A loose, painful, uncemented hinge; disruption of the extensor mechanism; and our earlier experience with parapatellar incisions and early mobilization soon convinced us to change to our present technique. This involves a gently curved medial parapatellar incision with detachment of the vastus medialis insertion. Intra-articular adhesions are divided to allow lateral eversion of the patella. In severely damaged knees with long-standing loss of motion, division of the collateral ligaments and cruciates is often necessary to allow flexion of the knee to 90°.

At this stage the cruciates are excised, if present, and the intercondylar notch of the femur is cleared to allow resection of the distal femur followed by resection of the proximal tibia. Sufficient bone is resected to allow correction of flexion deformity plus the thickness of the prosthetic components. The horizontal plane of resection is at right angles to the shaft of the tibia, correcting varus-valgus deformities and restoring the normal 7° of femoral valgus alignment. The amount of bony stock resected must be sufficient to allow easy extension of the knee without peroneal nerve stretch. Supporting the weight of the leg with a hand under the calf should allow full passive extension if sufficient bone has been resected. The posterior femoral condyles and the posterior flare of the tibia are resected to allow full, unrestricted flexion.

Meticulous hemostasis is obtained after deflating the tourniquet before final insertion of the components. After the components are cemented in place and the hinge-pin inserted, a final assessment of alignment and range of motion are made and necessary revisions carried out. The incision is closed in layers with nonabsorbable sutures following insertion of suction catheters. A bulky dressing and soft splint are used to immobilize the extremity for 24 hours.

Quadriceps setting exercises, started preoperatively, are reinstituted in the recovery room. The suction catheters are removed at 24 hours and gentle quadriceps exercises begun. At 48 hours the dressing is changed, the incision is inspected, and active assisted range-of-motion exercises are started. When the patient has achieved 60° to 70° of flexion with active muscular control, ambulation with crutches is begun using a three-point partial–weight-bearing gait. At the time of suture removal at 2 weeks, most patients have achieved 90° of motion, are independent in ambulation and activities of daily living, and can be discharged. Protected weight bearing is maintained for 3 months.

RESULTS

The average length of follow-up in this series was 30 months. An assessment was made of pain relief, range of motion, and functional improvement.

Pain

Pain relief was essentially complete in 90% of patients. Six percent had mild discomfort attributable to patellofemoral disease, slight loosening, or synovitis. Four percent had severe pain associated with gross loosening. One patient, whose Walldius prosthesis was not initially cemented, developed pain that was relieved by reinsertion of the components with methacrylate fixation.

Range of motion

Average flexion was 85° preoperatively and 88° postoperatively. Patients with the Guepar prosthesis averaged 115° of flexion postoperatively. The average flexion deformity was 23° preoperatively and 5° postoperatively. Ninety per-

AMBULATORY CAPACITY

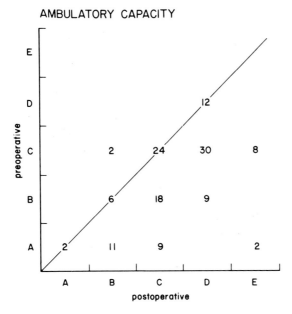

Fig. 30-1. Functional status of 133 knees available for evaluation. Preoperative and postoperative status are represented on two ordinates. Points on 45° line represent no change from preoperative status, points to right of line represent improvement, and those to left represent deterioration in functional level. Distance of point from line represents amount of change in that knee. (*A*, Bedridden; *B*, bed-chair/wheel chair [minimal ambulation]; *C*, indoor ambulation; *D*, some outdoor ambulation [1 or 2 blocks]; *E*, extended outdoor ambulation.)

cent of patients achieved 60° or more of flexion, 75% achieved 80° or more, and 90% had less than 15° of fixed flexion deformity.

Functional results

There is no widely accepted rating scheme for the knee because of the difficulties and inaccuracies of assessing functional results in a single joint without being unduly influenced by the presence or absence of disease in adjacent joints and distant joints. Rating systems also necessarily ignore progression of the disease process in the patient. For these reasons, we have made no attempt to assess functional improvement by any numerical rating system. Rather, we have used a simple scheme involving readily determined parameters of ambulation: bedridden, bed to chair/wheelchair or minimal ambulation, indoor ambulation, limited outdoor ambulation (1 to 2 blocks), and extended outdoor ambulation. Of the 133 knees available for functional evaluation, 2 were worse, 44 showed no change, and 87 were improved. These results are shown in Fig. 30-1.

COMPLICATIONS

Major complications are shown in Table 30-1.

Table 30-1. Major complications in 144 hinge arthroplasties

Complication	Number	Percentage
Death	1	0.5
Avulsion of patellar tendon	1	0.5
Synovitis (requiring hospitalization)	4	3
Major loosening (requiring revision)	6	4
Sepsis	10	7
TOTAL	22	15

Synovitis

Persistent synovitis has been an infrequent but ominous complication. In four patients in this series, synovitis (as judged by effusion and warmth with or without discomfort in the operated knee) was persistent and worrisome enough to warrant hospitalization for diagnostic purposes. These patients were studied for possible infection by repeated aspiration, with analysis and culture of the joint fluid, and arthrography.

The joint fluid in these patients has been grayish in color with metallic particles evident after centrifugation and microscopic examination. All cultures were negative, and arthrography has not revealed loosening at either bone-cement or metal-cement interfaces. Joint fluid sugar levels have been low (0 to 70 mg/100 ml) on several occasions; white blood cell counts have ranged from less than 300 to more than 50,000. In spite of these parameters, normally associated with infection, four of seven patients have not developed obvious sepsis thus far, although three patients have—at intervals of 2, 11, and 20 months after "sterile" synovitis was detected.

Loosening

Major loosening requiring revision occurred in six knees (4%). One has not been revised because of the poor condition of the patient; furthermore, this patient recently sustained a fracture of her femur proximal to the femoral stem and the outcome is not known yet. Of the five that have been revised, one was an uncemented Walldius prosthesis revised to a cemented type and the other four were cemented Walldius prostheses converted to Guepar prostheses. Of these, a satisfactory outcome has been achieved in four; the unsatisfactory result is a Walldius converted to a Guepar prosthesis that is now loose secondary to a massive osteolytic reaction in the tibia. The final outcome of this knee has not been determined.

In addition to these six cases, there are six others that are known to be loose but functioning satisfactorily with minimal symptoms. The exact number of minor degrees of loosening is not known, as this is easily confused with the normal amount of laxity that occurs at the hinge-bolt interface. It is clear that minor loosening per se is still compatible with satisfactory function.

Table 30-2. Postoperative sepsis

Patient	Diagnosis*	Onset	Previous surgery	Organism	Treatment†	Outcome
1	RA	Immediate	—	Gram-negative	Débridement	Ambulatory; no drainage
2	RA	Immediate	Hemiarthroplasty	Gram-negative	Arthrodesis, skin grafts	Ambulatory; solid fusion after 16 mo
3	RA	Immediate	Hemiarthroplasty	S. aureus	Débridement	Minimally ambulatory; draining at 24 mo
4	RA	3 mo	Hemiarthroplasty	S. epidimidis	Aspirations	Ambulatory at 42 mo
5	RA	9 mo	—	S. aureus, enterococcus	Arthrodesis	Ambulatory; solid fusion after 6 mo
6	OA	12 mo	Hemiarthroplasty	S. aureus	Aspirations	Ambulatory; no drainage; died of unrelated causes
7	OA	Loose at 18 mo, septic at 22 mo	—	S. aureus	Arthrodesis	Ambulatory (pseudarthrosis) at 15 mo
8	OA	Loose at 18 mo, septic at 30 mo	—	S. epidimidis, gram-negative	Arthrodesis	Solid at 26 mo after 4 operations; now ambulatory
9	RA	24 mo	—	S. aureus	Débridement, arthrodesis	Pseudarthrosis
10	RA	48 mo	—	S. aureus	Hip disarticulation for concomitant ipsilateral septic girdlestone	Healing

*RA = Rheumatoid arthritis; OA = osteoarthritis.
†In addition to antibiotics, which were administered in all cases.

Sepsis

Sepsis occurred in 10 of 144 knees (7%). In three patients there was immediate sepsis associated with failure to achieve primary wound healing, and in seven the onset of sepsis was delayed. Wound breakdown in the immediate postoperative period was usually associated with an excessively curved incision producing a zone of impaired blood supply just medial to the superior pole of the patella. Rheumatoid vasculitis and steroid-induced skin atrophy may have been further contributing factors.

The seven delayed infections became apparent over a time period ranging from 3 months to 48 months. Two of the seven were preceded by a definite period of loosening without evidence of infection, followed by obvious sepsis. Three patients had persistent synovitis with negative cultures for periods ranging from 2 to 20 months before sepsis was documented. In at least one additional delayed infection, circumstantial evidence suggests hematogenous spread from an infected focus elsewhere. Four of the 10 patients who developed sepsis had previous surgery with metallic implants that failed, necessitating revision to a hinge replacement.

The primary organisms were *Staphylococcus aureus* in six patients, *Staphylococcus epidermidis* in two, and gram-negative organisms in two. Both of the gram-negative infections were in patients with wound breakdown and immediate infection.

The choice of treatment in these infected knees was determined by antibiotic sensitivity of the infecting organism, the general condition of the patient and the infected joint, and the presence or absence of loosening of the implant. In general, if loosening could not be demonstrated in a patient who was tolerating an infection with a sensitive organism, multiple aspirations and parenteral antibiotics were tried, with occasional success (Table 30-2).

DISCUSSION

Hinge replacement of the severely deranged knee provides either dramatic success or dramatic failure. Eighty-seven of 133 knees evaluated were functionally improved, 10 of these are capable of extended outdoor ambulation and function in a near-normal fashion, and 90% of the patients are essentially pain free.

Table 30-3. Incidence of reported complications

Author	Number in series	Cement	Infections (%)	Major loosening (%)	Operative revisions (%)
Jones[3]	120	No	10	5	10
Phillips and Taylor[7]	83	No	5	5	10
Bain[1]	100	Yes	10	4	10
Freeman[2]	80	Yes	5	5	10
Present series	144	Yes	7	4	11

Twenty-two knees sustained some sort of complication, necessitating operative revision in 16. Fourteen of the 22 knees with complications ended up with a stable, painless, functional extremity, leaving 8 knees (6%) in the unsatisfactory or failed category at final analysis.

Clearly the most significant complication is infection, seen in 7% in this series. The rate of infection in the major reported series has ranged from 5% to 10%, with loosening rates of approximately 5%, and the percentage of operative revisions approximately 10% (Table 30-3). Whether or not cement was used for fixation of the implant does not seem to affect the incidence of any of these complications.

With the number of therapeutic modalities now available for reconstruction of the severely destroyed knee, hinge replacement should be relegated to salvage of knees that cannot be reconstructed with metal-to-polyethylene unconstrained prostheses. Such metal-to-polyethylene replacements appear to have a significantly lower rate of complications, especially infection. At present, our indication for use of a metal hinge arthroplasty of the knee is a fixed flexion deformity of 45° or more, valgus or varus deformity of more than 25°, complete loss of medial or lateral collateral ligaments, or salvage of an unstable failure of a previous arthroplasty. Perhaps metal-to-polyethylene constrained prostheses can be used to salvage these knees equally well without the high percentage of complications associated with metal hinge replacement.

References

1. Bain, A. M.: Replacement of the knee joint with the Walldius prosthesis using cement fixation, Clin. Orthop. **94**:65, 1973.
2. Freeman, P. A.: Walldius arthroplasty: a review of 80 cases, Clin. Orthop. **94**:85, 1973.
3. Jones, G. B.: Total knee replacement—the Walldius hinge, Clin. Orthop. **94**:50, 1973.
4. MacAusland, W. R.: Total replacement of the knee joint by a prosthesis, Surg. Gynecol. Obstet. **104**:579, 1957.
5. Mazas, F. B., and GUEPAR: Guepar total knee prosthesis, Clin. Orthop. **94**:211, 1973.
6. Moeys, E. J.: Metal alloplasty of the knee joint. An experimental study, J. Bone Joint Surg. **36-A**:363, 1954.
7. Phillips, H., and Taylor, J. G.: The Walldius hinge arthroplasty, J. Bone Joint Surg. **57-B**:59, 1975.
8. Shiers, L. G. P.: Hinge arthroplasty of the knee, J. Bone Joint Surg. **47-B**:586, 1965.
9. Walldius, B.: Arthroplasty of the knee joint using an acrylic prosthesis, Acta Orthop. Scand. **23**:121, 1953.
10. Walldius, B.: Arthroplasty of the knee using an endoprosthesis, Acta Orthop. Scand. Suppl. 24, 1957.
11. Wilson, F. C.: Total replacement of the knee in rheumatoid arthritis. A prospective study of the results of treatment with the Walldius prosthesis, J. Bone Joint Surg. **54-A**:1429, 1972.
12. Young, H. H.: Use of a hinged Vitallium prosthesis for arthroplasty of the knee: a preliminary report, J. Bone Joint Surg. **45-A**:1627, 1963.

Index